MALE INFERTILITY

TO JIM AND ERLENE CUMMINS
With much gratitude for all their support, help and advice over the last decade.

MALE INFERTILITY

A GUIDE FOR THE CLINICIAN

ANNE M. JEQUIER
FRCS, FRCOG, FRACOG
Clinical Associate Professor, Department of Obstetrics & Gynaecology,
University of Western Australia, and Gynaecologist/
Andrologist & Head of Fertility Services,
King Edward Memorial Hospital, Perth, Western Australia

Blackwell
Science

© 2000
Blackwell Science Ltd
Editorial Offices:
Osney Mead, Oxford OX2 0EL
25 John Street, London WC1N 2BL
23 Ainslie Place, Edinburgh EH3
  6AJ
350 Main Street, Malden
  MA 02148 5018, USA
54 University Street, Carlton
  Victoria 3053, Australia
10, rue Casimir Delavigne
  75006 Paris, France

Other Editorial Offices:
Blackwell Wissenschafts-Verlag
  GmbH
Kurfürstendamm 57
10707 Berlin, Germany

Blackwell Science KK
MG Kodenmacho Building
7–10 Kodenmacho Nihombashi
Chuo-ku, Tokyo 104, Japan

First published 2000

Set by Excel Typesetters Co.,
Hong Kong
Printed and bound in Great Britain
by MPG Books Ltd, Bodmin,
Cornwall

A catalogue record for this title is
available from the British Library

ISBN 0-632-05129-9

Library of Congress
Cataloging-in-publication Data

Jequier, Anne M.
    Male Infertility: a guide for the
clinician/Anne M. Jequier.
        P.   cm.
    Includes bibliographical
references and index.
    ISBN 0-632-05129-9
    1. Infertility, Male.   I. Title.
    [DNLM: 1. Infertility, Male.
WJ 709 J54m 2000]
RCBB9.J473   2000
616.6'92 — dc21
DNLM/DLC
for Library of Congress 99-16293
                                          CIP-1

DISTRIBUTORS
  Marston Book Services Ltd
  PO Box 269
  Abingdon, Oxon OX14 4YN
  (*Orders*: Tel: 01235 465500
              Fax: 01235 465555)

USA
  Blackwell Science, Inc.
  Commerce Place
  350 Main Street
  Malden, MA 02148 5018
  (*Orders*: Tel: 800 759 6102
                      781 388 8250
              Fax: 781 388 8255)

Canada
  Login Brothers Book Company
  324 Saulteaux Crescent
  Winnipeg, Manitoba R3J 3T2
  (*Orders*: Tel: 204 837 2987)

Australia
  Blackwell Science Pty Ltd
  54 University Street
  Carlton, Victoria 3053
  (*Orders*: Tel: 3 9347 0300
              Fax: 3 9347 5001)

For further information on
Blackwell Science, visit our
website:
www.blackwell-science.com

Contents

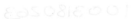

Preface

Library shelves contain many books on infertility, but very few are devoted solely to infertility in the male. Many of the books that do discuss the subject of male infertility relate to its scientific basis or to some specific aspect of clinical andrology rather than to male infertility in general.

With the application of microassisted fertilization to the management of many forms of male infertility, the problem of male infertility is increasingly in the hands of the gynaecologist. Many of these clinicians have had little training in either the examination or the investigation of the disorders of the male genital tract. With these problems in mind, I decided that a book that was concerned only with the clinical aspects of male infertility was indeed needed.

This book is concerned solely with the clinical aspects of male infertility and contains only basic information relating to the science of andrology. I make no apologies for this omission: the science of andrology is not the object of this book. This is a book by a clinician for clinicians, particularly for gynaecologists, who now often have to battle to understand reproductive pathology in infertile male patients. My intention was to inform the gynaecologists and others interested in the clinical management of infertile men and to provide such individuals with a 'hands-on' approach to a clinical problem. I have tried to include in the text a reasonable number of references so that any clinician who is interested can explore each aspect of male infertility in much more detail both clinically and scientifically.

In the writing of this book, I have many people to whom I owe a great deal. My thanks must go first to Gillian Walker-Northcott, photographers Philip Williams and Chris Labrooy and all the staff in the Audio-visual Department of the Queen Elizabeth Medical Centre in Perth, Western Australia, who were very patient with what were, at times, fairly excessive demands upon their time. I also wish to extend many thanks to Dr Ashley Murch of the Genetic Services Department in Perth for providing me with the karyotypes used to illustrate the chapter on genetics and male infertility in this book.

A heartfelt thank-you must also go to Brigitte Glockner and her colleagues in the library at King Edward Memorial Hospital for tracking down numerous references. Thanks are also due to my colleagues, Dr Roger Perkins and Associate Professor Jim Cummins, for all their helpful comments and criticisms of the manuscript.

Finally, I must thank all my staff at Fertility West in the Mount Hospital who have put up with all the stresses and strains that writing a book has, of necessity, induced in me. All I can now hope is that the effort has all been worthwhile and that this book will be of value to some of the clinicians involved in the management of the distressing condition of human infertility.

Anne M. Jequier
Perth, Western Australia
July 1999

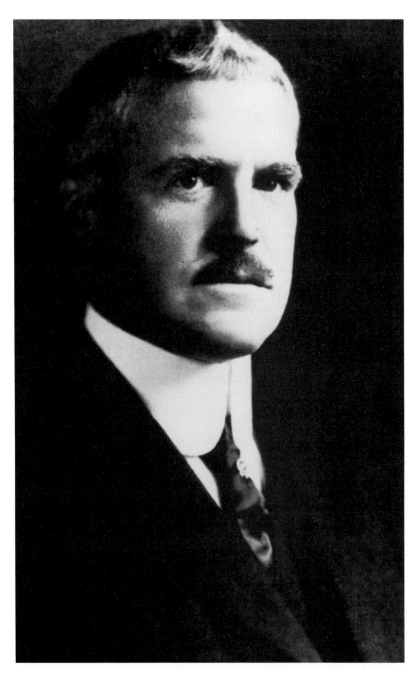

Edward Martin (1859–1938), The founding father of modern clinical andrology, who was also the first surgeon to carry out a vaso-epididymostomy.

1: What do we Mean by Male Infertility?

Traditionally, the definition of male infertility is based on one or more abnormalities within a semen analysis (WHO 1992). As we all know, there are several causes of infertility where the semen analysis can be, at least on superficial examination, perfectly normal. Thus, one must find another definition or series of definitions in order to describe the problem known as male infertility.

The semen analysis

The World Health Organization defines normal semen as having a sperm concentration greater than 20 million sperm per millilitre (WHO 1992) and a sperm motility of more than 50% (Table 1.1). This conclusion is in fact based upon little evidence but has been decided upon by consensus within a working group.

The concentration of semen in an ejaculate will, of course, depend upon the volume of the secretions of the accessory glands. These secretions can vary from day to day and this will thus vary the concentrations of the spermatozoa. If these differences are very marked, then the concentration can also vary greatly even though the number of spermatozoa within the ejaculate remains the same (Table 1.2). Thus, to define sperm numbers within an ejaculate in terms of the concentration is clearly untenable.

Many studies that examine the semen of men attending a clinic for vasectomy, all of whom had been fathers in the past, make it clear that the biological variation between individuals, in terms of sperm concentration, is very large. One of the first of such studies (and one of the largest) was reported from the Margaret Sanger Institute in New York. This institute demonstrated that more than half the patients attending for vasectomy had a semen analysis that would have deemed them to be infertile by present WHO standards.

It must also be remembered that sperm concentrations can vary greatly not only between individuals, but also at different times within an individual. As the sperm counts taken from one man over a long period of time have demonstrated (WHO 1992), the sperm count in a normal fertile man may, at times, fall well below that deemed to be normal by WHO. However, one important feature of this change in a fertile patient is that this fall in sperm count is not sustained (WHO 1992). Thus, fertility cannot be defined by a single sperm count but may be defined by the length of time that the sperm count remains low. Therefore, one of

1

Table 1.1 The WHO classification of a 'normal' semen analysis

Volume = 2 mL or more
  pH = 7.2–8.0
Sperm concentration = 20 million per mL or more
Motility = 50% or more that are also showing forward progression
Morphology = 30% or more normal forms
White blood cells = less than 1 million per mL

Table 1.2 An example of how increasing volumes of seminal plasma will alter the sperm concentration while the total numbers of spermatozoa in the ejaculate will remain the same

	Volume		
	2 mL	5 mL	10 mL
Concentration	25 million	10 million	5 million
Total sperm count	50 million	50 million	50 million

the parameters of semen quality that is seldom taken into consideration is that of time.

Another major difficulty in assessing fertility from a semen sample is the ever-present problem of artefact. Semen samples can be spilled at collection. As it is the first portion of the ejaculate that contains the spermatozoa and it is frequently the first portion of the ejaculate that is most commonly lost, the erroneous diagnosis of oligozoospermia may, thus, be made.

Another common problem is the contamination of the specimen that can occur at collection. This contamination may be the result of collection into an unsuitable container or pollution of the sample after it has been collected from the floor. Some patients who have problems producing semen samples by masturbation may opt to collect the sample in an ordinary condom during sexual intercourse. Ordinary condoms are made of latex, and the associated hydrocarbons are very toxic to sperm. Ordinary commercially available condoms are, of course, designed to be as spermicidal as possible and thus often contain a spermicidal powder that renders the sperm immotile. In such cases, a false diagnosis of male infertility may be made.

The collection of a sample of semen may also prove difficult for a patient because of the presence of another pathology. Patients who are impotent have great difficulties in producing a complete semen analysis, especially if they are uncircumcised. In the case of the patient presented in Table 1.3, the patient's wife presented alone at the clinic with infertility and she was told to ask her husband to produce a semen sample. At no time did any of the clinicians meet with this male patient, let alone did he ever come for a consultation. After a cursory glance at the results of a semen analysis and without even meeting with the patient, the gynaecological clinician at the

Table 1.3 The semen analyses from a man with erectile failure and who was also deemed to have oligozoospermia*

Specimen 1	Specimen 2
Volume = 7 mL	Volume = 5.5 mL
Concentration = 11 million/mL	Concentration = 3.0 million/mL
Motility = 60%	Motility 10%
Morphology = 30% abnormals	Morphology = 60% abnormals

*Careful history taking revealed that the anterior portion of the ejaculate containing the spermatozoa was being partially trapped in the foreskin. Note that the ejaculatory volume remains within normal limits. The wide variation in semen parameters is suggestive but not diagnostic of collection artefact. This case demonstrates the need for a clinical history always to accompany a semen analysis.

infertility clinic promptly lost interest in the female patient and packed the unfortunate husband off to the local andrologist.

At long last, however, it was discovered that the poor man was totally impotent and had been suffering from this problem for many years. On examining this male patient, it was clear that the semen was being trapped in a very long foreskin, and thus a proportion of the ejaculate was being repeatedly excluded from the semen sample. Thus, with the help of a clinical history and examination, the cause of this particular couple's infertility was being properly evaluated.

The above comments, as well as the case illustrated here, make it very clear that semen samples cannot be judged for their quality or their fertility when divorced from the clinical history and examination. Comments by pathology departments at the bottom of semen analysis reports and pompous remarks concerning the fertility of a semen sample by scientists who frequently do not have access to any of the clinical history must always be totally ignored. At all times, the semen analysis must be related to the clinical history and the clinical examination of the infertile male patient or grave mistakes will be made in the management of a couple's infertility.

It must also be remembered that very high counts may also be a cause of infertility. If sperm numbers in an ejaculate are excessive, the energy sources in semen are rapidly exhausted and sperm movement can be totally lost as a result of a low fructose concentration (Amelar *et al.* 1979). This situation can be rectified by adding either fructose or glucose to the semen sample and using it for artificial insemination. Thus, to determine fertility in relation to a lower limit of sperm concentration is clearly not helpful.

One way to express fertility in terms of semen quality was suggested by Eliasson in 1971, and it is a remark that makes a great deal of sense (Eliasson 1971). Eliasson commented that a reduction in semen quality may not render a man sterile but will simply reduce the probability of pregnancy. It may thus be best for us to discuss the probability of infertility with the patient rather than its inevitability.

Sperm function as a parameter of infertility within a semen analysis

It is, of course, possible to have reasonable quality seminal fluid in terms of a semen analysis but have infertility resulting from poor sperm function. Thus, abnormalities of sperm function are indeed a parameter by which we can measure fertility.

A wide variety of sperm function tests have been devised in an attempt to predict the potential fertility of a semen sample. Examples of simple tests include the postcoital test and the sperm invasion test, both of which correlate well with fertility, although this correlation is not absolute. More complex tests include the acrosome reaction ionophore challenge test (Cummins *et al.* 1991), the hemizona binding test (Burkeman *et al.* 1988) and the hamster egg penetration test (Rogers *et al.* 1979), but these have not shown to be more predictive than some of the more simple tests. It is thus clear that the 'perfect' sperm function test has yet to be devised.

These tests are, however, of value in attempting to avoid the devastating problem of total fertilization failure at *in vitro* fertilization (IVF). This problem is not, however, totally avoided as some fertilization failure is caused not by abnormalities of the spermatozoa but rather by disorders of the oocyte. The use of sperm function tests does at least avoid some of the distress caused by fertilization failure during an expensive cycle of assisted conception.

The clinical history and clinical examination as a parameter of male infertility

The clinical history may not only alert the clinician to the presence of infertility in the male but also provide many clues as to its cause.

It must also be remembered that severe forms of infertility can exist in patients in whom there is no history that is suggestive of the presence of an abnormal semen analysis and in whom even a careful clinical examination will reveal no abnormality. A good example of such an abnormality is the condition known as germinal aplasia, which renders the patient azoospermic. In this condition, despite the azoospermia, there is frequently no past history to suggest the presence of pathology and the clinical examination can show no abnormality.

Endocrine changes as indicators of male infertility

If there are obstructive lesions present and sperm production is normal, then severe changes may occur in semen quality, but there will be no alteration in either the serum testosterone or the serum levels of the gonadotrophins. It is also possible to have a total ablation of all sperm production together with an apparent total loss of spermatogonia, as is seen in the condition known as germinal aplasia, in which the gonadotropins remain resolutely within the normal range (Jequier *et al.* 1984). This probably occurs because much of the feedback to the pituitary in relation to follicle-stimulating hormone (FSH) secretion comes from the Sertoli cell and its products. Thus, should Sertoli cell function be normal then so will be the secretion of FSH.

The Leydig cells, however, are much more resistant to injury than is the spermatogenic epithelium and, as a consequence, testosterone secretion is often normal. Occasionally, however, it is clear that the Leydig cells are being 'pushed' to function normally by luteinizing hormone (LH), as occasionally one can see a raised serum level of LH in the presence of normal serum testosterone level. However, gonadotrophin levels are useful as an indicator of malfunction of the spermatogenic epithelium, but that correlation is not absolute.

Testicular histology as an indicator of the presence of male infertility

Histological examination of testicular tissue is a poor indicator of the presence of infertility and frequently cannot be used to differentiate between a mild, a moderate or a severe reduction in sperm production. This is because, in many circumstances, the changes that occur in the testis are not only focal but can vary in different parts of the testis. These pathological changes may even differ between contiguous seminiferous tubules and, because only a very small area of testicular tissue is being examined, this tissue may not be representative of all of the other areas of the gonad. The semen sample, however, represents a summation of all of these changes within not just one but both testes. Indeed, because of the focality of these changes within the testis, a testicular biopsy can even appear to be normal in a man with severe and clinically obvious spermatogenic failure simply through sampling artefact.

In men with obstructive lesions, the testicular histology will usually be completely normal, although the presence of an obstructive lesion of the immediate excurrent ducts of the testes can induce a small amount of oedema in the interstitial tissue of the testis.

Thus, testicular biopsy is not a very good method of diagnosing male infertility and indeed its use diagnostically can be a very frustrating way to diagnose any form of genital tract pathology.

Male infertility — as it interacts with problems in the female partner

Male infertility can become more profound depending upon the manner in which it interacts with any problems that may coexist in the female partner. High fertility in the female partner may overcome the presence of relatively poor semen quality (Steinberger & Rodrigues-Rigau 1983); however, the presence of even minor abnormalities in the fertility of the female can, in the presence of abnormalities in semen quality, give rise to prolonged periods of childlessness.

Thus, in the assessment of male infertility, the evaluation of the female partner is very important. There is indeed no place for a clinician to say we must resolve the infertility of one partner before we turn our attention to his partner. Too often we hear the gynaecologists say to the andrologist 'I am not going to carry out a laparoscopy until you have cured this man's oligozoospermia'. Need one say again that infertility is a disorder of a couple, not of an individual, and the treatment of a couple's infertility is the evaluation of this childlessness in relation to both these individuals.

Fertility factors in each patient may of course interact in many different ways and one of these factors may simply be time. If, for example, a man only produces reasonably fertile semen for 1 month each year and his female partner only ovulates once in every year, the mean time to conception will be 12 years. If, however, this man finds himself another partner who ovulates every month, then the mean time to conception will be 12 months. This latter situation cannot even be defined as infertility even in the presence of an obvious seminal abnormality (Fig. 1.1). Thus, male fertility cannot be defined in relation to sperm count alone but must be defined in relation to the status of fertility in the partner and in relation to the length of time that these abnormalities occur in these patients.

It is often stated that infertile women frequently marry infertile men, and it is suggested that there is some selection process at work in order to preordain this situation. This, of course, is not the case as this is simply the effects of 'double pathology' presenting itself in this situation. It is again the effect of a second lesion rendering infertile a man who would, if attempting conception with a fertile partner, much more easily achieve a pregnancy. If one divides the male and female population each into three groups, one can see that pregnancy will only with certainty be achieved in one of these nine groups of individuals: in four of these nine groups, double pathology, i.e. infertility factors in both partners, would be present (Fig. 1.2).

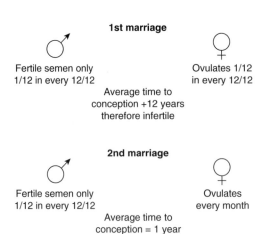

1st marriage

Fertile semen only
1/12 in every 12/12

Ovulates 1/12
in every 12/12

Average time to
conception +12 years
therefore infertile

2nd marriage

Fertile semen only
1/12 in every 12/12

Ovulates
every month

Average time to
conception = 1 year
therefore fertile

Fig. 1.1 Time plays an important role in the assessment of infertility, apparent male infertility can be nullified by enhanced fertility in the female. As the above example shows, decreased frequency of a fertile semen sample will induce infertility much more obviously in a woman with a decreased frequency of ovulation than in a woman who ovulates every month. These factors make the definition of male infertility very difficult indeed.

Fig. 1.2 With the population of each gender being designated sterile, infertile or fertile it can be seen that, by random selection, pathology would be present in both partners in four out of the nine groups of couples and in four of the eight groups of couples with infertility.

MALE				
Fertile	Fertile	Infertility	Possible infertility	Fertile
Infertile	Infertile	Infertility	Possible infertility	Possible infertility
Sterile	Sterile	Infertility	Infertility	Infertility
	Sterile	**Infertile**	**Fertile**	

FEMALE

As the fertility status of the male is, from the examples above, dependent upon the fertility status of his partner and vice versa, the definition of male infertility (and for that matter the definition of female infertility) becomes very difficult. It is clear that definite answers concerning prognosis for pregnancy and time to pregnancy are virtually impossible to provide to the patients. It is also abundantly clear that it is almost impossible to define what we mean by male infertility either in terms of pathology or in relation to semen quality or sperm function.

With all this in mind, it is now time to examine the many different types of pathology that may occur in relation to infertility in the male and the attempts, in terms of treatment, that may be used to overcome them.

References

Amelar, R.D., Dubin, L., Quigley, M.M. & Schonfeild, C.C. (1979) Successfull management of infertility due to polyzoospermia. *Fertility and Sterility* **31**, 521–524.

Burkeman, L.J., Coddington, C.C., Franken, D.R., Kruger, T.F., Rosenzaks, Z. & Hodgen, G.D. (1988) The hemizona assay (HZA): development of a diagnostic test for the binding of human spermatozoa to the human hemizona pellucida to predict fertilization potential. *Fertility and Sterility* **49**, 688–697.

Cummins, J.M., Pember, S., Jequier, A.M., Yovich, J.L. & Hartmann, P.E. (1991) A test of human sperm acrosome reaction following ionophore challenge (ARIC): relationship to fertilization and other seminal parameters. *Journal of Andrology* **12**, 98–103.

Eliasson, R. (1971) Standards for the investigation of human semen. *Andrologie* **3**, 49–64.

Jequier, A.M., Ansell, I.D. & Bullimore, N.J. (1984) Germinal aplasia: how it may mimic obstructive azoospermia. *British Journal of Urology* **56**, 537–539.

Rogers, B.J., van Campen, H., Ueno, M., Lambert, H., Bronson, R. & Hale, R. (1979) Analysis of human spermatozoa fertilizing ability using zona free ova. *Fertility and Sterility* **32**, 664–670.

Steinberger, E. & Rodrigues-Rigau, L.J. (1983) The infertile couple. *Journal of Andrology* **14**, 111–118.

World Health Organization (1992). *WHO Laboratory Manual for the Examination of Spermatozoa and Sperm–Cervical Mucus Interaction*, 3rd edn. Cambridge University Press, Cambridge.

2: The Anatomy and Physiology of the Male Genital Tract

In order to understand the basis of infertility in the male, it is important to have a reasonable knowledge of the anatomy of the male genital tract together with the sources of the seminal fluid.

The scrotum

The scrotum is a cutaneous sac containing the testes and the lower parts of the spermatic cord. It is divided into two halves by a fibromuscular septum. The wall of the scrotum is made up of hair-bearing skin, containing the nonstriated cutaneous muscle known as the dartos. Contraction of this muscle gives the scrotal skin its corrugated appearance. Subcutaneous fat is absent.

Each half of the scrotum is lined by an isolated portion of the peritoneum known as the tunica vaginalis. The tunica vaginalis covers the scrotal cavity and also covers the testis and the epididymis (Fig. 2.1).

The testes

Each testis is an ovoid organ that lies in the scrotum on either side of a septum that divides the scrotum into left and right halves. Each normal testis has a volume of 15 mL or more and should measure around 5 cm in length.

The outer covering of each testis consists of a thick and somewhat rigid fibrous capsule called the tunica albuginea (Davis *et al.* 1970). This covering has very little distensibility and thus any disease or injury of the testis that will induce oedema could impair testicular blood flow. Ischaemia induced in this way might thus result in either temporary or even permanent damage to the spermatogenic elements within the testis (Fig. 2.2). In the capsule of the testis, there are also numerous mast cells that may play a part in control of the testicular blood flow (Nistal *et al.* 1984).

Immediately beneath the tunica albuginea is a vascular layer called the tunica vasculosa, which contains many blood vessels suspended in a loose connective tissue. It is this layer that bleeds when the tunica albuginea is incised, as occurs during operations such as testicular biopsy. Arising from the outer tunica albuginea and extending down through the substance of the testis are a series of fibrous septa that divide the interior of each testis into lobules. Lying within the confines of these lobules are several looped or blind-ended seminiferous tubules and it is from the epithelial lining of

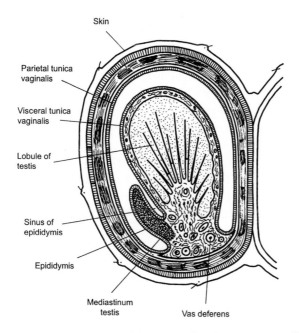

Fig. 2.1 Diagrammatic representation of the testis within the scrotum as well as its relationship to the epididymis.

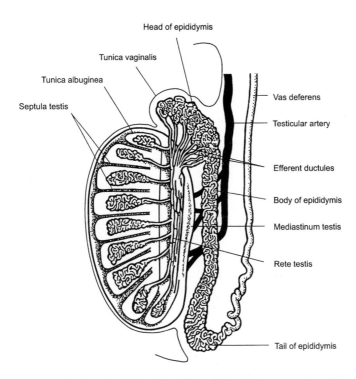

Fig. 2.2 Drawing showing the relationship of the tubules to the rete testis and the efferent ductules that lead out of the testis and form the epididymal duct. It should be noted that the branches of the testicular artery enter the testis behind the epididymis.

these tubules that the development and the production of the spermatozoa takes place.

Along the posterior border of each testis, the fibrous tunica albuginea becomes thickened and indents into the substance of the testis to become the mediastinum testis. Within the mediastinum, there is a complex network of channels known as the rete testis into which enter the terminal segments of the seminiferous tubules.

Each testis contains some 200–300 seminiferous tubules. Their total length may amount to some 1–2 m, providing an enormous area for spermatogenesis (Bascom & Osterud 1925). Each tubule is highly convoluted and forms either a loop within the lobule when the two ends of this loop join together close to the mediastinum or, alternatively, the tubule may simply be blind-ended (Fig. 2.3). Very tight convolutions of the seminiferous tubules may result in their incomplete obstruction. Close to the mediastinum, these convolutions are lost and the tubules straighten out to form the tubuli recti (also known as the straight ducts), which drain into the network of channels that make up the rete testis.

Between the seminiferous tubules lies the interstitial tissue that is made up of loose connective tissue in which are suspended the Leydig cells. It is these Leydig cells that secrete testosterone. In man, the interstitial tissue makes up around 5% of the total testicular tissue.

The rete testis is lined by a ciliated epithelium. The rete testis may contribute fluid to the sperm suspension leaving the seminiferous tubules that will assist sperm transport into the epididymis (Hees *et al.* 1987). The presence of myoid elements around the channels of the rete may result in the

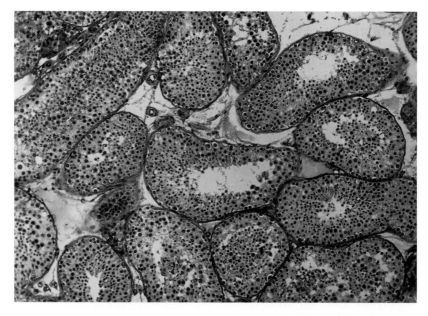

Fig. 2.3 Histological section of a normal testis. Note that all the stages of development of the male gametes from the spermatogonia to the spermatozoa are present in the tubules.

active expulsion of the spermatozoa from interior of the testis. Apart from its channel system, the function of the rete testis is not known but it may certainly become blocked and can therefore be a site for infertility (Guerin *et al.* 1981).

The epididymis

The epididymis lies along the posterolateral border of each testis. It is made up of convoluted tubules that are packed together within loose connective tissue. Although the epididymis is divided into many different segments for scientific reasons, clinically the human epididymis can be divided into three main regions. These consist of the proximal caput (head) at the upper pole of each testis, the middle corpus (body) and the distal cauda (tail) which is situated at the lower pole of each testis (Fig. 2.2). However, more structurally and functionally related subdivisions have been suggested in the past (Glover & Nicander 1971), but these are certainly not used in the clinical field.

Each epididymis contains three main contiguous duct systems. At the upper pole are the 12–20 ductuli efferenti through which the sperm exit the testis. These ductuli efferenti become highly convoluted and make up the bulk of the caput of the epididymis. The ductuli efferenti are very fine and their walls are composed of myoid cells which undergo frequent autonomous contractile activity and which are overlaid by a highly ciliated columnar epithelium for maximal absorption of water. It is at this point that a major concentration of the spermatozoa takes place (Brooks 1983).

The efferent ductuli then all converge to form a single, highly convoluted duct called the epididymal duct, which lies tightly coiled up alongside the posterolateral border of the testis and which comprises most of the corpus and the cauda of the epididymis. The epididymal duct is some 6 m in length and its walls are made up of myoid cells and some inner circumferential smooth muscle cells.

The epididymal duct is also lined by a columnar epithelium that has a very important secretory activity. This epithelium is complex and is made up of several cell types that vary in their proportions in different parts of the epididymal duct (Hamilton 1975). On the luminal surface of these cells are microvilli known as 'stereocilia' because of the absence of an axoneme (Fig. 2.4).

The passage of sperm down the epididymis usually takes around 8–10 days. Interestingly, this journey may vary among different populations of sperm (Orgebin-Crist 1965) and this transport time will, of course, differ among different species. During their journey down the epididymal duct, the spermatozoa undergo an important maturational process, acquire motility and can now achieve fertilization (Overstreet & Bedford 1974). The cauda of the epididymis (Fig. 2.5) is also an important site for sperm storage prior to ejaculation.

11

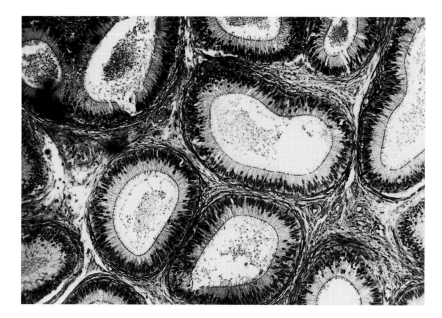

Fig. 2.4 Histological section taken through a normal caput epididymis. Note the dense microcilia that are present on the surface of the epithelium to enhance absorption and the relative absence of spermatozoa in the lumen of the duct. The activity of the myoid cells in the wall of the duct within the caput rapidly move the sperm on down the duct towards the cauda epididymis.

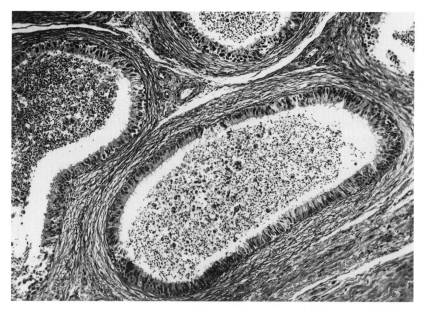

Fig. 2.5 Histological section through the cauda of the epididymis. The epithelium is now less densely endowed with microcilia and copious numbers of sperm are now seen in the lumen of the duct. The caput is an important storage area for sperm prior to ejaculation.

Within the cauda of the epididymis, the epididymal duct increases in diameter but remains convoluted to form the vas deferens. The vas deferens forms within the cauda of the epididymis, and it is in the most proximal portion of each vas deferens that the majority of the now mature sperm are stored prior to ejaculation (Fig. 2.5).

The vas deferens

After each vas deferens has emerged from the tail of the epididymis, it loses its convolutions and as a straight duct it passes upwards and out of the scrotum within the spermatic cord. In man the vas measures some 25 cm in length. Each vas can be divided into three anatomical parts: the proximal segment, the distal section and the terminal vas. The proximal segment involves that part of the vas that is contained within the scrotum. The distal vas involves that part within the inguinal canal while the terminal vas is that part of the vas within the abdominal cavity.

The vas is powerfully contractile and has a thick muscle coat. It contracts vigorously and propels the sperm out throughout its length at ejaculation. The epithelium of each vas is crenellated and also bears stereocilia, but the distribution of these stereocilia is patchy and they are much less dense than in the epididymal duct (Fig. 2.6). It is the scrotal or proximal portion of the vas, at the upper border of the epididymis, that is transected during the operation of vasectomy.

Each vas deferens passes up through the inguinal canal and enters the pelvis. The vasa then pass forwards and medially to reach the back of the bladder where each vas arches over the ureter. At this point each vas dilates

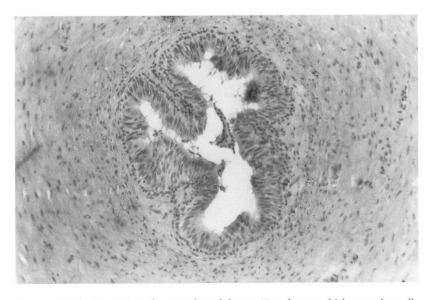

Fig. 2.6 Histological section of a normal vas deferens. Note the very thick muscular wall and the persistence of microcilia on the surface of the luminal epithelium.

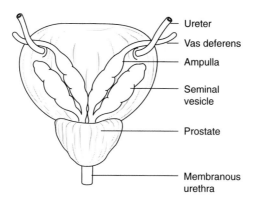

Ureter

Vas deferens

Ampulla

Seminal
vesicle

Prostate

Membranous
urethra

Fig. 2.7 Diagrammatic representation of the distal ends of the vasa deferentia and their relationship with the seminal vesicles. Note that the duct of the seminal vesicles joins with the terminal portions of the vas to form the ejaculatory ducts.

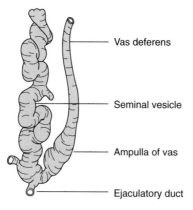

Vas deferens

Seminal vesicle

Ampulla of vas

Ejaculatory duct

Fig. 2.8 A drawing of the seminal vesicle showing its coiled structure. Its relationship with the ampulla and the terminal portion of the vas deferens is also shown.

to form a chamber known as the ampulla of the vas deferens. It is in the ampulla as well as in the cauda epididymis that sperm are stored prior to ejaculation. Each ampulla is around 2 cm in length and, distal to the ampulla, the duct narrows substantially (Fig. 2.7).

The seminal vesicles

These structures were so named because early investigators believed that the seminal vesicles were the storage point for the spermatozoa. The seminal vesicles lie behind the bladder. Each seminal vesicle is a sacculated pouch of about 5 cm in length. Each vesicle consists of a tube coiled up upon itself which contains several blind-ended diverticula (Fig. 2.8). The seminal vesicles have a thick muscular wall that contracts powerfully at ejaculation. They are lined by a columnar mucus-secreting epithelium containing many goblet cells.

The ejaculatory ducts

The junction of the duct of the seminal vesicle and the now narrowed portion of the vas deferens distal to the ampulla forms the ejaculatory ducts. Each duct is some 2 cm in length. The walls of the ducts are thin and

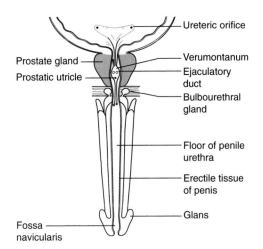

Fig. 2.9 A drawing of the prostate and the penile urethra. Note the position of the openings of the ejaculatory ducts on the verumontanum as well as their relationship to the prostatic utricle.

are made up of smooth muscle myocytes and are lined by a columnar epithelium. From the base of the prostate, each ejaculatory duct runs antero-inferiorly between the median and the lateral lobes of the prostate. Each duct skirts the prostatic utricle to open as two slit-like orifices in the prostatic urethra on a protrusion in the prostatic urethra known as the colliculus seminalis (Fig. 2.9).

Appendages of the testis and epididymis

There are a number of aberrant structures that can be found close to the testis and the epididymis. The most common is the appendix epididymis, which is found at the upper end of the epididymis. It is a vestigial remnant of the müllerian duct system, whose development has been suppressed in the male. It resembles the distal end of a fallopian tube and also contains a large number of oestrogen receptors.

Aberrant ductules may be found at either end of the epididymal duct and are likely to represent remnants of the now regressed mesonephros.

The prostate

The prostate gland is a glandular organ that surrounds the proximal portion of the urethra. It is enclosed within a muscle coat that contracts at ejaculation. The prostate is conical in shape, the base of the prostate being largely contiguous with the base of the bladder. The prostate is divided into three lobes, namely the two lateral lobes and a median lobe. The secretions of the prostate are expelled into the urethra at ejaculation. The secretions enter the urethra by means of a series of small ducts that drain the main part of the gland. The prostatic secretions from both the submucosal and mucosal areas of the prostate drain through small ducts that surround the urethra (Fig. 2.10).

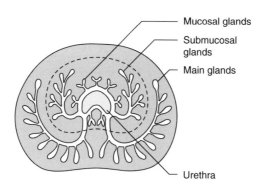

Mucosal glands

Submucosal glands

Main glands

Urethra

Fig. 2.10 A diagrammatic representation of the prostate gland showing the arrangement of the ducts that drain the prostatic acini.

The prostate is made up of glandular acini and stroma that contains a lot of fibrous tissue (Aumuller 1989). Concretions and calculi are often seen within the gland and these are also occasionally seen in the seminal fluid.

The bulbourethral and urethral glands

The bulbourethral glands are two small lobulated glands that secrete mostly mucus. They open into the membranous urethra. The urethral glands are very small mucus-secreting glands that open into the roof of the penile urethra and are particularly numerous in a dilation of the distal portion of the penile urethra known as the fossa navicularis.

The secretions that make up semen

Semen is a grey opalescent fluid that is formed at ejaculation and emission. Although semen contains spermatozoa, it is far from solely testicular in origin: indeed only a very small proportion of semen is derived from the testes themselves.

The contribution of the testes to the ejaculate only makes up about 5% of the total volume while the seminal vesicles and prostate gland together contribute around 90% of the total ejaculate (Lundquist 1949). The remaining 5% of the ejaculatory volume is formed by the bulbourethral and urethral glands. These volumes are outlined in Table 2.1.

Semen is thus largely made up of the secretions from the accessory glands of the male genital tract. Volumetrically, only a small proportion of the ejaculatory volume comes from the testes. However, the secretions of the accessory glands contain substances which have an important effect on sperm function. Thus, even minor changes in the volume and the constituents of the secretions that go to make up seminal fluid will have a profound effect, not only upon the concentration of the sperm in a semen sample, but also on the function of the sperm within the ejaculate. As will be demonstrated in later sections, reproductive failure can be the result of pathology in one of the accessory glands rather than the result of any abnormality of sperm production.

Table 2.1 The percentage contribution of each of the secretions that make up the seminal fluid

Source of secretion	Ejaculate (%)
Testes and excurrent ducts	5
Seminal vesicles	46–80
Prostate	13–33
Bulbourethral and urethral glands	2–5

From Lundquist (1949).

Each of the contributions that make up semen is individually propelled into the posterior urethra in a set order. The propulsion of these secretions into the posterior urethra is known as emission. The ejection of the semen out of the penile urethra is known as ejaculation. Thus, during ejaculation each of the components of the ejaculate are discharged from the urethra in a predetermined sequence. Therefore, by carefully collecting semen as it is discharged, it is possible to separate out the secretions that make up an ejaculate. Semen collected in this way is known as a split ejaculate. Using split ejaculates it is possible to examine each of the components of the ejaculate individually and this can be of great value diagnostically as it can provide useful information concerning the malfunction of the accessory glands, particularly in relation to infection.

It must also be remembered that mixing of the components of the ejaculate thus does not take place until after ejaculation, and loss of any part of the semen sample during ejaculation can result in an artefactually induced abnormality in a semen analysis.

It is now of value to consider each of the components of an ejaculate in more detail.

The testicular contribution

As the testicular component contains the sperm, it is of course very important to the fertility of the ejaculate. However, in terms of volume, it only makes up around 5% (or 0.2 mL) of the total semen sample. Thus, no significant reduction in semen volume is noticed by the patient following a vasectomy.

The fluid that emerges from the testis and enters the efferent ductules is known as rete testis fluid. This fluid contains the spermatozoa but is also rich in testosterone, much of which is bound to the androgen-binding protein produced by the Sertoli cells. Here, the testosterone is released for uptake by both the efferent ductules and the epididymal duct for this is their main source of androgen that is essential for their normal function. Contained in rete testis fluid is the hormone inhibin and the enzyme transferrin, both of which are also produced by the Sertoli cells (Skinner & Griswold 1980). The copper-carrying protein ceruloplasmin has also been shown to be produced by the Sertoli cells (Skinner & Griswold 1983). A reduction in the concentrations of both inhibin and transferrin has been demonstrated in semen from men with epididymal obstruction. However, it must be remembered that low levels of these substances will also be found in the semen of infertile men with severe abnormalities of Sertoli cell function.

Contained in the sperm is an enzyme called lactate dehydrogenase (LDH) C_4, which that is released from sperm when they die or break up. This enzyme can be easily measured and its presence in semen may indicate that the sperm are being damaged during their passage through the epididymal duct.

As the rete testis fluid passes through the efferent ductules, a large proportion of the water is reabsorbed. Thus, water reabsorption results in a considerable concentration of the spermatozoa within the rete testis fluid. Because of the contractile activity of the myoid cells that make up the walls of the efferent ductules and the proximal portions of the epididymal duct, the concentrated sperm suspension is rapidly propelled out of the caput of the epididymis.

During the passage of sperm down the epididymal duct, many substances are added to the sperm suspension. The substances that can be of diagnostic importance include L-carnitine and glycerophosphorylcholine, both of which have been used as indicators of epididymal functions. However, as both these substances have been shown to be secreted in other parts of the genital tract, their use diagnostically is limited (Table 2.2).

Table 2.2 Important chemical substances that are present in each of the contributions to the ejaculate

Source	Important biochemical substances
Testes and excurrent ducts	Testosterone
	Inhibin
	LDH C_4
	L-Carnitine
	Glyceryophosphorylcholine
Seminal vesicles	Fructose
	Prostaglandins
	Substrate for semen clotting
Prostate	Acid phosphatase
	Citrates
	Proteases
	Pepidases
	Hyaluronidase
	Vesiculase
	Spermine
	Zn, Ca, Mg
Bulbourethral and urethral glands	Mucoproteins
	IgG

The seminal vesicles and their secretions

In terms of volume, the seminal vesicles are the most important contributors to the seminal fluid as the secretions from these glands make up between 40% and 60% of the total ejaculatory volume. Aside from their volume, the secretions of the seminal vesicles are very important diagnostically. They profoundly affect the function of the sperm and the physical properties of the seminal plasma. The seminal vesicular secretions tend to be slightly alkaline and thus their exclusion from an ejaculate will lower the pH of the seminal plasma.

The best-known substance contained in these secretions is the sugar fructose, which is an important energy source for the spermatozoa. Interestingly, this sugar is absent from the seminal vesicular secretions in some mammals, examples of which are the dog and the horse.

Exclusion of the seminal vesicular component from the ejaculate will result in almost completely immotile sperm. Disorders of the seminal vesicles that result in diminished fructose secretion will also give rise to reduced sperm motility. The seminal vesicles are also a major source of prostaglandins (PG), which are mainly those of the PGE and 19-OH PGE groups. The role of these prostaglandins is uncertain, but they may play a role in maintaining sperm motility after ejaculation and may even act as calcium ionophores.

The seminal vesicles also secrete a fibrinogen-like substrate that is acted upon by the prostatic enzyme vesiculase to induce the clotting that occurs in seminal plasma.

The prostatic fluid

The prostate secretes its contribution to semen straight into the urethra by means of multiple ducts that surround the verumontanum in the prostatic urethra. The prostate gland is the second largest contributor to the ejaculate, for the prostatic contribution makes up around 10–30% of the total seminal plasma volume.

The prostatic secretion is biochemically very active. It contains large numbers of enzymes which are involved with semen clotting and liquefaction. The enzyme vesiculase induces clotting by its action on a substrate similar to fibrinogen and which is present in the seminal vesicular fluid. Prostatic fluid also contains a number of proteases and peptidases and hyaluronidase, which are all enzymes that breakdown this clot. Thus, both clotting and liquefaction of the clot are induced by substances secreted by the prostate.

The prostatic secretions also contain the bacteriostatic amine called spermine, which will crystallize out in semen as spermine phosphate. This phenomenon may be seen when a semen sample is left on the bench for any length of time and the pH of the seminal plasma is allowed to fall.

However, these crystals are not uncommonly seen on the routine microscopy of semen.

The prostatic secretions also contain large amounts of the enzyme acid phosphatase which is an important marker of prostatic function. This enzyme is very stable and for this reason is commonly used in forensic medicine as a marker of the presence of semen stains on clothes.

Citrates are also abundant in prostatic secretions and can be used as an indicator of prostatic function.

Zinc and magnesium are also present in prostatic fluid but their function is unknown. At one time zinc was thought to be important in the maintenance of sperm motility, but this is now doubtful. Zinc may, however, be of value in the protection of the condensed chromatin within the sperm head. Calcium is also present in high concentration in prostatic fluid.

Secretions of the bulbourethral and urethral glands

These mucus-secreting glands open into the urethra proximally and the volume of their combined secretions is small, often totalling less than 0.2 mL. The fluid they produce is rich in mucoproteins and the role of these glands is solely to lubricate the urethra and to facilitate the ejaculation of the seminal fluid. These glands also produce the secretory immunoprotein immunoglobulin G (IgG). Although the secretions of these glands is of little significance in the normally fertile patient, the immunoglobulins can on occasions be directed against the sperm as antisperm antibodies, and in this situation these secretions could, therefore, be a cause of infertility.

Seminal fluid is thus made up not only of sperm but also contains a wide range of different chemical substances. It should therefore be clear that any change in one or more of the secretions that make up semen could produce major changes in both the physical and chemical properties of semen and in the function of the sperm within it. The differing role that each of these secretions may play in producing an abnormality in semen must also be remembered during the performance of a semen analysis. As will be seen later, such a thought process when applied to a semen analysis, may be extremely helpful diagnostically. As diagnosis is the most important factor in determining the correct management of an infertile patient, the laboratory may, therefore, play a vital role in the successful treatment of an infertile couple.

The endocrinology of the testis

The endocrinology of the testis is complex. There are two major areas of hormone secretion in the testis, namely the Leydig cells, which secrete testosterone, and the Sertoli cells, which lie within the seminiferous tubules.

Like the ovary, the endocrine secretions of the testis are largely controlled by the pituitary gonadotrophins, namely luteinizing hormone (LH) and follicle-stimulating hormone (FSH). Both LH and FSH are glycoproteins produced by the anterior pituitary and are produced in response to the secretion of the hypothalamic hormone, gonadotrophin-releasing hormone (GnRH).

The gonadotrophin LH has its main action on the Leydig cells, which respond to LH by secreting the androgenic steroid testosterone. The gonadotrophin FSH has its main action on the Sertoli cells, where it stimulates the production of androgen-binding protein (ABP), a protein that has a very high affinity for testosterone. A concentration gradient for testosterone thus exists between the interstitial tissue and the interior of the Sertoli cell. As a consequence, testosterone passes across the tubular basement membrane to form an ABP–testosterone complex within the Sertoli cell (Fig. 2.11). This provides a supply of androgen to the process of spermatogenesis. The ABP–testosterone complex also enters the lumen of the seminiferous tubules by a process of exocytosis (Palliniemi *et al.* 1981). The Leydig cells, via the Sertoli cells, thus provide a supply of testosterone to the rete testis, the efferent ductules and the proximal portion of the epididymal duct. Testosterone also enters the general circulation and by its action on the pituitary is the major negative feedback for LH on the pituitary–hypothalamic axis.

In response to stimulation by FSH, the Sertoli cells also produce the hormone inhibin, which is the major negative feedback for FSH secretion. Inhibin is produced in two forms, namely the α-subunit and the two β-subunits known as β-A and β-B. The subunit β-B is present only in male serum. There is known to be an inverse relationship between inhibin B and FSH in male sera but no such relationship exists between inhibin A and FSH levels in the serum of male patients. Damage to the Sertoli cell will thus reduce inhibin B production and therefore will cause an increase in FSH secretion.

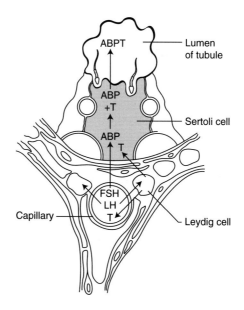

Fig. 2.11 The relationship between the pituitary gonadotrophins and the Sertoli cells within the tubule and the Leydig cells in the interstitial tissue of the testis. Note that the androgen-binding protein complex passes into the lumen of the tubule whence it passes to the excurrent duct system of the testis. This is an important source of androgen for the efferent ductules.

If the two β-subunits are joined, they form another hormone known as activin, which stimulates the production of FSH. A variety of activins exist as this dimeric hormone can be formed by various combinations of the β-subunits, e.g. β-A–β-B, β-A–β-A or β-B–β-B.

It is also now known that the Sertoli cells produce an additional substance called follistatin. This hormone, like inhibin, suppresses FSH secretion, but it is much less potent than inhibin and its biological relevance is unclear. These FSH suppressing substances may also have a minor suppressive action on LH secretion. There is also now some evidence that the Sertoli cells produce a substance that acts on the Leydig cells to modulate the production of testosterone.

There is thus a complex interrelationship between the Sertoli cells and the pituitary–hypothalamic axis and between the Sertoli and Leydig cells.

As can be seen, the hormonal activity of the testis is still poorly understood. However, an understanding of the process of sperm production as well as the basic features of testicular endocrinology is essential in order to understand some of the changes that occur in male infertility and in the associated changes that take place in the seminal fluid of these patients.

Spermatogenesis and the development of the spermatozoon

Spermatogenesis in the human was first studied and the cell cycle elucidated in 1963 by Clermont in Montreal (Clermont 1963). The cells that make up the precursors of the spermatozoa lie between the Sertoli cells within the epithelium that lines the seminiferous tubules. These cells can be grouped into five main categories.

Spermatogonia

Spermatogonia are the stem cells from which all sperm are generated and are descendants of the primordial germ cells that migrate to the gonadal ridge from the yolk sac in early intrauterine life.

There are three basic groups of spermatogonia, known as dark type A, pale type A and type B. They can be recognized by their dimensions, their large nuclei and their position on the seminiferous basement membrane. Dark type A cells divide to maintain their own numbers while others differentiate into pale type A, which differentiate into type B, which are the immediate precursors of the spermatocytes. Thus, the dark spermatogonia form a reservoir of resting cells while the pale type A cells divide into type B cells, which in turn divide into the primary spermatocyte.

Primary spermatocytes

These diploid cells are characterized by their nuclear appearance in which chromatin condensation is conspicuous. The primary spermatocytes divide by meiotic division into the secondary spermatocytes. Primary spermatocytes may be resting or may be in the various stages of meiotic division and can be seen in the proleptotene, leptotene, zygotene, pachytene or diplotene stages.

Secondary spermatocytes

The secondary spermatocytes now undergo the second meiotic division to spermatids. The process of sperm development from the spermatogonium to the formation of the secondary spermatocyte is known as spermatogenesis.

Spermatids

Spermatids do not undergo further division but gradually mature into spermatozoa by changing their shape. The nuclei becomes oval and eccentric and the cytoplasm elongates. Spermatids are often described as 'round' or 'oval' and may also be called 'early' or 'late'. Finally, the spermatids develop into the mature spermatozoa. The change from spermatocyte to the formation of mature spermatozoa is known as spermiogenesis (Fig. 2.12).

Spermatozoa

Each sperm breaks free from the Sertoli cell, probably aided by the action of the Sertoli cell cytoskeleton. It may carry with it a small piece of cytoplasm from the Sertoli cell, which is called a cytoplasmic droplet. The process of release of the spermatozoa from the Sertoli cell is called spermiation.

The spermatogenic cycle

It is clear that, at any point along the seminiferous tubules, the development of the germinal cells and the associations between the different cell types pass through a cycle. The stages and the length of this cycle vary in different species, but in man it is made up of six stages and lasts around 16 days. Each region of a tubule passes through a cycle of changes and then begins again. In the human testis, different areas of a single tubule will show the epithelium at different stages of a cycle. Not even all four quadrants of the epithelium inside a single tubule will necessarily be at the same stage of a spermatogenic cycle.

The stages of a spermatogenic cycle in the human are defined in six sections known as stages I–VI.

Stage I: In this stage, two generations of spermatids are seen. The

23

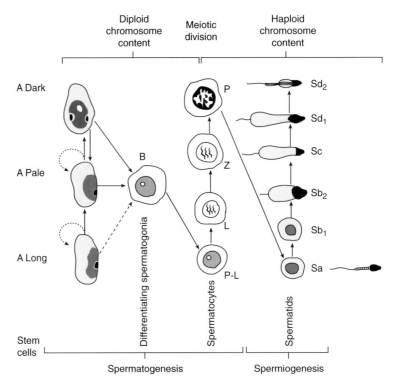

Fig. 2.12 A diagram showing the maturation of the sperm from the spermatogonia.

primary spermatocytes are entering the long pachytene stage of meiotic division to form secondary spermatocytes. Pale type A and type B spermatogonia are present on the tubular basement membrane.

Stage II: Spermatid maturation is also seen in this stage but is more advanced, the older spermatids now nearing the change to mature spermatozoa. Type B spermatogonia are present in increased numbers.

Stage III: Spermiation is now seen together with large numbers of spermatids. Younger primary spermatocytes are now present both in the resting phase and in the proleptotene stage while some older cells in the pachytene stage can be identified. Type A spermatogonia, both dark and pale, now predominate in the lower part of the spermatogenic epithelium.

Stage IV: Spermatid nuclei are becoming oval, the older primary spermatocytes are moving into the pachytene stage while the younger ones are moving from the resting to the leptotene stage.

Stage V: The spermatids now show very eccentric nuclei and the cells are becoming elongated. The primary spermatocytes are now in the late leptotene stages.

Stage VI: Primary spermatocytes are now at the pachytene stage and some are dividing to form secondary spermatocytes. Type A spermatogonia again are seen in large numbers on the basement membrane of the tubule. In this way undulating changes in the spermatogenic epithelium take place, but because of the patchy nature of the spermatogenic cycle in the human these cyclical changes are difficult to identify in a testicular biopsy. Although the spermatogenic cycle takes only 16 days to complete, the total length of time for sperm maturation, from spermatogonium to a mature spermatozoon, is around 70 days. As it takes a further 10–14 days to undergo spermiation and to travel down to the cauda of the epididymis, the whole process of sperm maturation from spermatogonium to the presence of sperm in an ejaculate will take at least 80 days.

It is clear that sperm production is a complex process. However, in order to understand semen and its analysis more clearly, a working knowledge of the process of sperm production is essential.

References

Aumuller, G. (1989) Morphologic and regulatory aspects of prostatic function. *Anatomy and Embryology* **179**, 519–531.

Bascom, K.F. & Osterud, H.L. (1925) Quantitative studies of the testicle. Pattern and total tubule length in the testicles of certain mammals. *Anatomical Record* **31**, 159–169.

Brooks, D.E. (1983) Epididymal functions and their hormonal regulation. *Australian Journal of Biological Science* **36**, 205–221.

Clermont, Y. (1963) The cycle of the seminiferous epithelium in man. *American Journal of Anatomy* **112**, 35–51.

Davis, J.R., Langford, J.A. & Kirby, P.J. (1970) *The Testicular Capsule in the Testis* (eds A.D. Johnson, W.R. Gomes & N.L. Vandermark), pp. 281–337. Academic Press, New York.

Glover, T.D. & Nicander, L. (1971) Some aspects of structure and function in the mammalian epididymis. *Journal of Reproduction and Fertility Suppl.* **13**, 39–50.

Guerin, J.-F., Cyza, J.-C., Perrrin, P. & Rollet, J. (1981) Les obstructions congenitales ou aquises de l'epididyme humain: etude de la mobility des spermatoides en amont de l'obstruction. *Bulletin de l'Association Des Anatomistes* **65**, 297–306.

Hamilton, D.W. (1975) Structure and function of the epithelium lining the ductuli efferentes, ductus epdidymis and ductus deferens in the rat. In: *Handbook of Physiology* (eds D.W. Hamilton & R.O. Greep), pp. 259–301. American Physiological Society.

Hees, H., Wrobel, K.H., Kohler, T., Leiser, R. & Rothbacher, I. (1987) Spatial topography of the excurrent duct system in the bovine testis. *Cell and Tissue Research* **248**, 143–151.

Lundquist, F. (1949) Aspects of the biochemistry of semen. *Acta Physiologica Scandinavica* **19** (Suppl. 66), 7–105.

Nistal, M., Santamaria, L. & Paniagua, R. (1984) Mast cells in the human testis and epididymis from birth to adulthood. *Acta Anatomica* **119**, 155–160.

Orgebin-Crist, M.-C. (1965) Passage of spermatozoa labelled with thymidine ^{3}H through the ductus epididymis. *Journal of Reproduction and Fertility* **10**, 241–251.

Overstreet, J.W. & Bedford, J.M. (1974) Transport, capacitation and fertilizing ability of epididymal sperm. *Journal of Experimental Zoology* **189**, 203–214.

Palliniemi, L.J., Dym, M., Gunsalus, G.L., Muslo, N.A., Bardin, C.W. & Fawcett, D.W. (1981) Immunocytochemical localisation of androgen binding protein in the male rat reproductive tract. *Endocrinology* **108**, 925–931.

Skinner, M.K. & Griswold, M.D. (1980) Sertoli cells synthesise and secrete a transferrin-like protein. *Journal of Biology and Chemistry* **255**, 9523–9525.

Skinner, M.K. & Griswold, M.D. (1983) Sertoli cells synthesise and secrete a ceruloplasmin-lie protein. *Biology of Reproduction* **28**, 1225–1230.

3: The Structure and Function of the Human Spermatozoon, Sperm Transport and Fertilization

The spermatozoon is a highly specialized cell with considerable powers of movement. In order to complete its task of fertilization of the oocyte, it must be capable of complex biochemical and structural changes. An understanding of both its structure and the physiological changes that it must undergo to achieve fusion with the oocyte is important to the clinician, as some of these changes form the basis of commonly used sperm function tests.

The structure of the human sperm

The structure of the spermatozoon is complex (Fawcett 1975). Each sperm can be divided into four parts and these consist of the head, the neck-piece, the midpiece and the tail (Fig. 3.1).

The head

Each sperm head is shaped like a thickened paddle making it rounded posteriorly but flattened at its tip. There is, however, very considerable variation in the shape of the head amongst human spermatozoa and it is uncertain what degrees of differences in head shape result in either fertile or infertile sperm.

Each sperm head measures approximately 4.4 μm in length, 3 μm in width but is only on average some 1.5 μm thick. A sperm head is thus only about half the size of a red blood cell. Each sperm head is made up of two main parts: the nucleus and the acrosome.

The darkly staining nucleus contains the whole nuclear DNA of the sperm. As the sperm head is relatively small, a special packaging mechanism exists in the sperm head so that the DNA will fit into such a small space. In the human sperm, the DNA is not stored in the helical form in which it exists in all other cells. The nuclear DNA of the sperm is fixed to a small annulus from which the layers or sheets of DNA are tightly folded. On decondensation within the oocyte, these folds penetrate the inner cell membrane to unfold outside the sperm head. Moreover, unlike the normal cell nucleus, the sperm DNA is swaddled in protamines rather than histones. Thus, at fertilization, these histones have to be replaced, a process that may take 12–18 h. Only very scanty cytoplasm is present in the sperm head that is enclosed in a plasma membrane.

Covering the anterior two-thirds of the sperm head is the sac-like struc-

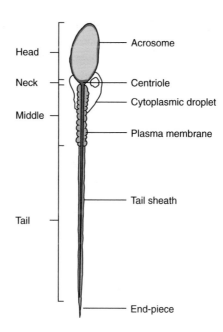

Fig. 3.1 A diagrammatic representation
of a human spermatozoon together with
its anatomical subdivisions.

ture known as the acrosome. The acrosome ends at the equatorial segment,
which that is a specialized area for egg penetration. The acrosome is made up
of an outer and an inner acrosomal membrane, between which is stored the
enzymes which aid the penetration of the zona pellucida. These enzymes
include hyaluronidase and a number of proteinases. At the posterior limit of
the acrosome on the sperm head is a ridge known as the equatorial ring. Posterior to this ring and behind the acrosome, the nuclear and the plasma
membranes fuse to form a relatively dense post-acrosomal lamina. This
region of the sperm head is usually known as the post-acrosomal region. The
acrosome is anchored to the nucleus by the perinuclear theca, a structure
thought to play a key role in the activation of the egg at fertilization.

The neck

The head is joined to the neck by a very short structure known as the basal
plate, posterior to which lies the proximal centriole. The proximal centriole
is thought to be important in the generation of normal sperm movement.
Malformation of the proximal centriole may result in absent sperm movement and thus can be a cause of infertility. The centriole is also passed on to
the oocyte at fertilization and is a critical organelle involved in the first cell
division.

The axoneme

The axoneme is a structure that forms the centre of the neck, middle piece
and most of the tail of each sperm. It is the central contractile element of the
sperm that generates movement. The axoneme consists of nine doublet

27

microtubules giving the well-known '9 + 2' configuration (Fig. 3.2). This arrangement of the microtubules continues throughout the midpiece and the tail to terminate at the terminal segment. Each doublet has an outer coarse fibre that is thought to strengthen the axoneme and to contribute mechanical effects to the flagellar wave.

The outer doublets of tubulin consist of two subunits known as A and B. Subunit A is a complete tubule while subunit B is incomplete and has its two ends joined to subunit A. Each subunit A is joined to its neighbour by arms that are made up of the protein dynein, a substance which can convert chemical energy into contractility. Abnormalities of these dynein arms or even their total absence are well-known causes of poor or absent sperm movement. An association between the absence of these dynein arms in all the cilia in the body constitutes the disorder known as Kartagener's syndrome, in which immotile sperm are associated with sinusitis, bronchiectasis and not infrequently with situs inversus. Also arising from subunit A are the nexin links which connect the adjacent outer doublets.

The single tubules in the centre of the axoneme are surrounded by a central sheath, which itself is connected to each outer doublet by a radial link. The normality of these structures and their arrangement is vital for normal sperm, and thus for normal fertility. The normality of the axoneme can only be assessed in detail using transmission electron microscopy, preferably using special stains such as tannic acid.

The midpiece

The neck leads into the midpiece, which measures some 10 µm in length. In this section of the sperm, the axoneme is surrounded by a closely packed winding helix of mitochondria, making a total of some 10–12 coils that are all contained within a fibrous sheath. The close anatomical relationship between the tubules and the mitochondria is important as it allows for the easy transfer of energy to the contractile microtubular system of the axoneme.

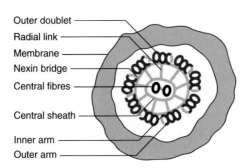

Outer doublet
Radial link
Membrane
Nexin bridge
Central fibres

Central sheath

Inner arm
Outer arm

Fig. 3.2 A drawing of the axoneme of the human spermatozoon showing the 9 + 2 arrangement.

The tail

The sperm tail is relatively long and measures around 50 μm in length. Each sperm tail is made up of a long principal piece that forms about 90% of the tail and a much shorter terminal segment.

Each principal piece contains the central axoneme only. The helical mitochondria are lost, but the fibrous sheath persists over the principal piece to give it a slightly ribbed appearance. In the small terminal segment, the axoneme is covered only by a thin plasma membrane and is where the coarse fibres terminate. There is a close association between the architecture of the tail components and the efficiency of sperm movement.

The cytoplasmic droplet

Attached to the posterior portion of the head, to the neck and to the middle piece may be found a small portion of cytoplasm that has been derived from the Sertoli cell at the site where each sperm separated at the time of spermiation (Fig. 3.3). This cytoplasmic droplet is normally lost as the sperm ages. Its presence is of relevance in a semen analysis as it is an indication that a spermatozoon is relatively young or has not matured correctly. It is also known that cytoplasmic droplets in the neck region may be the site of

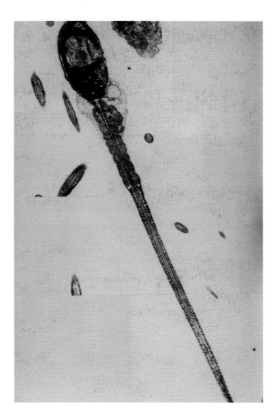

Fig. 3.3 Transmission electron microscopy of a human spermatozoon. A cytoplasmic droplet is clearly visible.

formation of peroxides and other reactive oxygen species that are harmful to sperm function (Aitken 1995).

Changes in sperm function that occur prior to ejaculation

Major functional changes occur in the spermatozoa as they pass through the excurrent ducts of the testis, in particular as they pass through the epididymal duct and during their time in the female genital tract. These physicochemical and morphological changes that take place during this time are collectively known as capacitation and this process is not complete until just prior to fertilization.

As the sperm leave the rete testis and enter the efferent ductules, the first change that takes place is a massive reabsorption of water, which markedly concentrates the sperm in this area. In the rat, around 90% of the water leaving the rete testis is reabsorbed by the efferent ductules before the sperm enter the epididymal duct. Interestingly, this feature of epididymal function is oestrogen dependent. This concentration in sperm numbers because of water reabsorption continues, but to a lesser extent, as the sperm pass down the epididymal duct.

The epididymal duct itself also secretes substances such as the sugar inositol, the energy source L-carnitine and several amino acids, in particular taurine and tryptophan. There are also large numbers of proteins, lipids and phospholipids that are present in abundance in the epididymal duct, where they are converted into glycerophosphorylcholine.

Testosterone is essential for the normal function of the epididymal duct. Testosterone arrives in the upper epididymis via the rete testis in the form of a testosterone–androgen-binding protein complex that has been exocytosed by the Sertoli cells. Here, the testosterone is freed from this protein complex and is converted to the more potent 5α-dihydrotestosterone by the enzyme 5α-reductase. However, the epididymal epithelium is itself capable of synthesizing small amounts of testosterone from cholesterol. The epididymal duct is thus biochemically very active, and there also exists a powerful blood–testis barrier that probably protects the spermatozoa from substances in the blood that may have an adverse effect upon their function.

During their passage down the epididymal duct, the sperm acquire motility. Sperm taken from the caput show little motility and are infertile while sperm from the cauda are motile and can achieve fertilization. How sperm motility is initiated in the epididymal duct is uncertain, but a sperm motility protein has been demonstrated in both the corpus and the cauda of the epididymis. A sperm immobilization protein may also be present in the epididymal duct. Sperm motility also relates to the availability of ATP: indeed the frequency of and the amplitude of the tail movements of the sperm relate closely to the dephosphorylation of ATP.

The cauda of the epididymis, which includes the very proximal portion of the vas deferens, is an important storage place for sperm and it is here that the majority of the sperm await ejaculation. In most species, the cauda epididymis lies below the testis and thus occupies the coolest part of the scrotum. The purpose of this positioning of the site of storage of the sperm may be to reduce the oxygen requirements of the sperm and thus conserve their motility for as long as possible.

Ejaculation and emission

Ejaculation is a complex process in which the secretions from the testis and the epididymis, together with the secretions from the seminal vesicles and the prostate, are expelled into the posterior urethra. From here they are propelled down the penile urethra and into the vagina in a process known as emission.

The secretions that make up the ejaculate enter the posterior urethra in a specific order. The first fraction of the ejaculate to arrive in the posterior urethra are the spermatozoa with the accompanying epididymal fluid. This is rapidly followed by the secretions of the prostate and then the secretions of the seminal vesicles. Thus, if during the collection of a semen sample the first portion is lost, then it may appear that the patient is producing sperm in reduced numbers.

The secretions of the bulbourethral and the urethral glands, however, reach the vagina first as they are secreted further down the urethra. Thus, the secretions that make up the whole ejaculate only come into contact with each other on arrival in the female vagina as, on contact, coagulation of the semen will occur and this coagulum will take 2–15 min to liquefy. Only after liquefaction can true mixing of the ejaculate occur.

Transport of the sperm through the female genital tract

The first problem that will face the sperm within a liquified ejaculate is the very low pH of the midcycle vagina. At midcycle, the secretions of the vagina are extremely acid and may reach a pH as low as 3.5 or 4. However, the high protein content of semen acts as a powerful buffer that protects the sperm from this hostile environment. With this protection, the sperm can leave the seminal fluid and enter the cervical mucus, which is secreted in great quantities at midcycle and with which the semen is in direct contact.

Both the quantity and the quality of the cervical mucus are controlled by oestrogen. Close to ovulation, the oestrogen secretion is maximal and in response to this high level of oestrogen, the cervical glands secrete mucus that is very fluid and has a high ionic content. On contact with the cervical mucus, the motile sperm progress into the mucus in columns. The ability of the sperm to migrate into the cervical mucus is dependent upon their movement patterns. When the spermatozoa arrive in the cervical mucus there is a massive influx of white blood cells into this area. This phenomenon may be used as a means of removing the dead sperm, but the possible immunological role of the sperm in inducing some form of tolerance to paternal antigens must also be considered.

Abnormalities of the cervical mucus can thus cause infertility. This may relate to poor oestrogen secretion or premature progesterone production. Operations on the cervix such as large cone biopsies may also greatly reduce the production of this mucus by removing the endocervical glands. The production of antisperm antibodies that may enter the cervical mucus is discussed elsewhere.

On leaving the cervical mucus at the internal os, the sperm now find themselves suspended in the small volume of fluid secreted by the endometrium within the uterine cavity. Their presence within the uterine cavity may also induce further leucocytosis. How movement of the sperm through the uterine cavity is achieved is still not clear but their progress towards the cornua of the fallopian tubes is probably aided by the segmental contractions of the myometrium, the movement of the cilia on the endometrium and the motility of the spermatozoa themselves. Some sperm may be convulsively transported to the tubes within minutes, but studies in rabbits suggest that these sperm are simply a moribund population.

On entering the tubes, the progress of the sperm towards the ampullary region is probably aided by both contractions of the tubes and the ciliary action of the tubal epithelium. Certainly, many sperm can be found in the peritoneal cavity among fertile women, and their absence from the peritoneal fluid among infertile women has been cited as a cause of that infertility.

How many spermatozoa are required for fertilization in the ampulla of the fallopian tube is unknown but this is probably in the hundreds or thousands. Likewise, their lifespan in the fallopian tube is also unclear, although the author has seen conception occur 1 month after a serious gang rape of a young girl.

The capacitation of sperm

This phenomenon was first described by Chang and by Austin (Chang 1951; Austin 1952). Capacitation confers to the sperm an ability to fertilize an intact oocyte. It consists of a variety of functional and structural changes in the sperm, many of which are poorly understood. One of the most important discoveries leading to the development of IVF was the ability of scientists to induce capacitation of spermatozoa *in vitro*.

In the patient, the process of capacitation begins as the sperm enter the cervical mucus. There are several changes in the sperm that are recognized as being part of the process of capacitation (Yangamachi 1988).

The most obvious of these is the change in sperm movement known as hyperactivation (Yanagamachi 1970). Sperm showing hyperactivation *in vitro* demonstrate a great increase in the bending of the sperm tail, resulting in an increase in the curvilinear velocity that results in a great increase in the lateral (or side-to side) movement of the sperm head. Such sperm have limited forward progression but have a very greatly increased thrust. Such hyperactivated sperm movement may enhance the ability of the sperm to manoeuvre through the extensive folds in the tubal mucosa during its progression down the Fallopian tube, and also greatly increases the ability of the sperm to penetrate the zona pellucida of the oocyte. Hyperactivation is seen in humans and its definition in terms of the changes that indicate its presence have been explored among human spermatozoa (Mortimer *et al.* 1997).

Capacitated sperm are also capable of undergoing the acrosome reaction. The acrosome reaction occurs in sperm prior to their penetration of the cumulus that surrounds the newly ovulated oocyte. The acrosome reaction occurs as the result of an influx of calcium into the sperm. This influx can be produced by follicular fluid, by progesterone and by one of the proteins produced by the protein in the zona pellucida, known as zona pellucida protein 3 (ZP3) (Saling *et al.* 1979; Bleil & Wassarman 1980). The acrosome reaction is also dependent upon the presence of cyclic AMP and may also be controlled by the intracellular pH.

The acrosome reaction is a fairly complex event that results in a major structural change to the sperm. The first event in the acrosome reaction consists of a fusion between of the plasma membrane with the outer acrosomal membrane of the sperm head. Vesiculation now occurs within these fused membranes, after which they break down to release the contents of the acrosome. The acrosome contains enzymes such as hyaluronidase and proteinases that may assist in separating the cells of the cumulus and also assist the sperm in penetrating the zona pellucida. There is some evidence that surface enzymes such as hyaluronidase may act prior to the acrosome reaction and thus assist penetration of the cumulus.

Binding of the sperm to the zona pellucida

The release of the contents of the acrosome during the acrosome reaction is associated with tight binding of the sperm to the zona pellucida. This binding is thought to relate to the presence of zona pellucida protein 2 (ZP2) within the zona pellucida. Binding of the sperm takes place on the zona pellucida in the region of the post-acrosomal area of the sperm head that is close to the equatorial ring.

It must be remembered that the acrosome reaction can occur spontaneously in sperm long before such sperm come in contact with any of the stimuli that normally induce this change. The spontaneous acrosome reaction may take place in around 10% of sperm in an ejaculate, but such sperm are almost certainly infertile and take no part in any aspect of fertilization.

Sperm–egg fusion

Once the sperm has penetrated the zona pellucida and arrived in the perivitelline space, it now fuses with the plasma membrane. This fusion appears to be dependent upon the presence of a substance, known as pH-20, that mediates this event although its presence in the human has not been confirmed. The substance pH-20 is a glycoprotein that consists of two subunits known as α and β. The α-subunit is markedly hydrophobic and thus will assist in the fusion between the sperm surface and the plasma membrane of the oocyte (Phelps & Myles 1987; Lanthrop *et al.* 1990). The β-subunit of pH-20 also assists sperm binding to the oolemma as well as its recognition by the sperm surface.

As soon as the sperm has bound to the oolemma, there occurs a phenomenon known as the 'cortical reaction' in the egg. In this change, the contents of a large number of secretory granules are released into the perivitelline space. This reaction begins at the point of fusion between the egg and the sperm and rapidly spreads all over the surface of the egg. It produces a block to any further sperm binding and prevents any penetration by any other sperm. This reaction is therefore an important method of preventing polyspermy. The cortical reaction is caused by calcium oscillations over the egg surface. These changes may also induce completion of meiosis and the expulsion of the second polar body so that a haploid female pronucleus can be formed.

Fertilization of the human egg

Fertilization is normally thought to begin as soon as the sperm enters the oocyte. After fusion with the oolemma, the sperm, including its tail, is engulfed by the oocyte. As soon as this fusion has occurred, sperm movement disappears.

After its inclusion in the cytoplasm of the oocyte, the sperm head undergoes decondensation. A new nuclear membrane is formed around the DNA in the sperm head and a male pronucleus is formed. The male and female pronuclei approach each other, their individual nuclear membranes are lost and the chromosomes are released into the cytoplasm of the oocyte. The first cleavage division of the zygote is then initiated.

Thus, the sperm components that contribute to the process of fertilization include the proximal centriole, which contributes to the formation of the spindle together with the perinuclear theca and the calcium oscillation. The roles of the mitochondria, the α-tubulin and the plasma membrane of the spermatozoon are unknown.

It is thus clear that the sperm have a major task in achieving fertilization. First, they have to overcome the hostile environment of the midcycle vagina. The sperm then have to make a major journey from the cervix to the ampulla of the fallopian tubes, a distance that, if converted into human terms, may be equivalent to some 100 miles. Each spermatozoon now has to penetrate the cumulus of the oocyte and the zona pellucida to enter the oocyte. It is important that, for the clinician, the process of fertilization in the human is understood as this is of great value in the understanding of many causes of infertility in the human male.

References

Aitken, R.J. (1995) Free radicals, lipid peroxidation and sperm function. *Reproduction, Fertility and Development* **7**, 659–668.

Austin, C.R. (1952) The capacitation of the mammalian spermatozoa. *Nature* **170**, 326.

Bleil, J.D. & Wassarman, P.M. (1980) Synthesis of zona pellucida proteins by denuded and follicle enclosed mouse oocytes during culture in vitro. *Proceedings of the National Academy of Sciences of the USA* **77**, 1029–1033.

Chang, M.C. (1951) Fertilizing capacity of spermatozoa deposited in the Fallopian tubes. *Nature* **168**, 697–698.

Fawcett, D.W. (1975) The mammalian spermatozoon. *Developmental Biology* **44**, 394–436.

Lanthrop, W.F., Carmichael, E.P., Myles, D.M. & Primakoff, P. (1990) cDNA cloning reveals the molecular structure of a sperm surface protein, pH20 involved in sperm–egg adhesion and the wide distribution of this gene among mammals. *Journal of Cell Biology* **111**, 2939–2949.

Mortimer, S., Schoevaert, D., Swan, M.A. & Mortimer, D. (1997) Quantitative observation of the flagellar motility of capacitating human spermatozoa. *Human Reproduction* **12**, 1006–1012.

Phelps, B.M. & Myles, D.G. (1987) The guinea pig sperm plasma membrane protein, pH 20, reaches the surface via two transport pathways and becomes localised to a domain after an initial uniform distribution. *Developmental Biology* **123**, 63–72.

Saling, P.M., Sowinski, J. & Storey, B.T. (1979) An ultrastructural study of epididymal mouse spermatozoa binding to zonae pellucidae *in vitro*: sequential relationship to the acrosome reaction. *Journal of Experimental Zoology* **209**, 229–238.

Yanagamachi, R. (1970) The movement of the golden hamster spermatozoa before and after capacitation. *Journal of Reproduction and Fertility* **23**, 193–196.

Yangamachi, R. (1988) Mammalian fertilization. In: *The Physiology of Reproduction* (eds E. Knobil & J.D. Neill), pp. 135–185. Raven Press, New York.

4: The History and Clinical Examination of the Infertile Man

The history and clinical examination form a very important part of the evaluation of the infertile male. Without the history and the clinical examination, no diagnosis can be made, and thus no rational treatment can be instigated nor a prognosis given to the patient. A semen analysis can only very occasionally provide the clinician with a diagnosis because many of the changes that occur in the semen of infertile men are nonspecific.

Contrary to popular opinion, a careful history and examination can often reveal the cause of a patient's infertility and may provide clues as to appropriate therapy. A good history and clinical examination may thus avoid the need to resort to the various types of advanced reproductive technology.

Infertility is a disorder of a couple, not of an individual. For this reason, both partners must be involved in the investigation of infertility as factors that may contribute to their problem of childlessness can interact in many often fairly subtle ways. Thus, both partners must be equally involved in all the facets of their problem. It is therefore important to take the history and carry out the clinical examination of both the male and the female partners at the initial clinic visit.

Another aspect of patient treatment involves the number of clinicians that may be involved in the decision making concerning treatment. Most patients do not like being treated 'by committee' with numerous clinicians, each with expertise in only one small field of infertility, having an input into the problem but none able to take overall decisions. It is therefore important that clinicians who are involved in the treatment of infertility should have competence in disorders of both the partners, i.e. in disorders of the male as well as the female. Thus, one must not forget that the history and the clinical examination of the infertile male is as important as the history and the examination of the infertile female.

The history

The history is taken from the infertile man in the presence of his partner. The consultation must be carried out in a quiet, calm environment that also provides privacy. There must be no apparent constraints on the clinician's time and both partners must be allowed or indeed encouraged to question the clinician at all times.

Firstly, it is important to determine the patient's age, although this is not so important in the infertile man as it is in the infertile woman. The length of the infertility must also be determined and details of any previous pregnancies, together with their outcomes, need to be ascertained.

Any recent severe illness or surgery will result in stress and can interfere with sperm production. Some anaesthetic agents can temporarily suppress gonadotrophin secretion and concomitantly raise serum prolactin levels, both of which will interfere with sperm production.

A history of any surgery or injury to the testis is important as surgery, particularly operations on or around the epididymis, can cause obstruction. Genital trauma may cause testicular oedema and this can result in loss of spermatogenesis, probably by causing varying degrees of testicular ischaemia. Significant genital trauma in childhood is also suspected of causing infertility in adult life (Finkelhor & Wolak 1995). Hernia repair can occasionally result in damage to the vasa deferentia; each vas is especially vulnerable during herniotomy operations in children as, at that age, the vas is small and can easily be damaged. Testicular maldescent is a well-known cause of spermatogenic abnormalities, especially when it is associated with episodes of testicular torsion (Jequier & Holmes 1993). Mumps, a very overemphasized cause of male infertility, will cause spermatogenic failure only when it occurs in the adult and is associated with a bilateral (not unilateral) orchitis.

Past genital tract infection can also result in infertility. Chlamydial epididymitis is now a common disease (Grant *et al.* 1987) and may frequently result in obstruction of the duct system within the epididymis. Gonococcal infection is also relevant to male infertility but interestingly, as a result of simple and frequently prompt treatment, this infection only rarely causes obstruction. Tuberculous infection may also causes infertility in a number of different ways (Ferrie & Rundle 1983) but is rarely seen in the Western world today. In tropical areas, leprosy and even bilharzia (Mitry *et al.* 1986) can cause infertility in the male. Malaria is a common problem worldwide but it remains uncertain whether this disease is a cause of male infertility. However, such an association between the two disorders is probable.

Enquiries must be made concerning the general health of the male patient. General symptoms such as fatigue and weight loss may indicate a number of generalized disorders. Even anorexia nervosa can occasionally occur in the male patient. Many general medical disorders including liver disease and renal failure may give rise to infertility.

A history of chronic chest disease, particularly bronchiectasis, or a long history of sinusitis is associated with a number of causes of male infertility, especially obstruction of the excurrent ducts from the testes in the condition known as Young's syndrome (Young 1970).

Current medication can also result in changes in semen quality. Agents such as salazopyrine, used in the treatment of ulcerative colitis, and the H_2 antagonist cimetidine may impair semen quality, while other drugs such as the hypotensives can act by interfering with ejaculation and potency. Most antimitotic agents also damage sperm production.

A sexual history is also important in the evaluation of the infertile male.

The frequency of intercourse and any history of potency problems must be elicited. Loss of libido or infrequent intercourse may be an indicator of a variety of different endocrine disorders, including hyperprolactinaemia, that can result in reduced testosterone production and infertility.

The presence of retrograde ejaculation or ejaculatory failure is indicated by an absence of ejaculate or a reduction in its volume. Such abnormalities in ejaculation may occur following surgery to the para-aortic region, including retroperitoneal node dissection and lumbar sympathectomy. In men with retrograde ejaculation, cloudy urine may be observed postcoitally.

The occupation of the patient is also relevant to his infertility. The ingestion of toxins, particularly pesticides and herbicides, as well as exposure to heat or radiation may also damage the spermatogenic epithelium and give rise to infertility.

Substance abuse can also cause infertility in the male. Chronic alcoholism, especially when associated with significant liver dysfunction, can result in infertility. Marijuana smoking may cause infertility in a number of different ways including a reduction in LH secretions and reduced testosterone production (Kalodny *et al.* 1974). There is, however, some evidence that cigarette smoking will reduce sperm concentration but little evidence to date that it will cause infertility in a previously fertile man. However, if a cause of infertility is already present, the so-called 'cofactor' effect may be seen that can worsen a sperm count in a man who already as a lesion causing oligozoospermia (Peng *et al.* 1990).

The examination

In the evaluation of the infertile male, a general examination may be as helpful as the examination of the genitalia. The signs of hypoandrogenization, such as a reduction in beard growth, changes in body hair distribution and an absence of androgen-dependent balding, may indicate reduced testosterone secretion, which can occur in many of the endocrinopathies and any condition where there is damage or malfunction of the Leydig cells.

Examination of the chest in an infertile man may indicate the presence of a number of abnormalities. Bronchiectasis may be associated with certain forms of epididymal obstruction such as that in Young's syndrome (Young 1970). Dextrocardia and situs inversus, also in association with bronchiectasis, may signal the presence of a condition known as the immotile cilia syndrome (Afzelius *et al.* 1975).

On the examination of the abdomen, evidence of surgical procedures, especially in the groin, may indicate past herniotomy operations or orchidopexies that may have been forgotten by the patient.

Examination of the genitalia is, of course, the most important part of the examination of an infertile man. The penis must be inspected and the normal position of the external urethral meatus must be confirmed. Phimosis and meatal strictures must also be excluded.

The size of the testes must be estimated as testicular volume is important diagnostically. Testis size is usually ascertained by comparision of testis size with an orchidometer, such as the one designed by Prader (Fig. 4.1), which provides the clinician with a testicular volume measured in millilitres (Prader 1966). It is not sufficiently accurate to guess the size of the testes, as their volume is important diagnostically. In certain abnormalities of the testis, reduced sensation to gentle squeezing of the testes may indicate the presence of certain forms of spermatogenic failure.

When there is an obstruction in the epididymis, it is possible to palpate the upper epididymal distension that such a lesion will induce. When such distension is palpable, this finding is known as 'Bayle's sign' after the French andrologist who first described it (Bayle 1952). In tuberculous epididymitis, nodularity of the testis may be present and this nodularity is enhanced when calcification is present.

It is also important to palpate the vasa deferentia as congenital absence of the vas is a common cause of ductal obstruction. The absence of the vasa will thus confirm the diagnosis and save the patient from any unnecessary attempts at remedial surgery.

The presence of a varicocele is best detected with the patient in the standing position. The varicocele, if large, can often be easily palpated, but smaller varicoceles can also be demonstrated very easily on distension by the Valsalva manoevre. Venous bruit and in particular the reversal of flow in the pampiniform plexus caused by the Valsalva manoeuvre can also be detected by using Doppler ultrasound.

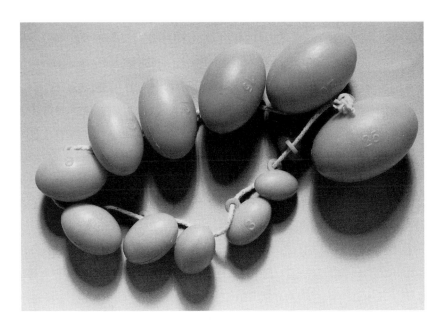

Fig. 4.1 The Prader orchiometer that is used for estimating testicular volume. These are usually manufactured in plastic but the more 'up-market' versions can even be made in wood.

Rectal examination also occasionally provides useful information. The presence of ejaculatory duct cysts may be detected this way and when these or other similar lesions cause ejaculatory duct obstruction, the seminal vesicles will distend and may be palpable. An enlarged or inflamed prostate may cause abnormalities in semen, particularly an increase in the numbers of leucocytes present in the semen.

The history and clinical examination of the infertile man are vital to the evaluation of the infertile man. Without clinical assessment, very few diagnoses can be made and thus no rational treatment can be instituted. Once a diagnosis is made, this can be confirmed or refuted by a variety of different investigations. Only when a diagnosis is made can the appropriate management of the infertile male patient be planned and carried out.

References

Afzelius, B.A., Eliasson, R., Johnsen, O. & Lindholmer, C. (1975) Lack of dynein arms in immotile human spermatozoa. *Journal of Cell Biology* **66**, 225–235.

Bayle, H. (1952) Azoospermia of excretory origin. *Proceedings of the Society for the Study of Fertility* **4**, 30–38.

Ferrie, B.G. & Rundle, J.S.H. (1983) Tuberculous epididymo-orchitis. A review of 20 cases. *British Journal of Urology* **55**, 437–439.

Finkelhor, D. & Wolak, J. (1995) Nonsexual assaults to the genitalia in the youth population. *New England Journal of Medicine* **274**, 1692–1697.

Grant, J.B.F., Costello, C.B., Sequiera, P.J.L. & Blacklock, N.J. (1987) The role of *Chlamydia trachomatis* in epididymitis. *British Journal of Urology* **60**, 355–359.

Jequier, A.M. & Holmes, S.C. (1993) Primary testicular disease presenting as azoospermia or oligozoospermia in an infertility clinic. *British Journal of Urology* **71**, 731–735.

Kalodny, R.C., Masters, W.H., Kolodner, R.M. & Toro, G. (1974) Depression of plasma testosterone after chronic intensive marihuana use. *New England Journal of Medicine* **290**, 872–874.

Mitry, N.F., Satti, M.B., Tamini, D.M. & Metawaa, B. (1986) Testicular schistosomiasis. *British Journal of Urology* **58**, 721–727.

Peng, B.C., Tomashevsky, P. & Nagler, H.M. (1990) The co-factor effect: varicocele and infertility. *Fertility and Sterility* **54**, 143–148.

Prader, A. (1966) Testicular size assessment and clinical importance. *Triangle* **7**, 240–243.

Young, D. (1970) Surgery of male infertility. *Journal of Reproduction and Fertility* **23**, 541–542.

5: The Analysis of Semen

Although infertility must be the most common reason for a semen analysis, it must be remembered that there are other indications for this procedure. Semen analysis is used to ensure sterility after vasectomy and semen may also be examined prior to use for artificial insemination or cryopreservation. Men whose future fertility is threatened by irradiation therapy or surgery may also wish to have their semen examined with a view to storage for future insemination. Semen analyses are also used in research involving the development of either treatments for infertility or during the development of new contraceptives. The role of environmental toxins and their effects on semen quality are now under increasing scrutiny and such studies will, of course, rely very much on the results of semen analyses.

Whatever the reason for a semen analysis, it must always be remembered that, at least for some patients, the production of a sample by masturbation may be distasteful, difficult and embarrassing. The distress caused by such an experience is not only unpleasant for the patient but is likely to lead to fear of further investigation and to poor attendance at the clinic. Such stress may also cause inadequate ejaculation resulting in the production of an incomplete semen sample and the erroneous diagnosis of male infertility.

For these reasons, it is essential that the production of a semen sample can take place in a private and secure environment, in surroundings that are comfortable both emotionally and physically for the patient. If the patient lives within three-quarters of an hour from the laboratory and the climate is not extreme (neither too hot nor too cold), there is no reason why the patient cannot produce his sample at home and bring it into the laboratory under controlled conditions. Indeed, it is known that samples produced at home and brought to the laboratory in this way are of better quality than those produced by the same man in unfamiliar or hostile surroundings. For all these reasons, it is clear that the collection of semen samples must be organized by experienced and understanding hospital staff.

The collection of the semen sample for laboratory analysis

The production of a semen sample must take place under controlled conditions and these will be considered individually.

Length of abstinence

The length of abstinence from sexual activity or ejaculation prior to production of a semen sample alters the quality of the semen (Mortimer *et al.* 1982): a short interval between ejaculations reduces sperm numbers while prolonged abstinence reduces the motility. A normal male produces around 80 million sperm per day, but this may vary greatly between individuals and may be very much less than this figure in an infertile man. Frequent ejaculation will deplete the stores of sperm and result in reduced sperm numbers in a subsequent ejaculate (Eliasson 1965). Conversely, long periods of abstinence will allow the build-up of sperm numbers in storage at the lower end of the epididymis, but their ageing during this time may result in a reduction in motility. However, provided that the semen sample is not produced within 24 h of a prior ejaculation and the length of abstinence is known, a period of abstinence of 2–3 days is adequate for the accurate assessment of semen quality. As in normal circumstances sexual intercourse usually takes place every 2–3 days, then the length of abstinence before the production of a semen sample for analysis is also best maintained at 2–3 days.

Site of production of the semen sample

There is no doubt that the production of a semen sample at the laboratory is by far the easiest option for the staff; the specimen can be brought straight to the bench for analysis. However, it must be remembered that semen analyses are not carried out for the benefit of the laboratory staff but for the benefit of the patient.

As has already been pointed out, the production of a semen sample can be a major problem for some men, and for this reason the patient must be allowed, within reason, to choose where he wishes to produce his sample. If he prefers to produce the sample at home, so be it. If, however, he lives a long way away and is happy to produce the semen sample at the laboratory then he must be provided with a room in that laboratory which is quiet, secluded and where total privacy is guaranteed. It must be remembered that inadequate ejaculation may give rise to an erroneous diagnosis of infertility where in reality no such pathology may exist.

Time of production of a semen sample

A semen sample is usually best produced in the morning for, as will be seen later, a number of sperm function tests may need to be carried out on that sample and these may take several hours to complete. However, if this proves to be difficult for the patient, then a sample produced later in the day will have to suffice. Indeed, what may be gained by pressuring a patient to produce a sample at an inconvenient time may be lost in the misinformation that may result from the production of an inadequate sample.

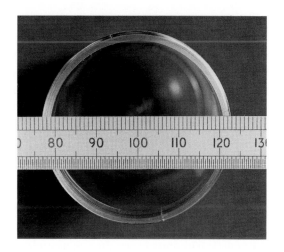

Fig. 5.1 A plastic sperm collection pot with a diameter of between 4 and 7 cm.

Journeys to the laboratory during working hours may jeopardize employment or at least induce a fear of job loss. For this reason, an appointment system for semen analyses must be handled sensitively and the presence of a 'deadline' for the delivery of a semen sample is best avoided.

Container for semen samples

All patients must be provided with containers for their semen samples. Jars obtained at home by the patients have frequently been washed in detergent which, even in minute amounts, is very toxic to sperm and can seriously reduce sperm motility. Such containers may also be wet and tap water with its low osmolality is equally toxic to sperm. Semen may also require culture, and thus the containers should initially be sterile.

Each semen jar should be wide necked with a minimum diameter of 5–7 cm (Fig. 5.1): if narrow-necked containers are used, it is easy for part of the sample to be lost at ejaculation. The jar can be made of either plastic or glass, but it is important that it is not made of a substance that is toxic to sperm. There must be no rubber lining to the lid as the hydrocarbons in the rubber are also very toxic to sperm. Above all, the container must be clean and dry and must not have been used for any other purpose. It is also important that each specimen jar is clearly and correctly labelled.

Method of production of the semen sample

There are several ways in which a semen sample can be produced by the patient.

Manual masturbation

There is no doubt that the production of the semen sample by masturbation usually results in a specimen that is complete and uncontaminated. Some

43

patients, however, may use talcum powder for lubrication during masturbation and crystals of talc can occasionally find their way into the semen sample. It is important that the technologist is aware of this possibility. If the patient is provided with too small a container for the semen sample, it is not uncommon for part of the ejaculate to be lost.

There are nevertheless some patients who find masturbation difficult or who have religious objection to it; for these men, other methods of collecting semen have been devised.

Coitus interruptus

This method, also often known as the 'withdrawal' method, involves the use of sexual intercourse to stimulate ejaculation. Just prior to orgasm, the penis is withdrawn from the vagina and ejaculation takes place into the container provided for the semen.

During collection of the semen in this way, the withdrawal may be mistimed and, as a result, part of the semen sample is frequently lost. Also, the semen sample can become contaminated by vaginal secretions. This method of collection also has the disadvantage that intercourse has to take place during laboratory hours, which may be inconvenient to both partners.

Silastic condoms

Ordinary rubber contraceptive condoms must never be used to collect a semen sample. Because of the volatile hydrocarbons that are present in the interstices of the rubber, the condom is very toxic to sperm. Many condoms are also lined with spermicidal powder that swiftly obliterates all sperm motility. Many of these spermicidal powders have characteristically shaped crystals that can easily be identified during microscopy of semen.

Silastic condoms (Apex Medical Technologies Inc.), which are completely nontoxic to sperm, are easily obtainable but are reasonably expensive. It is, however, important that a laboratory that carries out semen analyses does have at least a few of these silastic condoms available for the few patients that do have problems with, or a religious objection to, masturbation.

Despite the nontoxicity of these condoms, it is nevertheless easy for a patient to lose a portion of the ejaculate when such a condom is used for the collection of a semen sample, and this should be remembered when a semen sample collected in this way proves to be abnormal.

Transport of a semen sample to the laboratory

Maintenance of temperature

Sperm can easily be damaged by both excessive heat and by excessive cold. Semen samples should therefore not be exposed to direct sunlight nor should they be transported to the laboratory in a handbag or an outside pocket where they will be allowed to cool.

After production of the semen sample, the lid is replaced on the container and tightly closed. The container should then be wrapped in face tissues as paper is a good thermal insulator. The paper-covered container is now wrapped in kitchen foil, which will further prevent cooling and will protect it from the light. The semen can now be transported to the laboratory by the patient or his partner by carrying the paper and foil-covered container inside a layer of clothes, which will keep the sample closer to body temperature. The sample should arrive at the laboratory within 1–2 h of production.

The request form that accompanies the semen sample

Quite complex forms have been devised for use with semen samples, but all that is really required apart from the patient's name, address and date of birth is where the report is to be sent. However, it is also of value to know the time of production of the sample and whether the patient was aware of any loss of the sample at production. The length of time since this last ejaculation should also be recorded and an additional form containing these details is of value (Fig. 5.2).

The delivery of the semen sample from the laboratory reception desk to the bench

On arrival at the laboratory reception, a specimen of semen whose temper-

```
                        SEMEN COLLECTION
           Please complete the following at the time of semen production

    NAME: _ _ _ _ _ _ _ _ _ _ _ _ _ _ _ _ _ _ _ _ _ _ _ _ _ _ _ _ _ _ _ _ _ _ _ _ _
    ADDRESS:  _ _ _ _ _ _ _ _ _ _ _ _ _ _ _ _ _ _ _ _ _ _ _ _ _ _ _ _ _ _ _ _ _ _ _

    DATE OF BIRTH: _ _ _ _ _ _ _ _ _ _ _ _ _ _ _ _ _ _ _ _ _ _ _ _ _ _ _ _ _ _
    REFERRING DR: _ _ _ _ _ _ _ _ _ _ _ _ _ _ _ _ _ _ _ _ _ _ _ _ _ _ _ _ _ _

    DATE:_ _ _ _ _ _ _ _ _ _ _     TIME OF PRODUCTION: _ _ _ _ _ _ _ _ _ _ _.

    PLACE OF PRODUCTION: HOME/LABORATORY

    DAYS SINCE LAST EJACULATION:  _ _ _ _ _ _ _ _ _ _ _ _ _ _ _ _ _

    DID YOU COLLECT THE WHOLE EJACULATE: YES/NO
        IF NO, ESTIMATE THE PERCENTAGE LOST _ _ _ _ _ _ _ _. %
           Please ensure that your specimen is wrapped in tissue and foil
                          and kept next to your skin
```

Fig. 5.2 A form that states details of the sperm collection and any problems that may arise should accompany a semen sample to the laboratory.

ature has been well maintained by the patient during transport to the laboratory can now be inadvertently allowed to cool. The time spent by semen samples in a cold corridor or an over air-conditioned laboratory bench is quite enough to have a profound artefactual effect on sperm motility. Ill-informed and overenthusiastic technologists have even been known to store such samples in a refrigerator. Thus, rapid transport of the sample to an incubator at 37 °C immediately upon its arrival in the laboratory will play an important part in preventing errors in the interpretation of a semen analysis.

The number of semen samples needed to diagnose male infertility

Certainly in the management of infertility in the male, a reasonably accurate evaluation of the fertility status of an individual can be achieved by assessing at least two samples of semen, especially when these analyses are examined in conjunction with a careful history and clinical examination.

It is well known that sperm may be found in subsequent semen samples from men who were initially azoospermic. As it is now possible using microassisted fertilization techniques to generate an embryo and create a pregnancy from a few dozen sperm, the presence of only a very small number of sperm in an ejaculate can be important to the clinician undertaking treatment of a couple. Thus, 'azoospermic' semen samples must be centrifuged and carefully examined for the presence of even a very small number of spermatozoa.

Artefacts that can occur during the production of a semen sample

In order to be able to identify some of the artefacts that occur during the production of a semen sample, it is useful to consider how these problems come about.

Low semen volume

Although there are many pathological causes of a low ejaculatory volume, this can also, of course, indicate loss of a portion of the ejaculate from the sample, especially when such a reduction in volume is also associated with a reduced sperm count. However, some men have very high ejaculatory volumes and in these men, even when a substantial volume of the sample has been lost, the volume of the sample may still be within the normal range.

Foreign bodies in semen

Many patients whose ejaculate has in part 'missed the pot' attempt to retrieve the semen from the floor. When this occurs the semen sample becomes contaminated with dust, fluff and even on occasions small insects can be found on microscopy.

When a semen sample has been produced in a contraceptive condom, spermicidal crystals can also be identified in the semen (Fig. 5.3) and the sperm are frequently totally immotile and nonviable.

Temperature extremes

Overheating or cooling a semen sample will dramatically reduce sperm motility, and this is one of the more common forms of artefactual change seen in a sample of semen. Semen that has been left in the sun or cooled will show considerable loss of movement, and even cell death can occur without there necessarily being any change in sperm morphology. Thus, the presence of normal sperm numbers and morphology in a sample of semen where motility is very low is suggestive of the presence of artefact.

Contaminants

The contamination of a semen sample with water, soap, detergents and many other chemicals can profoundly damage sperm movement as well as sperm function. The collection of semen in an ordinary household receptacle is an important cause of this artefact.

From the above it is clear that great care must be taken by both the clinician and the laboratory to ensure that a semen analysis is a true reflection

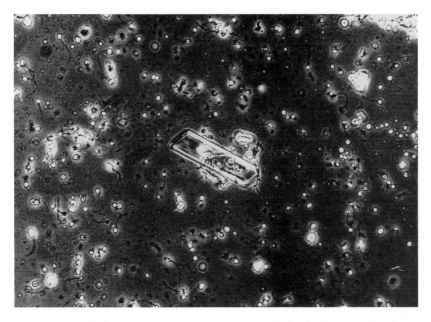

Fig. 5.3 A crystal of spermicidal powder in a semen sample that had been produced into a contraceptive condom.

of the patient's fertility. It must not be rendered invalid by either loss of part of the sample or its contamination during production or by physical or chemical damage during its transport to or its handling at the laboratory.

The physical properties of semen

The first task in performing a semen analysis involves the examination of the physical properties of the semen sample.

The colour of seminal fluid

Semen is normally an opalescent fluid. Its opacity is caused, for the most part, by its high protein content but this is also caused by the presence of the many millions of spermatozoa as well as some cellular debris contained within it. However, there are a number of pathological processes that will change the colour of semen, and it is important that the technologist as well as the clinician is aware of these possibilities.

Urine in seminal fluid

Semen samples can occasionally be contaminated with urine and this can be seen in men with abnormalities of bladder neck function or neurological disease as well as in men with retrograde ejaculation. Even relatively large amounts of urine in a semen sample only give the semen a faint yellow discoloration, but its presence is usually detected by the uriniferous odour that is present.

Because of the huge buffering power of the protein in seminal fluid, the pH of semen is usually unaltered by contamination even with large quantities of urine.

Urine is very toxic to sperm and contact with even a small amount of urine will rapidly render spermatozoa immotile (Crich & Jequier 1978). Thus, semen samples contaminated by urine will contain sperm that show either very poor motility or sperm that are completely immotile.

Blood in semen

The presence of blood in semen is known as haematospermia. The degree and type of discolouration of semen that is caused by blood will depend on both the amount of blood present relative to the seminal volume and the age of the blood in that sample. Small amounts of fresh blood will colour the sample pink while larger quantities of blood will render the sample bright red, often making the patient think that they are ejaculating blood alone. If the blood has been in the genital tract for some time then the semen will be coloured brown.

Most blood in semen arises from the prostate or seminal vesicles and can be the result of infection. It can also be generated by persistent müllerian tissue within the genital tract, as occurs among patients with müllerian duct cysts. More rarely, in the older patient, it may indicate the presence of a malignancy, which, most commonly, is a prostatic carcinoma.

However, in many patients the source of the blood may be difficult to identify. Split ejaculates can be used in an attempt to locate the source of such blood and abnormalities of the prostate and seminal vesicles may be identified by transrectal ultrasonography or by vasography.

Bilirubin in semen

Just as it will colour other tissues when it is present in excess, bilirubin can also change the colour of seminal fluid, and therefore in a deeply jaundiced patient the semen will also become bright orange in colour.

Interestingly the presence of bilirubin in semen seems to have little effect on sperm function. It is merely startling to a technologist who has not seen the phenomenon before but, if the jaundice is hepatocellular rather than obstructive, then both sperm numbers and sperm motility are likely to be reduced.

The volume of a semen sample

The normal volume of an ejaculate is said to lie between 2 and 6 mL.

The suffix 'spermia' relates to seminal fluid and not to spermatozoa. Thus, changes to seminal fluid volume are known by several names.

Aspermia means total absence of an ejaculate. The word aspermia is sometimes (but quite wrongly) used to describe lack of spermatozoa, for which the correct word is azoospermia.

A low seminal fluid volume, i.e. less than 2 mL, is known as hypospermia while an ejaculatory volume of greater than 6 mL is known as hyperspermia.

Causes of an abnormal ejaculatory volume

There are many causes of infertility that may be associated with an abnormal ejaculatory volume. Reduced volumes of an ejaculate may itself compound the infertility (Table 5.1).

Reduced ejaculatory volume

As the majority of the ejaculate comes from the seminal vesicles and the prostate, abnormalities of these glands can reduce their secretory powers.

Seminal vesiculitis may reduce the secretions of the gland and reduce the seminal volume. Inflammatory changes in this gland may also block the seminal vesicular ducts and exclude the seminal vesicular contribution to the ejaculate. The condition of bilateral congenital absence of the vasa

Table 5.1 The changes that may be seen in the semen of men with a variety of different cause of infertility

Genital tract lesion	Sperm concentration	Seminal volume	Seminal fructose
Bilateral epididymal obstruction	Azoospermia	Normal	Normal
Congenital absence of the vas	Azoospermia	Normal or reduced	Normal or reduced
Ejaculatory duct obstruction	Azoospermia	Reduced	Absent
Polyzoospermia	Very high	Normal	Reduced

deferentia is commonly associated with aplasia or hypoplasia of the seminal vesicles, and thus this condition is often associated with a reduced ejaculatory volume.

Prostatitis may also reduce the prostatic contribution to the semen but as the ducts from the prostate gland are numerous, these secretions are never totally absent.

Abnormalities of ejaculation may also result in a reduced or a total absence of the ejaculate. Poor ejaculation may occur in men who are nervous or uncomfortable about the prospect of producing a semen sample, but such problems can also result from neurological disease of various sorts. Retrograde ejaculation, a condition where most of the ejaculate passes back into the bladder, can also result in a loss of ejaculate. In this situation, the only part of the ejaculate that will end up in the semen sample container will be the secretions of the urethral or bulbourethral glands.

Testosterone is also essential for normal sexual function including ejaculation. Thus disorders of ejaculation and a reduction in the volume of the ejaculate may also be seen in men with endocrine disorders that cause hypo-androgenization.

Hyperspermia

Hyperspermia is a much less common disorder than hypospermia and its cause is largely unknown. It is probably only relevant to infertility where sperm numbers are small. A large ejaculatory volume may act as an added dilutional effect on sperm numbers and decrease the numbers of sperm that can come in contact with the cervical mucus.

The measurement of the ejaculatory volume

The recommended method of measuring semen volume is to draw the entire ejaculate up into a sterile (and warmed) graduated pipette after which the semen sample can be returned to its container. The volume is usually reported to the nearest 0.1 mL. It is important to remember, however, that all glassware used in semen analysis is scrupulously clean. For this reason it is usually best to use plastic disposable equipment.

It is also possible to measure semen volume by weighing the container together with the ejaculate. As most semen containers are plastic and vary very little in weight, the container and the ejaculate within it are weighed. The volume of the ejaculate in millilitres is the difference in grams between the weight of an empty container and that containing the semen sample. This is not, however, such an accurate method as is the direct measure of seminal volume.

The pH of semen

The pH of seminal fluid lies between 7.2 and 8.0. The pH should only be measured in fresh samples of semen as the pH will fall as the sample ages. The pH is best measured using litmus paper with a range between 6.0 and 9.0 (Fig. 5.4). It is best not to use a pH meter for this as such precision is not necessary and the proteinaceous nature of semen frequently blocks this expensive equipment.

The pH of semen can occasionally be of value diagnostically to the clinician. Because of its high protein content, semen is a very effective buffer and it is difficult to alter its pH. However, severe infection, particularly that of the prostate and seminal vesicles, can increase the acidity of semen and a low pH may be helpful in making such a diagnosis. Likewise, in men with bilateral congenital absence of the vas deferens where there is

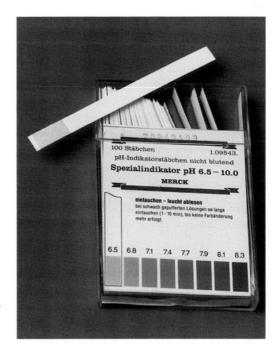

Fig. 5.4 Litmus paper used for the measurement of pH in semen.

often little or no secretion from the seminal vesicles, the pH is frequently reduced.

The viscosity of semen

The viscosity of semen relates to the protein content of semen and this may vary greatly between individuals and between samples from the same individual. Very viscous semen may cause infertility by creating difficulties for the spermatozoa to exit the seminal fluid and gaining access to the cervical mucus. It may also be a cause of a negative postcoital test. However, as around 10% of semen samples from normally fertile men show an increased viscosity (Crich, unpublished data), care must be taken not necessarily to blame the increased viscosity as the cause of a patient's infertility.

It is important to differentiate excessively viscous semen from semen that has failed to liquefy. Unliquified semen remains as a ball-like clot while viscous semen will flow over the bottom of the container, albeit fairly slowly. One can in fact quantify viscosity by measuring the time taken for a sample of semen of known volume to run out of a Pasteur pipette, but such measurements are never necessary for routine clinical practice.

The treatment of hyperviscous semen

Excessively viscous semen can easily be made more fluid both by mixing the semen with medium and also by forcing the seminal fluid down a narrow-gauge needle. The semen is first aspirated into a 5- or 10-mL syringe (with only a plastic or glass plunger as rubber is toxic to sperm) and then it is slowly forced using pressure down an 18 or 23 gauge needle. If the semen is driven too quickly down the needle, the sperm can be damaged and sperm motility reduced. Semen samples treated in this way, however, can then be used for cervical insemination.

The liquefaction of semen

In most mammals, semen is ejaculated in a liquid form and coagulates after emission. In the bull and the ram it remains liquid while, in the pig, the semen forms a firm gel after ejaculation. In the rodent, semen forms a very firm coagulum in the vagina that is often referred to as a 'plug'.

In the human, the semen forms a gel-like clot but within 5–20 min after ejaculation, liquefaction of the clot has occurred. The clotting of human semen is induced by a fibrinogen-like agent that is secreted by the seminal vesicles. This substance acts as a substrate and is first acted upon by the enzyme vesiculase, secreted by the prostate, which polymerizes the seminal vesicular substrate in a similar manner to that seen with fibrinogen in blood clotting. Liquefaction of this clot is then brought about by a series of proteolytic enzymes also produced by the prostate and these include pepsinogen and amylase together with hyaluronidase. Thus, both clotting and liquefaction are both brought about by the secretions of the prostate.

Absence of liquefaction will result in the containment of the sperm within the gel and is a well-known but not very common cause of both infertility and a negative postcoital test. However, it must be remembered that, if liquefaction is only partially impaired, normal fertility can still result.

Assessment of liquefaction

Liquefaction is usually assessed visually. A fully liquefied semen sample will be obviously fluid while a sample that is still clotted will remain a rounded gel-like coagulum. A partially liquefied semen sample can easily go unrecognized and may also contain many small gel-like clots that are best identified by holding the sample up to a good light source. As has been seen with hyperviscous semen, a partially liquefied semen sample may allow the liberation of sufficient sperm to achieve fertility.

Measurement of liquefaction

It is possible to quantify liquefaction by using the third fraction of an ejaculate and comparing the rate of liquefaction with that of a normal donor (Eliasson 1971). The third fraction of an ejaculate liquefies very slowly and in the absence of other fractions will take at least 1–2 h to complete the process. The third fractions of the abnormal semen sample and that of a normal ejaculate are each placed in a nylon mesh and are suspended in a 2–3-mL graduated tube at 37 °C. As a coagulum, the semen cannot pass though the mesh. However, as liquefaction occurs, the seminal fluid will drip into the graduated tube. The end point of the test occurs when the nylon mesh is empty. The rate of liquefaction of the slowly lysing fractions of the two samples can thus be compared and quantified. The absence of liquefaction is obvious on simply examining the semen, and if liquefaction has not occurred after 20 min it may be deemed to be abnormal. However, these tests are usually of little value from the clinical point of view.

The treatment of unliquefied semen

It has been known for a long time that spitting into a sample of clotted semen will cause it to liquefy (Bunge & Sherman 1954). This occurs because saliva contains the enzyme amylase. Spitting into a semen sample is not, however, the most hygienic way to manage this type of infertility.

Instead, a number of different enzymes have been used for this purpose. The best treatment of nonliquefaction of semen is the addition of 2–3 mL of a 0.2% solution of α-amylase (Sigma Chemicals) to the sample of unliquefied semen of average volume. Other enzymes that have been used for this purpose are α-chymotrysin, lysozymes and hyaluronidase. Contact between these enzymes and the semen must be limited or the cell membranes of the spermatozoa can become damaged by proteolytic activity. As soon as liquefaction is complete, the semen sample should be washed in medium, after which it can be used for cervical insemination.

The estimation of the sperm concentration

The determination of the numbers of sperm in a semen sample forms an important part of a semen analysis.

Several terms are used to describe sperm numbers in semen with which the clinician must be familiar. The sperm concentration describes the number of sperm in millions that are present per unit volume of seminal fluid. The unit volume used is usually a millilitre, but in some centres the sperm concentration may be reported as the number of spermatozoa per litre.

However, the sperm concentration takes no account of the total number of sperm in an ejaculate, which is probably a better indicator of fertility potential than is the sperm concentration alone. For example, a sperm concentration of 10 million sperm in a seminal volume of 5 mL will provide a total of 50 million sperm in an ejaculate, while a sperm concentration of 10 million in an ejaculatory volume of 0.5 mL will provide a total of only 5 million sperm.

Thus, in reporting the number of sperm, the volume must be taken into account. Thus the total sperm count is defined as the total number of sperm in an ejaculate and is obtained by multiplying the sperm count in millions per millilitre by the ejaculatory volume. It is important that both these values are indicated on the semen analysis report.

Other more generalized terms are used to describe both the sperm count and the total sperm count. Azoospermia describes the total absence of sperm in an ejaculate. The word oligozoospermia refers to a reduced number of sperm in a semen sample and is usually used to describe a sperm concentration of less than 20 million per mL or a total sperm count of less than 40 million. The word oligospermia is also used in this context, but this is incorrect.

Polyzoospermia denotes an increased number of sperm in semen and usually refers to a sperm concentration in excess of 350 million per mL (Amelar *et al.* 1979). The word normozoospermia can also be used to describe a semen sample that contains both a normal concentration of sperm and a normal total sperm count.

Methods of measuring the sperm concentration

Spermatozoa are very small and for this reason a microscope with good definition and capable of high magnification is needed. Phase contrast optics can also very useful. As only an aliquot of semen will be used to carry out the sperm count, complete liquefaction and good mixing of the sample is essential. Dead or immotile sperm will tend to sink to the bottom of the container and thus can easily be inadvertently excluded from the count. Sperm concentration can be assessed in a number of different ways.

Visual assessment on a glass slide

The application of a drop of well-mixed semen is made onto a clean glass slide, the application of a cover-slip and its examination at a magnification of ×400 will give an approximation of the sperm concentration. The numbers of sperm in one microscopic field is very roughly the same as the number of sperm in millions that are present in 1 mL of seminal fluid. This technique will also identify any gross abnormality such as sperm agglutination.

For many clinicians who practise a long way from a laboratory, this can be a useful way to identify gross abnormalities in a semen sample.

The improved Neubauer counting chamber (haemocytometer)

This chamber is probably the most commonly used method of estimating sperm concentration. The major advantage of this chamber is that it is cheap and can be found in most laboratories. However, this counting chamber is certainly less popular than it was and many laboratories are now purchasing the newer types of chambers that have been specifically designed for conducting sperm counts. Its major disadvantage is that it is more difficult to use than the newer chambers and because of the necessity for dilution of the semen, it is a method that is subject to considerable error.

Dilution of the semen

The usual dilution of semen needed for its analysis in this chamber is 1 in 20 or 1 part of semen to 19 parts of diluent (volume/volume). Thus a 50-µL aliquot of semen needs to be diluted in 950-µL aliquots of diluent. For semen samples containing very low numbers of sperm a 1 in 10 dilution can be used instead. Conversely, in samples with a very high concentration of sperm a 1 in 50 dilution may be used.

All dilutions are carried out in a small test tube. An automatic pipette is used to minimize errors in the dilution. White cell pipettes must never be used for this purpose. The tube containing the semen and diluent is then applied to a vortex to ensure mixing.

Diluent

The diluent used is a 0.5% solution of Gentian violet in buffered 3.5% formol saline (Table 5.2). Such staining of sperm will aid their identification during the sperm count. If this stain is not deemed to be necessary, the sperm can be immobilized by dilution in simple tap water.

Table 5.2 The formulation of buffered formol saline for use as a semen diluent

NaHCO$_3$	5.0 g
35% Formalin	1.0 mL
Gentian violet	5.0 mL
Distilled water	To a final volume of 100 mL

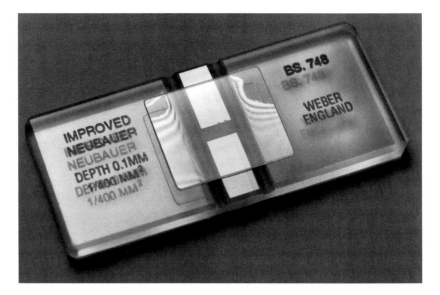

Fig. 5.5 An improved Neubauer counting chamber. The cover-slip is in place and the birefringent Newton's rings can easily be seen.

Loading the chamber

The haemocytometer must be very clean and prior to use must have been washed in distilled water and carefully dried with a lens tissue. To prepare the chamber, the clean, dry cover-slip is pressed onto the glass base and, using the thumbs, the cover-slip is then slid gently forward over the counting grids. Pressure is maintained on the cover-slip until the birefringent rings, also often known as Newton's rings, become clearly visible. Only when these rings are visible is the chamber ready for use (Fig. 5.5).

The diluted semen is now applied to the chamber. At this point it must be remembered that the sperm in the diluent are now all dead and careful mixing at this point is very necessary. Thorough vortexing of the mixture is thus needed just prior to the application of the sperm to the chamber. Using a Pasteur pipette, a small drop of the sperm diluent mixture (around 10 µL) is applied to the outer edges of the cover-slip on each side of the central trough. The diluted semen will quickly spread out under the cover-slip to fill each section of the counting chamber. Each chamber is then viewed at a magnification of ×200.

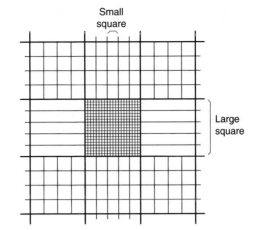

Small
square

Large
square

Fig. 5.6 One of the grids in an improved Neubauer counting chamber showing the arrangement of the small and the large squares.

The sperm count

When viewed down the microscope, each chamber is made up of nine large squares that cover an area of 9 mm². The central square is divided up into a further 25 smaller squares (Fig. 5.6). Of these 25 smaller squares only five are used in the sperm count, and it is traditional that the four corner squares and the central square are selected for this purpose. In reality, any square can be selected for use as long as none of these squares used in the sperm count are touching each other.

The total sperm numbers in these five squares are now counted. Those sperm touching the upper and left sides of each square are excluded from the count while those touching the lower and the right sides of the square are included. This counting procedure is then repeated in the second chamber.

Calculation of the sperm concentration

For the Neubauer haemocytometer, the sperm concentration is then calculated in the following manner.

Each large square = 1 mm².

As each large square contains 25 small squares, then,

each small square = $1/25$ = 0.04 mm².

Therefore,

5 small squares = 5×0.04 mm² = 0.2 mm².

The number of sperm/mm² = sperm count $\times$ 5

Therefore, the 'sperm count' in 1 μL (as the depth of the chamber is 10 μm)
= the 'sperm count' in 5 squares × 10.

If the dilution was 1 in 20, then

The sperm concentration per μL of neat semen = 'sperm count' per μL × 20.

Therefore, the sperm concentration/mL is the 'sperm count' per μL × 1000.

A more simple way of looking at this calculation is given below.

Sperm count in 5 small squares × 20 (dilution)
    × 5 (1/5 mm² is the area in which sperm are counted)
    × 10 (depth of chamber) × 1000 (to convert mm³ to mL³)
    = Number of sperm/mL.

For good precision and accuracy at least 200 sperm must be counted in both chambers and a mean obtained. If this total is not achieved then the dilution must be adjusted until this target is reached. The sperm concentration from two separately diluted aliquots of semen should differ by no more than 15%.

The Makler counting chamber

This counting chamber, unlike the haemocytometer, is designed specifically for counting sperm in semen (Makler 1980). The great advantage of the Makler chamber (Sefi Medical Instruments) is that no dilution is required (Fig. 5.7). The absence of the need for dilution saves time and greatly improves accuracy and reproducibility of the results. Motility can also be assessed at the same time as the sperm count.

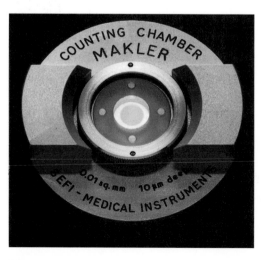

Fig. 5.7 The Makler counting chamber.

The structure of the Makler chamber

The Makler counting chamber is made up of two parts. The main lower section is made up of a flat metal ring base and two metal 'handles'. On the upper surface of the metal ring is fixed a glass disc onto which the semen is placed. Arising from the surface of the glass disc are four quartz-coated pins which rise up exactly 10 μm above the surface of the disc and which will support the second section of the chamber (Fig. 5.8).

The second section of the Makler chamber forms the upper portion and is the cover glass. It consists of a glass disc mounted within a metal ring. On the undersurface of the glass disc is marked a grid which overall measures 1 mm² (Fig. 5.9). This grid is subdivided into some 100 squares each measuring 0.1 mm². Thus, when the cover glass is placed on the four pins, the space that is bounded by these two surfaces and included within 10 of the small squares provides a volume of 0.001 mm³ (or 1 millionth of a mL). Thus, the number of sperm that are counted within 10 of these small squares equals the number of sperm in millions that are present in 1 mL of seminal fluid. Thus, using this chamber, no difficult calculations are needed to determine the sperm concentration.

Using the Makler counting chamber

Firstly, it is important to ensure that the chamber is absolutely clean. This is best achieved by rinsing it in distilled water and by careful drying with a

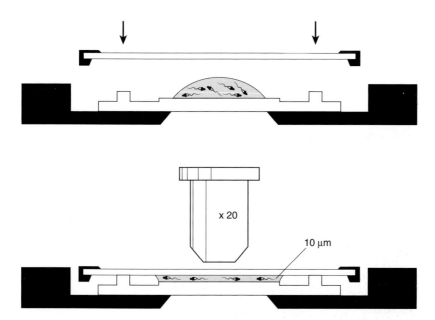

Fig. 5.8 A diagrammatic representation of the Makler counting chamber (reproduced by kind permission of Dr A. Makler and Sefi-Medical Instruments).

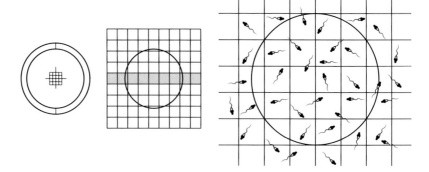

Fig. 5.9 The grid of the Makler counting chamber (reproduced by kind permission of Dr A. Makler and Sefi-Medical Instruments).

lens tissue. As this chamber will also be used to assess motility, and as water destroys sperm movement, it is important that it is completely dry.

Using a quill or a Pasteur pipette, a small drop of semen is now placed on the central glass disc in the lower portion of the chamber. It is important that the semen does not fill this area. It is also important to avoid the presence of air bubbles in the seminal fluid as this will reduce the volume of semen in which the sperm will be counted. The cover glass is then placed over the semen onto the four pins and is pressed down while looking for the appearance of the birefringent rings (Newton's rings) that appear around each of the pins. The presence of these rings indicates that there is a close contact between the pins and the cover glass and will ensure the automatic spread of the semen to a thickness of 10 µm.

The chamber is now lifted by its handles onto a microscope stage and viewed under phase contrast optics at a minimum magnification of ×200. On examining the semen through the grid it is first important to ensure that the sperm are evenly distributed; an uneven distribution of sperm will indicate that the semen sample has been inadequately mixed. The semen on this grid is undiluted and the sperm are therefore motile. The numbers of sperm in 10 squares is now counted and this is repeated in another set of 10 squares. The count is then repeated using another aliquot of neat semen and the result expressed as a mean of these four counts. The variation should not exceed 15%.

Other sperm counting chambers

Other chambers designed exclusively for semen analysis are also on the market, and these include the Microcell, available with depths of 12, 20 and 50 µm (Fertility Technologies, Natick, MA, USA), and the Chartpak Slide, which has a depth of 32 µm (Chartpack, Leeds, MA, USA).

Despite their relatively high price, these chambers save a great deal of time, have a high degree of accuracy and should certainly be recommended for any laboratory that performs more than one or two semen analyses each day.

Computer-assisted estimation of sperm numbers

Using computer-assisted sperm image analysis (CASA), it is now possible to estimate sperm concentration using a computer. These image analyser systems are very costly and are of little value today in routine clinical work, but are of course very useful for research, particularly in relation to sperm movement.

The counting of sperm in polyzoospermia

If sperm are present in very large numbers and are therefore difficult to count they can be immobilized. This is best carried out by putting an aliquot of semen into a test tube and incubating it at 50–60 °C for 5 min. Alternatively, the aliquot can be put in a refrigerator for 5–19 min. Semen so treated can then be used for the estimation of sperm numbers without the need for dilution and all the errors that may be incurred by such a procedure.

The assessment of sperm motility

In order to achieve fertilization, spermatozoa have to be motile and be capable of forward progression. Where the number of sperm showing motility is reduced the semen is said to show asthenozoospermia.

Sperm movement is a complex process. As the result of contractions of the fibres contained in the axoneme, a paddle movement is induced. The head turns from side to side while undulations of the tail cause the sperm to move forward (Fig. 5.10). Tail movement occurs in two planes: the amplitude of the tail wave being greater in the flat plane of the head than in the

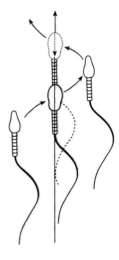

Fig. 5.10 A diagrammatic representation of the paddle movement made by spermatozoa that are undergoing good forward progression.

narrow plane of the head. If the sperm are correctly illuminated and, especially if phase contrast optics are used, light is reflected off the flat surface of the head in a phenomenon known as the light reflex. As the sperm carries out its paddle movement, the light reflex is temporarily lost until the flat surface of the sperm head becomes visible again. An absence of the 'turning on and off' of the light reflex is a sign of abnormal sperm movement.

Since the advent of computer-assisted imaging techniques and the ability to track sperm movement frame by frame on a video system, it is now possible to examine a variety of different parameters concerning sperm movement, including their velocity. Normal progressive sperm movement can be divided into a number of components. the track made by sperm and the speed at which it travels can now be computed and is known as the curvilinear velocity (V_{c-l}). From this, the straight-line velocity (V_l) can also be calculated. The head movement can also be tracked and the lateral head displacement (LHD) can be measured and it is now known that a lateral head displacement of less than 4μm is associated with significant infertility.

There are two types of normal movement exhibited by sperm. One type of movement is linear and the other is known as hyperactivation.

Normal linear movement is forward and progressive. Lateral head displacement is small and the amplitude of the flagella beat is relatively small. Under stimulation by the presence of substances such as the follicular fluid and as the result of an influx of calcium into the sperm, its movement will change to that known as hyperactivation (Fig. 5.11). Lateral head displacement is greatly increased and the flagellar movement forms a figure-of-eight pattern. This considerably reduces forward movement and straight-line velocity of the sperm but massively increases the thrust thus enhancing the ability of the sperm to penetrate the zona pellucida and enter the oocyte.

The tracks made by each type of sperm movement are therefore very different. There is some suggestion that hyperactivated sperm movement occurring in proximal parts of the genital tract such as the cervix may result in abnormal sperm transport within the female genital tract and could thus, in itself, be a cause of infertility.

Estimation of the percentage motility and the quality of sperm movement

During a routine semen analysis, the number of motile sperm can be counted on the Makler counting chamber and are expressed either as a concentration per mL or the total motile sperm count in the ejaculate. However, as sperm movement is much affected by temperature, it is best to carry out this estimation using a heated microscope stage.

As fertility tends to relate to the total number of motile sperm rather than their percentage of the total, the total numbers of motile sperm in an ejaculate are probably the more important diagnostically.

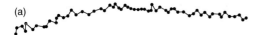

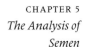

10μm

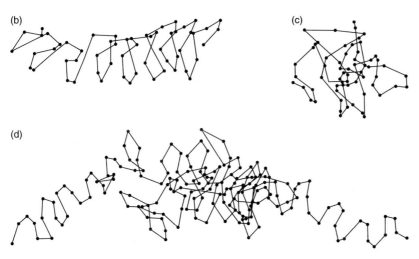

Fig. 5.11 This illustrates the changes in head tracks made by a spermatozoon passing from normal progressive forward movement (a), through progressive but hyperactivated movement (b) and then into nonprogressive hyperactivated sperm movement (c). The lower track (d) demonstrates the ability of a sperm to switch between nonprogressive hyperactivated and progressive hyyperactivated sperm movement. (Published by kind permission of Dr Sharon Mortimer.)

The quality of sperm movement is more difficult to assess without resorting to computer-assisted imaging. Nevertheless, sperm movement can be graded into four major categories according to the movement exhibited by the majority of sperm in the ejaculate. More accurately, again using the Makler chamber, the number of sperm showing each type of movement can be counted.

Sperm movement is usually graded as 0–4 according to the quality of forward progression (progressive activity) in the majority of the sperm in an ejaculate. Movement can be assessed descriptively as well on the 0–4 basis, with 0 showing no movement while 4 indicates vigorous forward progression (Table 5.3). In the measurement of motility, again at least 200 sperm must be counted from two aliquots of semen.

Hyperactivated sperm movement

It is now known that capacitated sperm can undergo a complete change in the pattern of their movement and undertake a form of movement known as hyperactivation (Mortimer *et al.* 1997). In response to an influx of calcium, the curvature of the sperm flagellum is increased greatly and results in a large increase in lateral head displacement (Fig. 5.11).

Table 5.3 One method of describing the quality of the forward movement (progressive activity) of sperm for a semen analysis

Definition	Description
0 None	A total absence of forward progression
1 Poor	Weak or sluggish forward progression
2 Moderate	Definite forward progression
3 Good	Good forward movement with progression
4 Excellent	Vigorous rapid forward progression

This change in movement pattern greatly increases the thrust of the sperm, which is likely to enhance its ability to penetrate the zona pellucida and achieve fertilization. However, this change also impairs forward progression, but as this alteration in movement is likely to occur close to the oocyte and indeed is induced by the zona proteins, forward progression may not be needed at this site.

Assessment of sperm vitality

If a sperm is showing no evidence of motility, it is difficult to know whether it is 'alive' and this problem can be overcome by the use of vital stains or by the application of the hypo-osmotic swelling test.

Eosin Y-test

For this test, one drop of fresh semen is mixed with one drop of a 0.5% solution of Eosin Y (C.I. 45380) in saline. An aliquot of this mixture is then placed on a slide and covered with a cover-slip. After 2 min the slide is examined at a magnification of ×400. The live sperm remain unstained while those that are nonvital are coloured pink. The proportion of live or dead sperm in this preparation can then be estimated (Fig. 5.12).

A large proportion of live but immotile cells in a semen sample may indicate the presence of an abnormality in the axoneme.

Eosin–nigrosin stain

For this test, one drop of the semen is mixed with one drop of a 1% solution of Eosin Y solution in distilled water. After 30 s, a drop of a 10% solution of Nigrosin (C.I. 50420) is added and a drop of this mixture is placed on a clean slide where it is allowed to air dry. The Nigrosin produces a dark background that enhances the colour difference between the sperm and the surrounding seminal plasma.

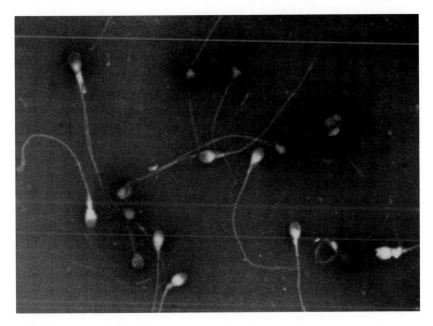

Fig. 5.12 A semen sample that has been stained with eosin to indicate the presence of dead and live sperm. The darker sperm heads show the uptake of stain that indicates nonviability.

Hypo-osmotic swelling test

This test is based on the ability of a live cell to swell under hypo-osmotic conditions (Jeyendran *et al.* 1984). A 1-mL aliquot of a freshly prepared and warmed solution containing 0.735 g of sodium citrate and 1.351 g of fructose in 100 mL of distilled water (which gives an osmolality of 150 osmol/kg) is added to 0.1 mL of neat semen and the mixture is incubated at 37 °C for 30 min. The sperm are then examined under phase contrast microscopy. Swelling and curling of the tails indicate the presence of live sperm.

Assessment of sperm morphology

Human sperm are not only pleomorphic but also tend to show large numbers of obvious abnormalities that may be associated with infertility. These differences may involve the head, midpiece or the tail and makes the assessment of what might be considered abnormal a very difficult task. It is also known that more than one abnormality may coexist in a single sperm. It is known that the greater the numbers of abnormalities present in each sperm (teratozoospermic index) relates closely to abnormalities in sperm function (Jouannet *et al.* 1988) and the presence of infertility. Thus, the identification of the different types of abnormalities among a population of spermatozoa within an ejaculate forms an important part of a semen analysis.

The variations in morphology that may be seen among human sperm involve the head, midpiece and tail. An oval head is deemed to be normal but many shape and size variations can be seen in an ejaculate, and these include large, small or tapering heads. Amorphous heads are now known to be associated with chromosomal anomalies and a sperm may even show the presence of a double head.

Another anomaly of sperm morphology that is occasionally seen is the abnormality known as globozoospermia. In this condition, the sperm head lacks an acrosome and, as a consequence, the head of each spermatozoon becomes rounded (Fig. 5.13).

The midpiece can be absent or not inserted into the head (to form the so-called 'broken neck') and there can also be abnormalities of the mitochondria in this area. A condition known as fibrous sheath dysplasia may also be present. It is also possible to see a cytoplasmic droplet present on the midpiece of the sperm just below the head. This small segment of cytoplasm is in fact a portion of the Sertoli cell from whence the sperm developed. These structures are important as they may generate reactive oxygen species that can damage sperm function by lipid peroxidation of the cell membrane.

The tails can be short stubby, hairpin and angulated. Double tails are also not infrequently seen in infertile samples (Fig. 5.14).

The morphology of spermatozoa can only be accurately assessed on a stained smear. A smear is made on a clean and dry microscope slide and the smear is then air dried prior to staining. The stains that can be applied to the

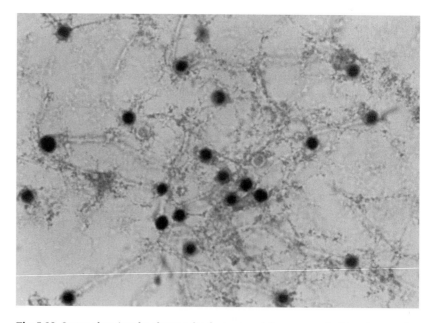

Fig. 5.13 Sperm showing the abnormality known as globozoospermia. Note the round heads of the spermatozoa and the absence of an acrosomal cap. The absence of the acrosome results in this rounding of the nuclear DNA.

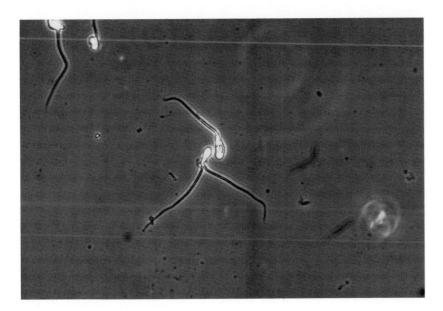

Fig. 5.14 A double-tailed sperm.

evaluation of sperm morphology vary in different laboratories but the most commonly used stain in semenology is probably a modification of the Papanicolaou stain used for cervical cytology. This stain is available in many laboratories and is often automated, making the staining of semen smears a simple task (Table 5.4). Other stains that can be used in a semen analysis

Table 5.4 A modification of the Papanicolaou stain that can be used to assess the morphology of human spermatozoa

The semen is spread thinly on a clean glass slide and air dried. The slide is then immersed for fixed times in the following solutions:	
1. Fix in methanol	20 min
2. 70% ethanol	1 min
3. Distilled water	1 min
4. Harris' haematoxylin	3 s
5. Running tap water	1 min
6. 1.5% acid–alcohol solution	15 s
7. Running tap water	1 min
8. 1.5% acid–alcohol solution	1 min
9. Absolute alcohol	1 min
10. Orange G	45 s
11. Absolute alcohol	1 min
12. Absolute alcohol	1 min
13. Papanicolaou EA 50	1.5 min
14. Absolute alcohol wash ×3	
15. Clear in two separate aliquots of xylene	
16. Mount in dibutylphthalate xylene	

include the May–Grünwald–Giemsa stain, the Shorr stain and the haematoxylin and eosin stain.

For the analysis of sperm morphology good optics are required and the semen smear is best evaluated at high magnification, i.e. under oil immersion. In carrying out an assessment of sperm morphology, at least 100 cells must be examined and categorized according to the anomalies present in the sperm. It is usual to divide each abnormality into head, midpiece or tail anomalies together with the presence of cytoplasmic droplets and express them as a percentage of the total.

In the original WHO method of classifying sperm, only the obviously deformed sperm were classified as abnormal, but in 1986 the Tygerberg system was introduced (Kruger *et al.* 1986), which demanded that there be very strict criteria for the definition of a normal sperm, and for a sperm to be considered normal it must fall within a strictly defined definition in terms of shape and size. Each head must be oval and must be 5.0–6.0 μm long. The midpiece must be completely normal and no cytoplasmic droplets of more than one-third of the size of the head must be present. The tail must also be normal. These strict criteria of normality thus allow for much greater numbers of sperm to be considered abnormal and, using the Tygerberg system, normal men will only show 14% or more of normal sperm.

The identification of germinal cells and white cells in seminal fluid

All semen samples will contain some round cells and these need identification. It is impossible to differentiate white cells from germinal cells without staining, and even then it can be difficult to identify white cells without resort to a special stain. Too often germinal cells are reported as white cells, for which the patient is subjected to unnecessary courses of antibiotics.

Leucocytes are present in most semen samples (Tomlinson *et al.* 1993) as are germinal cells. In a normal ejaculate, the number of germinal cells should not exceed 5×10^6/mL and the number of leucocytes should not exceed 1×10^6/mL.

To differentiate germinal cells from white cells, the semen smear must be subjected to a peroxidase stain. This stains all cells, producing peroxidase, a brown colour, while all the other cells including the germinal cells are stained pink. Using this staining technique on a semen smear, it is now possible to carry out a count on the number of white cells and germinal cells by comparing their number with that of the sperm. By using the sperm concentration which would be known, one can calculate the numbers of each of these cells present in 1 μL of seminal fluid.

Some useful sperm function tests

Although counting sperm and assessing their motility and morphology makes a very important contribution to the diagnosis of infertility, these parameters tell us very little about their function. There are some sperm function tests that can be used to help the clinician determine whether or not sperm in a given semen sample have the ability to penetrate and fertilize an egg. There are in fact many sperm function tests that can be utilized by a good andrology laboratory and some of the most useful and most commonly used will be outlined below.

Sperm–cervical mucus interaction tests

There are several ways in which the interaction between spermatozoa and cervical mucus can be demonstrated and such tests can be carried out either *in vivo* or *in vitro*.

The *in vivo* *postcoital test*

As cervical mucus undergoes cyclical changes within a menstrual cycle and becomes most easily penetrable by sperm when oestrogen secretion is at its height, the *spinnbarkeit* (the formation of a thread by cervical mucus) of the cervical mucus is maximal (Fig. 5.15) and the progesterone levels are still low. These tests are thus best carried out close to and just prior to ovulation. The couple are, after some 2 days' abstinence, asked to have intercourse when instructed by the clinic. The cervical mucus is then examined some 9–24 h later.

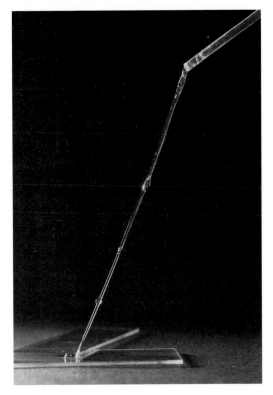

Fig. 5.15 Cervical mucus taken from a woman at mid-cycle showing marked *spinnbarkeit*.

A speculum is inserted into the vagina without lubrication and, using a pipette or a long tuberculin syringe attached to a quill, the seminal fluid is aspirated from the posterior fornix. Using a second clean syringe a sample of mucus is then aspirated from within the cervical canal. Both samples can now be placed separately onto a clean glass slide and covered lightly with a cover-slip. The slide is then examined at a magnification of around ×400 using phase contrast microscopy.

In the sample taken from the posterior fornix, all the sperm will be immotile as they will be killed by the low pH of the vaginal secretions at midcycle. The presence of sperm in the posterior fornix, however, at least indicates that intercourse has taken place. On examination of the cervical mucus sample, there should be a number of sperm present and some of these sperm should be motile.

In many fertile couples the postcoital test will show as many as 50 motile spermatozoa per high power field, but the test is deemed to be positive if there are five or more sperm showing poor or circular movement in each microscope field. A positive postcoital test gives a good prognosis for fertility at least in terms of sperm function. A negative postcoital test may indicate an abnormality of either sperm function or of an abnormality of the cervical mucus. It must be remembered, however, that low oestrogen levels or high progesterone levels, i.e badly timed postcoital tests, will frequently give a negative result. Postcoital tests will also very often be abnormal in anovulatory women.

The simplified slide test of sperm–cervical mucus interaction (also known as the Kurzrok–Miller test)

In this test the sperm–cervical mucus interaction is carried out in the laboratory. Such a test can also be carried out using donor sperm in parallel with the semen sample from the husband, and in this way one can isolate cervical mucus factors from those of the sperm.

Some cervical mucus taken from the cervix at midcycle is placed on a microscope slide and covered with a cover-slip. It is important to lie the mucus on the slide in a straight line. A drop of semen is then placed at the edge of the cover-slip and the preparation is incubated at 37 °C for 30 min. The slide and the cervical mucus is now observed using phase contrast microscopy. Very soon after their first contact with the cervical mucus, the sperm form phalanges within the mucus and most migrate into the mucus (Fig. 5.16).

The test is deemed to give a good result if most of the sperm penetrate the mucus and show definite forward progression. If few sperm enter the mucus and show circular or nonforward progression, then the test is deemed to give a poor result.

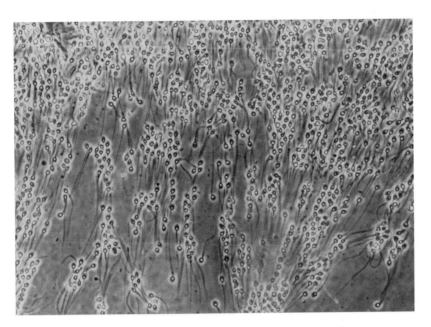

Fig. 5.16 The migration of spermatozoa into cervical mucus. Note how the sperm enter the cervical mucus in phalanxes or columns.

Hyaluronate migration test

This is a useful test as it examines the ability of sperm to migrate into an artificial mucus (Mortimer *et al.* 1990). It can thus be used in couples where the female partner is either anovulatory or has some pathology of her cervix.

Basically, this test uses a solution of the polysaccharide sodium hyaluronate contained in a capillary tube as a source of migration for spermatozoa. This solution is commercially known as Sperm Select (Select Medical Systems, Williston, VT, USA). The capillary tube containing sodium hyaluronate is dipped into a small 50-µL aliquot of neat liquefied semen, which is then incubated at 37 °C for 60 min.

The small capillary tube is then placed on a microscope stage and the advance of the sperm into the sodium hyaluronate solution is then examined at distances of 10, 20, 30 and 40 mm up the capillary tube and the numbers of sperm at each point are counted. The average number of sperm at each distance is then calculated. This test correlates well with the ability of sperm to penetrate cervical mucus.

The Kremer test

Another *in vitro* sperm invasion test that is sometimes used is the Kremer test (Kremer 1965). In this examination a capillary tube is filled with mucus which has an Insler score of at least 10. Flat tubes are best used for this purpose as they allow for easier microscopy of the mucus and the sperm

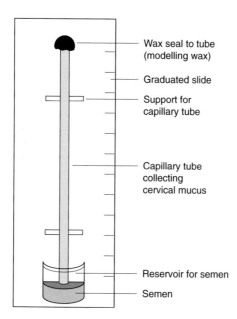

Wax seal to tube
(modelling wax)

Graduated slide

Support for
capillary tube

Capillary tube
collecting
cervical mucus

Reservoir for semen

Semen

Fig. 5.17 The apparatus needed for
the Kremer test.

that have migrated into the mucus. After the tube has been filled with
mucus one end is sealed.

The open end of the tube is then placed in a pool of liquefied semen and
incubated at 37 °C for 30 min (Fig. 5.17). The flat tube is then removed from
the aliquot of semen and examined microscopically. Using a magnification
of ×400, the tube is examined at 10, 40 and 70 mm from the open end and
the number of sperm counted in a field at these points. A score is then given
according to the number of sperm at these distances from the end of the
tube (Table 5.5).

Acrosome reaction ionophore challenge test (ARIC test)

The ability of sperm to undergo the acrosome reaction is a prerequisite of
fertilization. The acrosome reaction occurs as the result of an influx of
calcium and this can be induced using a calcium ionophore. It is known
that defective sperm function in terms of the sperm–oocyte fusion is associ-

Table 5.5 Method of scoring the Kremer test

No. of sperm/mm²	Score
0	0
1–30	1
31–60	2
61–120	3
121–200	4
>200	5

ated with an impaired acrosome reaction and that this may be a cause of fertilization failure at IVF.

This test thus examines the ability of sperm to undergo the acrosome reaction in response to treatment with a calcium ionophore, which provides a calcium influx (Cummins *et al.* 1991). This test correlates well with the fertility of sperm and can be used as a means of detecting abnormalities in sperm function in ejaculates that appear to be otherwise normal. It has the disadvantage, however, of being quite a complex test to carry out and the presence of motile sperm within the ejaculate are essential.

In this test motile sperm are separated from immotile sperm using the 'swim-up' technique. Ideally, the initial semen sample should contain at least 10 million motile sperm per mL or insufficient sperm will be harvested to complete the test. Basically, these motile sperm are then exposed to a solution of ionophore (A23187 in dimethylsulfoxide; DMSO) and stained for the presence or absence of the acrosome reaction.

Two 0.5-mL aliquots of the motile sperm preparation are placed in two small Falcon tubes. A 10-µL aliquot of DMSO is added to the control tube and a 10-µL aliquot of the ionophore in DMSO is added to the test tube. These mixtures are then incubated at 37°C for 60 min. The samples are now isolated from the ionophore by passage through a gradient and then fixed in 95% ethanol for 30 min. Smears are made of both the control and test sperm, which are then stained with fluorescein isothiocyanate-conjugated *Pisa sativum* (FITC-PSA). A cover-slip is then laid over the smear and the smear examined under ultraviolet light at a wavelength of 480 Å (48 nm) using an oil immersion lens. Light at this wavelength will cause the stained sperm heads to fluoresce (Fig. 5.18).

Four major staining patterns will be seen on the sperm. A fully stained acrosomal cap indicates the absence of an acrosome reaction while a par-

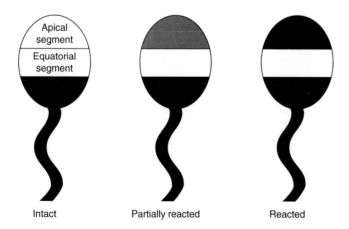

Fig. 5.18 A diagrammatic representation of the fluorescent acrosomal caps of sperm after treatment with a calcium ionophore. Those sperm with intact acrosomes can be differentiated from those whose acrosomes are partially reacted or are intact by an absence of fluorescence.

tially stained cap demonstrates an acrosome reaction in the process of completion. An absent acrosomal cap, however, indicates that a completed acrosome reaction has occurred. Abnormal sperm with deformed heads will also be seen.

The number of sperm showing a completed acrosome reaction are counted and expressed as a percentage of the total number of stained sperm. The ARIC test result is the difference between the percentage of completed acrosome reactions in the treated sperm and the percentage of completed acrosome reactions in the untreated sperm.

An ARIC test result of less than 5%, i.e. where the ionophore challenged sperm only increase their percentage of acrosome reactions over those in the unchallenged sperm by 5%, is highly predictive of infertility and of fertilization failure within an IVF programme. Such a test is thus useful in evaluating male infertility and also in the prediction of fertilization failure. Abnormal ARIC tests may also be found among patients with very normal looking semen analyses and this test should be performed on all patients with unexplained infertility and those undergoing IVF where the semen analysis is deemed to be normal or nearly normal.

Hamster egg penetration test (HEPT)

In natural circumstances, the fertilization of an oocyte by a sperm of a different species is prevented by the presence of the zona pellucida. Removal of the zona pellucida will allow penetration of the oocyte by sperm of a different species. In 1976, Yanagamachi and colleagues discovered that zona-free hamster eggs could be penetrated by human sperm (Yanagamachi *et al.* 1976), and Rogers and colleagues went on to develop this phenomenon as a test to predict the ability of a human sperm to fertilize an egg (Rogers *et al.* 1979).

It must be remembered, however, that this test in no way mimics natural human fertilization. It is a test that is performed *in vitro* and not *in vivo*. The oocytes are devoid of zonae and the oocytes are not human. The test has the disadvantage that it is extremely labour intensive and thus expensive. It is a test that cannot be performed in Australia, where the importation of hamsters is prohibited. However, it is possible to import freeze-dried hamster eggs if one would wish to perform this test (Charles River Professional Services, Wilmington, MA, USA).

The performance of this test is relatively simple to carry out. Female hamsters are first given 25 IU of human chorionic gonadotrophin (hCG) by intraperitoneal injection on day 1 of their 4-day cycle. Day 1 is identified by the presence of a slight white vaginal discharge. On day 3, a further intraperitoneal injection of hCG is given to induce follicular rupture.

Between 17 and 22 h after the second injection of hCG (the time seems to depend on the strain of hamster used), the animals are killed and their oviducts are dissected out. Attached to the ends of the oviducts is a mass of oocytes surrounded and stuck together by many cumulus cells. After separation from the oviduct these cells are placed in a 0.1% solution of hyaluronidase in a tissue culture medium. The cumulus cells will now rapidly dissociate leaving the oocytes free in the medium.

The next step is to remove the zonae, and to do this the oocytes are first washed in medium and then placed very briefly in a 0.1% solution of trypsin (30–60 s). As soon as the zona have disappeared, the zona-free eggs must be removed from the trypsin solution to prevent damage to the cell wall of the oocyte by the trypsin.

The eggs are then washed in medium and placed in groups of 30 under a drop of sterile mineral oil on a Petri dish. It is possible to obtain from each hamster only some 20–50 eggs for the HEPT procedure, so only one or two tests can be carried out using the eggs from one hamster.

The human sperm under test are first washed in medium and the motile sperm separated from the immotile ones using the 'swim-up' method. the motile sperm are now incubated for 1 h at 37 °C in an atmosphere of 5% CO_2 and 95% air. The concentration of sperm is now adjusted to 3.5 million/mL and a 50-µL aliquot of this suspension is then placed with the eggs under the droplet of mineral oil. The gametes are then incubated together in this way for 3 h.

The oocytes are now removed from the oil, washed in medium and examined using phase contrast microscopy. The oocytes can also be fixed and stained making the identification of the spermatozoa within each oocyte very simple. The number of sperm incorporated into each oocyte is now counted and expressed as a mean. Around 10 sperm per oocyte would seem to indicate fertility.

As can be seen from the above, this test is very time consuming and difficult to perform. With the advent of intracytoplasmic sperm injection, it has largely been abandoned but there are some centres that still use this test and knowledge of the existence of this test is still important.

Zona binding tests

Occasionally within an IVF programme, one will see oocytes that appear to be unable to bind sperm to their zonae. This phenomenon can be the result of abnormalities of either the sperm or of the oocyte. Some years ago, Burkman and colleagues devised a test using zonae from which the egg had been removed that tested the ability of the sperm to bind to their surface (Burkman *et al.* 1988).

Zonae are collected from discarded eggs within an IVF programme and can be stored almost indefinitely in concentrated salt solutions until ready for use. Either zonae or hemizonae can be used in this test. When required, the zonae are removed from their salt solution and placed under oil while an aliquot of motile sperm is prepared in a similar way to that for the HEPT. The zonae are then incubated with the spermatozoa and the number of sperm on their surface is then counted. The ability of the sperm to bind to the zona is thus ascertained.

However, it is now known that lack of sperm binding to the zona pellu-cida can be caused by many factors other than disorders of the spermato-zoa. For this reason as well as the fact that access to spare oocytes is rapidly becoming restricted, the zona binding assay has now largely been abandoned.

Some useful biochemical tests on seminal fluid

Seminal fluid contains a very complex mixture of many different biochem-ical substances that includes proteins, lipids and electrolytes. A limited number of these substances are produced, at least in the main, by one part of the genital tract and thus measurement of their concentration in semen may provide an indication of the normal or abnormal function of that segment of the genital tract.

The demonstration of the absence of a substance in semen or its pres-ence in reduced concentration can thus indicate pathology of a specific segment of the genital tract and can thus be of great value diagnostically (Table 5.6).

Fructose (normal concentration in semen ⩾ 13 μmol per ejaculate)

Fructose is present in large quantities in semen and is the main energy source for sperm. It is produced only by the seminal vesicles. In men with conditions such as bilateral congenital absence of the vas, where frequently the seminal vesicles are absent or hypoplastic, the fructose in the ejaculate will be absent or very low. The secretion of the seminal vesicles can also be obliterated as the result of severe infection, in particular that caused by tuberculosis. The seminal vesicular secretions and the fructose contained

Table 5.6 Some biochemical markers in semen and their sites of origin. The identification and measurement of these substances in a semen sample can be of diagnostic value to the clinician

Site of origin	Biochemical marker
Testis	Transferrin
	Inhibin
Epididymis	Carnitine
	Glycerophosphorylcholine
	Inositol
Seminal vesicles	Fructose
	Prostaglandins
Prostate gland	Citrate
	Acid phosphatase
	Zinc
Bulbourethral glands	Mucoproteins
	IgA

within it will also be excluded from the ejaculate in men with all forms of ejaculatory duct obstruction.

The concentration of fructose in a semen sample will fall as the sample ages because of its consumption by the sperm. For the same reason, men with very high numbers of sperm in an ejaculate will also rapidly reduce the concentration of fructose in the seminal plasma and this is of course the cause of the asthenozoospermia that so often accompanies sperm concentrations of over 350 million/mL.

Thus, the measurement of fructose can be helpful diagnostically and it can also be easily measured in most pathology laboratories. The method of measurement most frequently used is that of Seliwanoff using the resorcinol technique. However, as at least 1 mL of seminal plasma is required for the estimation of fructose, in some patients with very low ejaculatory volumes caused by conditions such as ejaculatory duct obstruction, it can sometimes be difficult to find a sample of semen of the required volume.

Acid phosphatase (normal concentration in semen ⩾ 200 units per ejaculate)

Acid phosphatase is secreted into the semen by the prostate gland and can therefore be used as a marker of prostatic secretion. It is a very stable enzyme and for this reason it is used by forensic laboratories as an indicator of the presence of semen in stains and on clothes. In a semen analysis it can also be used to demonstrate the presence of prostatic fluid in an ejaculate. However, it must be remembered that the secretions of the prostate pass into the posterior urethra through the many prostatic ducts, thus making it almost impossible to exclude the prostatic secretions from the ejaculate.

In men with ejaculatory duct obstruction the volume of the ejaculate is very reduced. The acid phosphatase in semen is therefore not diluted by the large volume of secretions from the seminal vesicles. In this condition therefore the concentration of acid phosphatase in the semen will be increased.

Acid phosphatase can be measured in most pathology laboratories. The method used is dependent upon the action of this enzyme on substrate at a reduced pH.

Citrate (normal concentration in semen ⩾ 52 μmol per ejaculate)

Citric acid and its salts are also present in semen and are produced by the prostate gland. Its measurement can also be used as a marker of prostatic secretory function. It is, however, less easy to find a laboratory that will measure this substance and thus if a prostatic marker is needed, acid phosphatase is a better compound to measure.

Zinc (normal concentrations in semen ⩾ 2.4 μmol per ejaculate)

A great deal of attention was at one time given to zinc levels in seminal fluid. Zinc is secreted by the prostate and stabilizes seminal proteins. Its role in the semen of the infertile male has yet to be established.

There are some other compounds in semen that may also be of value diagnostically.

Inhibin

Inhibin is a glycoprotein produced by the Sertoli cells within the seminiferous tubules. When inhibin enters the circulation it acts as the major negative feedback for FSH secretion by the pituitary. Inhibin is made up of an α- and β-subunit of which the β-subunits each exist in two forms. Inhibin is secreted into the semen and its concentration is reduced in men with spermatogenic problems and in men with bilateral obstructive lesions of the epididymis and the vasa deferentia.

Inhibin is measured using a radioimmunoassay. Its measurement in semen may one day prove to be a useful indicator of Sertoli cell function and of the presence of the testicular contribution in semen. However, the assay for inhibin is not yet available in many routine pathology laboratories.

Prostaglandins

The prostaglandins, and in particular the prostaglandin $PGF_{2\alpha}$, play an important role in the contractility of smooth muscle. All the prostaglandins are secreted by the seminal vesicles and are present in semen in high concentration. It has been suggested that prostaglandins play a role in the contractions of the urethral smooth muscle during ejaculation and emission. Their presence in semen may also stimulate contractions of the female genital tract after ejaculation and thus aid sperm transport through the female genital tract.

This group of substances may also enhance the penetration of the cervical mucus by the spermatozoa. The concentration of prostaglandins may be reduced in men with infertility but the mechanism of this reduction is not understood. When the role of prostaglandins in male infertility becomes clear, the measurement of prostaglandins may have some diagnostic value.

Transferrin

Transferrin is produced by the Sertoli cells and is released by them into the testicular component of the ejaculate. It acts as a carrier of protein in the Sertoli cell. It could thus be a useful marker for Sertoli cell function. However, transferrin in semen is only present in low concentrations and the normal assays used to measure this substance in blood are too insensitive to measure transferrin in an ejaculate. Using specially developed assays, seminal transferrin can be measured in semen, but whether it will ever have a major clinical value in semen analysis is at present very doubtful.

Glycerylphosphorylcholine

This substance is secreted by the epididymal epithelium and at one time enjoyed a role as an epididymal marker. However, it is also secreted in small amounts by the seminal vesicle and thus diagnostically its value as a marker of the presence of normally functioning epididymal epithelium is clearly limited.

Despite all these problems, the biochemical analysis of semen can be helpful diagnostically and should not be overlooked as an occasionally valuable parameter of a semen analysis.

References

Amelar, R.D., Dubin, L., Quigley, M.M. & Schoenfeld, C. (1979) Successful management of infertility due to polyzoospermia. *Fertility and Sterility* **31**, 521–524.

Bunge, R.G. & Sherman, J.K. (1954) Liquefaction of human semen by α-amylase. *Fertility and Sterility* **5**, 353–356.

Burkman, L.J., Coddington, C.C., Franken, D.A., Kruger, T.F., Rosenwaks, Z. & Hodgen, G.D. (1988) The hemizina assay (HZA): development of a diagnostic test for the binding of human spermatozoa to the human hemizona pellucida to predict fertilization potential. *Fertility and Sterility* **49**, 688–697.

Crich, J.P. & Jequier, A.M. (1978) Infertility in men with retrograde ejaculation; the action of urine on sperm motility and a simple method of achieving antegrade ejaculation. *Fertility and Sterility* **30**, 572–576.

Cummins, J.M., Pember, S., Jequier, A.M., Yovich, J.L. & Hartman, P.E. (1991) A test of the human sperm acrosome reaction following ionophore challenge: relationship to fertility and other seminal parameters. *Journal of Andrology* **12**, 98–103.

Eliasson, R. (1965) Effect of frequent ejaculations on the composition of human seminal plasma. *Journal of Reproduction and Fertility* **9**, 331–336.

Eliasson, R. (1971) Standards for the investigation of human semen. *Andrologia* **3**, 49–64.

Jeyendran, R.S., Van der Ven, H., Perez-Palaez, M., Crabo, B. & Zanefeld, L.J.D. (1984) Development of an assay to assess the functional integrity of the human sperm membrane and its relationship to other semen characteristics. *Journal of Reproduction and Fertility* **70**, 219–228.

Jouannet, P., Ducot, B., Feneux, D. & Spira, A. (1988) Male factors and the liklihood of pregnancy in infertile couples. I. Study of sperm characteristics. *International Journal of Andrology* **11**, 379–394.

Kremer, J. (1965) A simple sperm penetration test. *International Journal of Fertility* **10**, 2099–2105.

Kruger, T.F., Menkfeld, R., Stander, F.S.H. *et al.* (1986) Sperm morphologic features as a prognostic factor in *in vitro* fertilisation. *Fertility and Sterility* **46**, 1118–1123.

Makler, A. (1980) The improved ten-micrometer chamber for rapid sperm count and motility evaluation. *Fertility and Sterility* **33**, 337–338.

Mortimer, D., Mortimer, S.T., Shu, M.A. & Swart, R. (1990) A simplified approach to sperm–cervical mucus interaction using a hyaluronate migration test. *Human Reproduction* **5**, 835–841.

Mortimer, S., Schoevaert, D., Swan, M.A. & Mortimer, D. (1997) Quantitative observations of flagella motility of capacitating human spermatozoa. *Human Reproduction* **12**, 1006–1012.

Mortimer, D., Templeton, A.A., Lenton, A.E. & Coleman, R.A. (1982) Influence of abstinence and ejaculation-to-analysis delay on semen analysis parameters of suspected infertile men. *Archives of Andrology* **8**, 251–256.

Rogers, B.J., Van Campen, H., Ueno, M., Lambert, H., Bronson, R. & Hanson, F.W. (1979) Analysis of human spermatozoa fertilizing ability using zona-free ova. *Fertility and Sterility* **32**, 664–670.

Tomlinson, M.J., Barrett, C.L.R. & Cooke, I.D. (1993) Prospective study of leucocytes and leucocyte sub-populations in semen suggest that they are not the cause of male infertility. *Fertility and Sterility* **60**, 1069–1075.

Yanagamachi, R., Yanagamachi, H. & Rogers, B.J. (1976) the use of zona-free animal ova as a test system for the assessment of the fertilizing capacity of human spermatozoa. *Biology of Reproduction* **15**, 471–476.

6: Obstructive Lesions of the Male Genital Tract

Obstruction of the ductal system of the male genital tract is a common cause of infertility and may account for around 15% of all infertility in the male (Jequier 1986). Obstructive lesions can occur either in the ducts that lie within the testes themselves or in any part of the complex excurrent ductal system which ends in the urethra. If these obstructive lesions are both bilateral and complete then azoospermia will result. However, if the obstruction is unilateral or incomplete then only oligozoospermia will be present (Jequier *et al.* 1983). Also, if the ductal obstruction results in the exclusion of any of the secretions of the accessory glands of the genital tract (as would occur in ejaculatory duct obstruction), then profound changes will also occur in both the volume of the ejaculate and the biochemistry of the seminal fluid (Amelar & Hotchkiss 1963). Thus, ductal obstruction will cause a wide variety of different changes in sperm number, sperm motility and seminal biochemistry.

The symptoms, the clinical findings and the changes in the seminal fluid will depend upon the site of the obstructive lesion. In order to be able to restore patency, to treat the patient rationally and in particular to offer the infertile man a prognosis, it is vital to pinpoint the site of the obstruction with some accuracy, and to do this a very careful clinical evaluation is essential.

Obstructive lesions of the male genital tract can be congenital or acquired. It may now be helpful to consider the clinical presentation and the management of obstructive lesions that may occur in different parts of the genital tract.

Intratesticular obstructive lesions

Intratesticular obstruction is an uncommon cause of male infertility and probably makes up only around 2% of all the obstructive lesions in the male genital tract (Jequier 1986). There are two major sites of obstruction within the testis itself: one involving the seminiferous tubules themselves and the second where the obstruction occurs within the rete testis.

Intratesticular obstruction is likely to be a rare cause of ductal obstruction. The majority of patients who, at operation, appear to have intratesticular obstruction are, on the examination of their testicular biopsy, found to have some form of spermatogenic problem (Hendry *et al.* 1983).

Intratesticular obstruction is characterized clinically by the apparent absence, either on clinical examination or at operation, of any abnormality of the genital tract. As sperm production is normal, testicular size will not be reduced. As the obstruction is within the testes themselves, the excurrent ducts will also show no abnormality. As Sertoli cell and Leydig cell function is also normal, there will be no change in hormone levels. Depending on whether the obstruction is complete or incomplete, sperm will either be absent or will be in reduced numbers in a semen sample. However, this site of obstruction may be associated with the development of antisperm antibodies (Hendry *et al.* 1983) and their presence in semen may be of value diagnostically particularly in relation to obstruction of the rete testis.

Hypercurvature syndrome

This type of intratesticular obstruction was first described by Averback and Wight in 1979 (Averback & Wight 1979). Considerable controversy still exists as to whether this is a true clinical entity. As the aetiology of this condition is unknown, it is far from certain whether this condition is congenital or acquired.

In this condition the tubules are said to undergo a much increased tortuosity to a point where this change could induce obstruction. As there is no disorder of spermatogenesis in men who may have this condition, testis size and FSH levels will always be normal. However, it would appear that these obstructive lesions are never complete and thus patients who may have this disorder only show oligozoospermia in a semen sample.

The diagnosis can only be made by the examination of a testicular biopsy. The diagnosis was originally made using a Quantimet 720 Image Analysing modular computing system, which was applied to a testicular biopsy. In this condition, because of the increased tortuosity of the tubules, a higher number of tangential cuts were said to be present in the biopsy and the mean sectional area of the tubules was also increased. This computer system is much too costly to be generally available and thus the occurrence of this still theoretical cause of male infertility and its incidence has never been confirmed.

There is no way as yet known to treat this condition. If azoospermia is present, then the best management of this problem is IVF and intracytoplasmic sperm injection (ICSI) using sperm from the testis itself. Other methods of treatment of the infertility caused by this problem will depend upon the severity of the oligozoospermia.

Rete testis obstruction

Obstruction of the rete testis was first demonstrated histologically by Guerin and colleagues in 1981 (Guerin *et al.* 1981) and this disorder is now recognized as a cause of intratesticular obstruction.

In this condition, the network of channels that form the rete within the mediastinum are obliterated by fibrous tissue. If the obstruction of the rete is complete, which it usually is, then the semen will be azoospermic

On clinical examination, testicular size will of course be normal and no other abnormality will be found in the genital tract. If the obstruction is complete, then the semen will show azoospermia. As spermatogenesis in this condition is normal, testicular size and the levels of FSH will be normal. However, the presence of antisperm antibodies in semen is a frequent finding in this condition, and it has been suggested that rete testis obstruction may in fact be the result of some form of immune response (Hendry *et al.* 1983). No other aetiology has been suggested.

At operation, the epididymis and the excurrent ducts of the testis will be normal. As it is not possible to take a biopsy of the rete testis without provoking serious haemorrhage, histological confirmation of rete testis obstruction is impossible without performing an orchidectomy. For this reason, the presence of rete testis obstruction can only rarely be confirmed and its presence is usually only surmised. For these reasons its incidence among an infertile male population is basically unknown.

The histology of the testis among men with an obstructive lesion alone usually shows only normal testicular tissue even when the obstruction is within the testis itself, such as lesions that result in rete testis obstruction. However, it is not uncommon to see areas of interstitial oedema in such a testicular biopsy. The presence of diverticula of the seminiferous tubules has also been reported (Nistal *et al.* 1988).

There is no remediable therapy for this condition, which is now best treated by IVF and ICSI using spermatozoa harvested from the testis. Even if sperm are indeed present in the semen, the high titre of antisperm antibodies present in the semen may give rise to failed fertilization at conventional IVF. For these reasons, ICSI is best employed.

Epididymal obstruction

The epididymis is by far the most common site of all the obstructive lesions in the genital tract and makes up more that 50% of all such lesions in the infertile male population (Jequier 1986).

Causes of epididymal obstruction

The aetiology of epididymal obstruction would appear to be changing. Some 60 years ago, the French andrologist Bayle reported that the aetiology of the obstruction could be identified in all patients with this form of obstruction and that 65% of all epididymal obstruction was a result of gonococcal infection (Bayle 1952). However today, the aetiology of this condition frequently cannot be identified and gonococcal infection may account for less that 5% of all cases of epididymal obstruction (Jequier 1986).

There are, however, a number of well-known causes of epididymal obstruction, all of which need to be considered from both a diagnostic and a therapeutic point of view.

Nonjunction between the efferent ductules and the epididymal duct

This lesion is an uncommon but nevertheless well-recognized cause of obstruction and is caused by a failure of fusion between the mesonephric structures that make up the vasa efferentia with those of the testis (Hodges & Hanley 1966). Such abnormalities may also be seen alongside a cryptorchid testis (Heath *et al.* 1984). These lesions are usually bilateral and thus present with obstructive azoospermia. Except when it is in association with a maldescended testis, no abnormal physical signs will be present in men with this disorder. As spermatogenesis will usually be normal, testis size will likewise be normal.

This condition can only be diagnosed at scrotal exploration. At operation the epididymal caput is separate from the testis and lies free in the hemiscrotum, unconfined by the tunica vaginalis. The lower half of the epididymis, however, is normally attached by connective tissue to the postero-lateral border of the testis.

Therapeutically, there is little one can do surgically to correct this problem, but pregnancies can now be achieved by the aspiration of sperm from the rete testis and their use within an IVF programme. As spermatozoa from the rete testis are usually poorly motile, the problem really requires the application of ICSI.

Congenital absence of portions of the epididymis

This is in fact not an uncommon lesion among men with obstructive azoospermia (Wollin *et al.* 1987). It is also frequently associated with absence of the whole or of portions of the vas but can occur without there being any anomaly of the rest of the genital tract (Fig. 6.1).

This lesion can be difficult to diagnose clinically. Although the caput epididymis may be distended and easily palpable, a sign that suggests epididymal obstruction, no abnormal physical signs will be present if this anomaly affects the most proximal portions of the epididymis. In such patients, the diagnosis may have to be made at surgical exploration.

In this type of lesion it is may be possible to carry out a successful microsurgical epididymovasostomy (see below), but otherwise microsurgical epididymal aspiration of sperm will be indicated in association with ICSI.

Epididymitis

There are many infections that can involve the epididymis and many of these can obstruct the epididymal duct. Occasionally the sites of obstruction within the epididymis can be multiple. They can affect any part of the duct

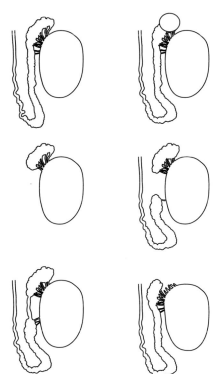

Fig. 6.1 Obstructive azoospermia can be the result of an absence of portions of the epididymal duct. The sites of these missing segments can be very variable and may involve different areas of the epididymis.

and even involve the efferent ductules and the rete testis if the infection is chronic. These lesions can also be caused by a wide variety of organisms.

Bacterial infection

Epididymal infection can be caused by a wide variety of organisms and these can include *Escherichia coli, Pseudomonas*, streptococci and even bacteria such as *Salmonella*. Predisposing factors in the generation of epididymitis include transurethral surgery, transurethral catheterization and recurrent urinary tract infection (Berger 1994).

Among men with obstructive lesions, there is frequently, but not invariably, a history of acute epididymitis, whose symptomatology includes pain, dysuria, scrotal swelling and fever. A severe episode of epididymitis may even give rise to an epididymal abscess. It must also be remembered that severe orchitis can be associated with an infective orchitis to produce an epididymo-orchitis. Such an infective process may severely impair spermatogenesis, and thus, in some men, epididymitis may induce a double pathology, where not only is the epididymal duct blocked but sperm production is also severely impaired. Recently, there has been a great increase in the incidence of *Chlamydia trachomatis* as a cause of epididymitis and this is especially frequent among men of less than 25 years of age (Grant *et al.* 1987). It must also be remembered that a suppurative epididymitis may, on rare occasions, even occur in a cryptorchid testis (Hassan & Chui 1985).

Tuberculous epididymitis is much less frequently seen today in the developed world than in the past, although such a pathology may still be seen in the developing countries. Tuberculous infection of the male genital tract causes major damage to the epididymal duct that is never amenable to surgery. On palpation, the epididymis is very thickened and calcification is often present and can be demonstrated radiologically. Tuberculous infection may also involve the seminal vesicles and the distal ends of the vasa deferentia producing multiple sites of obstruction. It must also be remembered that there is a very high incidence of tuberculous infection of the urinary tract in men with genital tuberculosis (Ferrie & Rundle 1983).

The sites of these obstructive lesions that are produced by epididymitis may either be single or multiple and most frequently involve the lower part of the epididymis. However, in some patients, the patency of the entire length of the epididymal duct can be obliterated and this may also include the efferent ductules and the rete testis. Certain infective lesions, particularly those that are the result of gonococcal infection, can also cause stricture of each vas deferens as well as the epididymal duct and so, in these patients, multiple sites of obstruction must be identified if any form of surgical remedy is to be successful.

Leprosy can induce lesions in the epididymis as well as in the testis (El-Shiemy *et al.* 1976; Pareek & Tandon 1985), but these are uncommon, even in areas of the world where leprosy is relatively common.

Very rarely, syphilitic infection can result in a gumma that is usually found in the testis but occasionally can occur in the epididymis and result in obstruction.

Viral infections

Epididymal obstruction can also be caused by viral infections. Smallpox is known to be associated with obstructive azoospermia and epididymal lesions (Phadke *et al.* 1973). Although smallpox has now been eradicated worldwide, there may still be adults, now of increasing age, who may present in certain parts of the world with this type of infertility (Hendry *et al.* 1983). Another virus that can occasionally cause epididymitis is the cytomegalovirus. However, how frequently this viral infection results in epididymal obstruction is unknown.

Unicellular organisms

In tropical countries, infection with either Bancroftian or Brugian filariasis can result in an acute epididymo-orchitis. This type of infection produces a severe disruption of the epididymis and results in obstructive azoospermia. Patients with this problem have inguinal lymphadenopathy, a thickened spermatic cord and epididymitis. The diagnosis is best confirmed by identifying microfilaria in a nocturnal blood film. Diethyl carbamazine is used in the treatment of this conditions but this drug will not reverse the epididymal damage and cure the patient's sterility. The epididymal obstruction caused by filariasis is not amenable to surgery. The other long-term effects of genital filarial infection are chronic hydrocele and scrotal elephantiasis.

Trauma

Trauma can occasionally be a cause of epididymal obstruction. It may occur as the result of injuries sustained in sport and is not infrequently seen in contact sports such as rugby football, but any injury to the scrotal area can cause this injury. The damage that occurs seems to be the result of a peri-epididymal or epididymal haematoma. In some patients, a stricture may result, producing a permanent epididymal obstructive lesion that may be unilateral or bilateral, but in other men the haematoma may resolve resulting in the return of spermatozoa to the ejaculate.

These types of injuries, however, can be associated with a concomitant testicular damage that may result in loss of sperm production. Thus, injury to the scrotal region may produce two types of injury, both of which can result in infertility.

Another type of injury that can result in epididymal obstruction is surgery. Operations for the removal of any of the epididymal appendages, especially if they have undergone torsion, may result in the inadvertent removal of a portion of the epididymal duct itself. Similar damage may also be caused during operations for the excision of a hydrocele and during the removal of a large spermatocele. Lack of understanding of the anatomy of the epididymis have even led surgeons to carry out epididymal biopsies; in infertile patients, it must always be remembered that removal of any portion of the epididymal duct will be as effective as a vasectomy in causing sterility. Thus, a history of scrotal surgery is important in the assessment of a man with obstructive azoospermia.

Infiltrations of the epididymis

The are some infiltrative diseases that can cause epididymal obstruction, although it must be remembered that they will only be seen very rarely in an infertility clinic.

Sarcoidosis

On rare occasions, the condition of sarcoidosis can be associated with obstruction of the epididymal duct (Winnaker *et al.* 1967). Sarcoid granulomata may be found in the epididymis and may produce a palpable mass within the scrotum. Corticosteroid therapy may resolve these epididymal granulomata and also resolve the epididymal obstruction. Sarcoid deposits can also occur within the testis itself and interfere with sperm production. Sarcoid infiltration of the hypothalamic area is well described and such lesions can result in a reduction of gonadotrophin-releasing hormone and hypogonadotrophic hypogonadism.

Fabry's disease

This rare X-linked metabolic disorder results in the defective activity of the enzyme galactosidase. As a consequence there is an accumulation of triglycosylceramide and diglycosylceramide in the tissues. Deposition of these substances may be seen within the Sertoli cells of the testis, within the rete testis and also in the walls of the epididymal duct (Nistal *et al.* 1983). Thus, Fabry's disease may cause infertility in several different ways, but it can also be a cause of epididymal obstruction.

Polyarteritis nodosa

Polyarteritic lesions of the epididymis were first described in a patient with Whipple's disease, which resulted in severe damage to the epididymal duct system in a previously fertile man (Middlekauf *et al.* 1987). The lesion was proved when the man underwent an orchidectomy for a suspected tumour. However, at a later date a swelling developed on the opposite side and resolved quickly after treatment with corticosteroids.

Polyarteritis nodosa must now be listed as a possible, although probably very rare, cause of epididymal obstruction. With careful evaluation, it is possible that many other disorders may also become recognized as a cause of infertility in the male.

Young's syndrome

This condition was first described more than 25 years ago (Young 1970) and was at one time a fairly common problem, but today this problem is much less frequently seen. The clinical syndrome consists of bronchiectasis, sinusitis and obstructive azoospermia. The site of the obstruction involves the epididymal duct and is found at the junction between the upper and middle thirds of the epididymis (Fig. 6.2). Young's syndrome must not be confused with Kartagener's syndrome (often also known as the immotile cilia syndrome), in which chest disease and heart disease are associated with large numbers of sperm in the ejaculate, all of which are immotile because of an anomaly of the sperm axoneme.

The cause of Young's syndrome is unknown, but it has been suggested that it may be the result of chronic mercury poisoning, although there is little positive evidence to support this possibility. The presence of a single gene for cystic fibrosis in men with this condition has also been described, but this relationship has not been confirmed and is probably coincidental. Electron microscopy of the microvilli of the bronchial mucosa in men with this condition shows the normal axonemal pattern (Hendry *et al.* 1978) as the tails of the sperm are removed from the epididymis in men with this

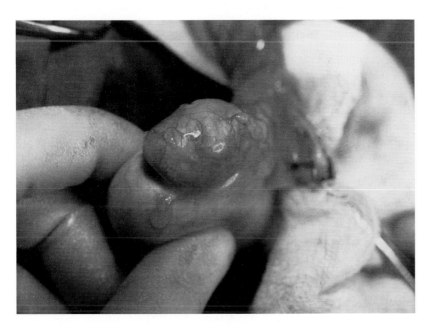

Fig. 6.2 An example of obstruction in the upper epididymis in a patients with obstructive azoospermia in Young's syndrome. The distension of the proximal portion of the epididymis is clearly seen. This distended upper epididymis can be detected clinically on palpation and is known as Bayle's sign after the well known French andrologist, Henri Bayle.

condition. The other major cause of chest disease in men is α_1-antitrypsin deficiency, but this disorder is not associated with infertility (Handelsman *et al.* 1984). Young's syndrome is, however, likely to be genetically determined as it has been described in identical twins (Teichtahl *et al.* 1987).

On examination of a patient with this condition, the chest disease is usually obvious and may even be incapacitating. Some of these patients have undergone lobectomy in the past and are often on long-term antibiotic therapy. As there is no associated testicular disease in these patients, testicular size is normal. However, on careful palpation, a distended caput epididymis may be felt alongside the testes, confirming the presence of obstruction in each epididymis. The presence of this distended epididymal caput is known as Bayle's sign after the andrologist who described it (Bayle 1952).

There are two ways in which this condition can be treated. The performance of a microsurgical epididymovasostomy can sometimes result in success, but this procedure seems to be less successful in Young's syndrome than in other causes of epididymal duct obstruction. The other way in which this infertility can be managed is by epididymal aspiration of sperm, IVF and ICSI. It must be remembered, however, that this disorder may be genetically predetermined and is associated with quite severe chest disease. Thus, the infertile couple must receive appropriate counselling about this problem before treatment.

Epididymal microcysts

These small cysts are probably an uncommon cause of epididymal obstruction and frequently represent small spermatoceles. They appear to be small diverticula that bud off the epididymal duct and obstruct the duct itself simply by pressure (Schoysman 1981). They may also cause incomplete obstruction that will present with oligozoospermia, but occasionally these cysts can be quite large.

The obstruction that these cysts cause can only reliably be diagnosed at scrotal exploration. Using magnification, their careful removal from the convolutions of the epididymal duct will often relieve the obstruction.

Dystrophic change

In some men with obstructive azoospermia, surgical exploration reveals that the epididymis has been replaced by fibrous tissue. The aetiology of this pathological change is unknown but this type of epididymal pathology seems to be more common in the older patient. Whether this is the result of ischaemic change is impossible to say.

The treatment of epididymal obstruction

The alleviation of obstruction of the epididymal duct can be carried out in two main ways. The obstruction can be relieved surgically by means of an epididymovasostomy, or the patient can have recourse to advanced reproductive technology.

It is the belief of the author that all such exploratory procedures performed on the infertile male should now be carried out close to an IVF laboratory so that all sperm and testicular tissue that is collected at the operation can be assessed and where indicated may be cryopreserved.

The operation of epididymovasostomy

This procedure consists of joining the epididymal duct proximal to the obstruction to the vas deferens. There are several ways in which this procedure can be carried out.

The fistula method

The first person to perform this procedure was Edward Martin from Philadelphia in 1902 (Martin *et al.* 1902), who was, of course, the first person to carry out any remedial surgery in the infertile male. He sutured the vas to the epididymis using silver wire and achieved very good results (Fig. 6.3). The life of Edward Martin has been reviewed in the past (Jequier 1991).

This method of performing such a by-pass procedure has been used

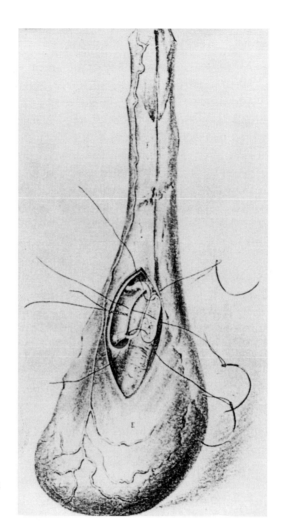

Fig. 6.3 The original drawing published by Edward Martin in 1902 of his operation of vaso-epididymostomy (Published by kind permission of the *International Journal of Andrology*).

Fig. 6.4 A schematic drawing of a vaso-epididymostomy performed by the fistula method. This technique is now seldom used in the management of epididymal obstruction.

almost up to the present day and modifications of this technique are still in use in some centres today. However, since the advent of microsurgery, better results are obtained using a tubule-to-tubule anastomosis and this is now a more commonly used procedure.

Fundamentally, the object of this operation is to create a fistula between the cut end of the vas deferens and either a loop or a series of loops of the epididymal duct (Fig. 6.4).

The first step in the performance of this procedure is to open the scrotum in the midline after infiltrating the area with local anaesthetic [usually 0.5% bupivacaine with 1:200 000 adrenaline (epinephrine)]. An alternative approach is to use the subpubic incision described by Kelami, in which the testis are each pulled up out of the scrotum, giving excellent access to both the epididymis and the vas deferens (Kelami 1978).

Holding each testis between finger and thumb, the parietal layer of the tunica vaginalis is now incised using a sharp scalpel blade. As the tunica is breached, a small amount of fluid that normally surrounds the testis escapes through the incision and indicates entrance to the cavity of the scrotum. During the opening of the tunica vaginalis, care must be taken not to incise the tunica albuginea of the testis itself. However, in many patients, especially those who have had several episodes of epididymitis in the past or any other procedure such as a testicular biopsy, quite dense adhesions may be present between the testes and the tunica vaginalis making access to the epididymis difficult. The testes are now delivered through the wound on each side and can be examined. The site of the obstruction can now be confirmed.

In a patient with intratesticular obstruction, the epididymis will not be distended and will appear normal at inspection. In this circumstance, a testicular biopsy may be taken to confirm the normality of sperm production histologically. Such a biopsy should also be cryopreserved as it may prove useful as a source of sperm that can be used later in an IVF programme. It may also be possible to collect sperm from the rete testis for storage.

If the obstruction involves the efferent ductules, it may be possible to perform a tubule-to-tubule anastomosis (see below), although most surgeons would find such a procedure a difficult operation to carry out. It may also be possible to collect sperm from this area for cryopreservation and use in a future IVF programme. In an epididymal obstruction, the epididymis is clearly distended above the point of the obstruction. In some men there may be some blue or brown discoloration in the distended segment and this is caused by the deposition of lipofuscin. The epididymal tubules proximal to the obstruction are dilated and contain a thick, yellow fluid that consists of inspissated testicular fluid, dead sperm and macrophages (Fig. 6.5). If, however, the obstruction is in fact in the vas deferens or even in the ejaculatory ducts, then the whole of the epididymis will be distended.

The first step in this procedure is to isolate the vas at the level of the of the epididymal caput. The vas is found in the posterior part of the cord and on palpation feels like a rather tough piece of partially cooked spaghetti. Using blunt dissection while holding the testis laterally and taking care not to disrupt the blood vessels in the cord, a loop of vas deferens about 2 cm in length is isolated from the spermatic cord. The lumen of the vas is now opened longitudinally. At this point in the operation, it is of value to carry out vasography to exclude a second stricture in the distal vas (Fig. 6.6). If such radiology cannot be arranged then a simple injection of saline into the vas and its free passage down the vas will also exclude a distal obstruction

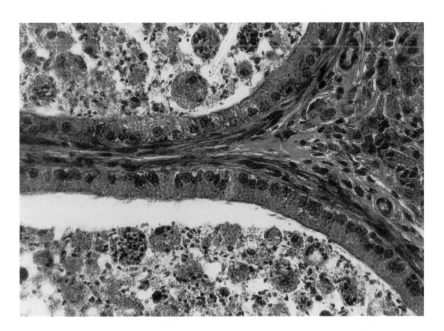

Fig. 6.5 A histological section of the epididymis proximal to an obstructive lesion. Note the large amount of debris in the lumen of the epididymal duct as well as the flattened epithelium and relative absence of the microcilia. The function of this epithelium is likely to have been severely compromised.

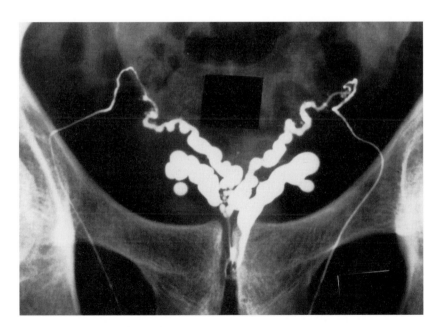

Fig. 6.6 A normal vasogram. This was carried out using an oily contrast medium that is now obsolete. This particular X-ray is included as this contrast provides very good anatomical detail.

but will not exclude the rare event of any other nonobstructive anomaly of the distal genital tract.

An ellipse of the epididymis above the level of the obstruction is now excised and the distended tubules under the tunica vaginalis are opened. The yellow, thick fluid will now ooze out of the cut surface of these distended tubules. The presence of spermatozoa is now confirmed by the application of a sterile microscope slide to these cut tubules and its examination by microscopy. The edges of the cut surfaces of the epididymal tubule are now apposed to the opened lumen of the vas deferens and, using a 6/0 nonabsorbable suture, the vas is now secured into position on the opened epididymal tubule. The testes are then returned to the scrotum and the incision is closed taking great care to ensure very adequate haemostasis. The scrotal skin is best closed using a subcuticular absorbable suture such as polyglycolic acid.

The results of the fistula method of epididymovasostomy have in recent years become poor and have now largely been replaced by the microsurgical tubule-to-tubule anastomosis.

Single tubule anastomosis

There are two main ways in which this procedure can be carried out, one involving an end-to-end anastomosis and the other in which an end-to-side anastomosis is performed.

End-to-end anastomosis

Some 20 years ago, Silber (1984) reported the use of a microsurgical end-to-end anastomosis between the cut end of the vas deferens and the epididymal duct (Fig. 6.7). The cut end of the vas is joined to the cut end of the epididymal duct where sperm had been shown to be present. However, in order to produce a good and accurate anastomosis, magnification is needed in the form of an operating microscope as well as some skill in its use.

Firstly, the scrotum is opened in the manner described for the fistula operation and both testes are delivered out through the wound. Vasogra-

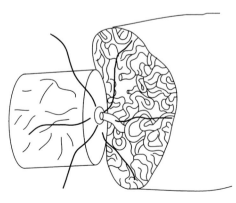

Fig. 6.7 A schematic representation of the end-to-end microsurgical method of vaso-epididymostomy.

phy is now carried out after identification and isolation of the vas deferens at a level compatible with the site of the obstruction in the epididymis. A demonstration of the patency of the distal vas prior to undertaking this procedure is important. If normality of the distal vas is demonstrated, the operation of epididymovasostomy can now begin. The first step is to incise the tunica vaginalis to expose the epididymis. The epididymis is then transected at a level just above that of the obstruction within the epididymis. This transection is often associated with quite a lot of bleeding, which must now be controlled using both bipolar diathermy and pressure. The proximal cut end of the transected epididymis is now touched with a sterile glass slide and the fluid that exudes from the tubules is now examined microscopically for the presence of spermatozoa. If spermatozoa are not identified, then the epididymis is again transected at a more proximal point until spermatozoa can be identified.

The proximal vas is now also transected at a point that will allow an easy anastomosis without tension. Using 9/0 nylon, the operating microscope and interrupted sutures, an end-to-end anastomosis is now performed between the vas and the patent epididymal duct that has been shown to contain spermatozoa. The muscle and the adventitial layers of the vas are then sutured in two layers to the surrounding epididymal tissue, again using interrupted sutures to ensure a stable and secure anastomosis.

Each testis is then returned to the scrotum, haemostasis is ensured and the wound closed in the same way as that for the fistula method.

This technique has produced excellent results in some hands, but this technique is difficult and has not been universally taken up by other reproductive surgeons.

End-to-side anastomosis

This operation described by Wagenknecht in 1982 (Wagenknecht 1982) is much simpler to perform but must also be completed using some form of magnification (Fig. 6.8).

The scrotum is first opened in the same manner as described for the fistula procedure. A small longitudinal incision is made in the tunica vaginalis, which covers the epididymis, to expose a small segment of the distended epididymal duct. This distended segment of the duct is now gently freed from its surrounding connective tissue so that it now bulges out through the small window that has been made in the tunica vaginalis. Using

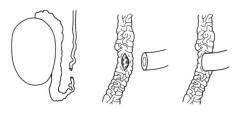

Fig. 6.8 A drawing of the end-to-side method of vaso-epididymostomy.

very fine scissors, a very small incision is made in the tubule at its most prominent point, which corresponds approximately to the diameter of the lumen of the vas deferens. The thick fluid that exudes from the duct is now examined for the presence of spermatozoa. If no sperm can be found, then the procedure is repeated in a more proximal part of the epididymis until sperm can be identified. A loop of vas is now isolated and transected at the level of the epididymal obstruction. In order to achieve stability during the anastomosis, the vas is first fixed to the tunica vaginalis covering the epididymis using 9/0 nylon interrupted sutures. A microsurgical anastomosis is now made between the cut end of the vas and the incision made in the epididymal ducts, again using 9/0 or 10/0 nylon interrupted sutures. Further stitches are now placed between the muscle of the vas and the tunica vaginalis, and a further layer between the adventitia of the vas and the tunica gives a good stability to the anastomosis. The wound is now closed in the manner described previously. In the author's hands, this is a much simpler procedure to carry out than the end-to-end technique.

Epididymo-epididymostomy

Good microsurgeons can also carry out the operation of epididymo-epididmostomy, in which the epididymal duct above the site of an obstruction is anastomosed to the epididymal tubule below the site of the obstruction (Fig. 6.9). This is naturally a difficult operation to carry out successfully and is performed by few surgeons today.

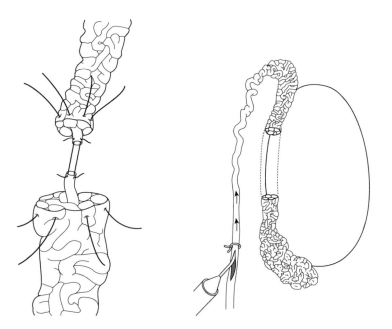

Fig. 6.9 A drawing depicting the operation of epididymo-epididymostomy. This is a technically difficult operation to carry out and is performed by a very small number of surgeons.

Crossed epididymovasostomy

Occasionally, obstructive lesions can occur at different sites on the two sides. For example, on one side there may be an epididymal obstruction and on the other a vasal obstruction may be present. In such a situation, a crossed epididymovasostomy may be performed, in which the lumen of the vas from one side can be joined by a single tubule anastomosis to the epididymis duct of the opposite side. Although in this situation only a single anastomosis can be performed, it is possible to achieve patency and even pregnancy in this situation (Silber 1984).

In any form of epididymal obstruction, the epididymal lumen, proximal to the obstruction, will become distended by dead sperm and debris and this area will show a considerable influx of white blood cells and macrophages. The damage that is done to the epididymal epithelium by the obstructive lesion is not infrequently irreversible.

Alloplastic spermatoceles in epididymal obstruction

The development of a reservoir to collect sperm from a fistulous opening in the epididymal duct was at one time an attractive option for patients with epididymal obstruction (Hamm & Kelami 1982). Indeed, prior to the advent of IVF, this was the only known treatment of infertility resulting from congenital absence of the vas deferens.

Many substances have been used in the past for this purpose, including saphenous vein grafts and even fetal amnion.

Artificial substances such as silicone were used at first, but later substances such as polypropylene and polytetrafluoroethylene were also employed. However, the pregnancy rates achieved after aspirating sperm from these spermatoceles were very poor and never exceeded 5%. Thus, for this reason, therapy of this type has now been completely abandoned in favour of epididymal aspiration of sperm and IVF.

Epididymal aspiration of sperm and IVF/ICSI in the management of infertility caused by epididymal obstruction

This is now the most commonly used treatment of the infertility caused by epididymal obstruction as it provides in most hands the best pregnancy rates of all. This will be described in detail in a subsequent chapter of this book.

Obstruction of the vasa deferentia

If the operation of vasectomy is excluded (vasectomy and its reversal are discussed in detail in Chapter 13), obstruction of the scrotal and inguinal portions of the vas deferens is far less common than obstruction of the epididymis. However, there are some well-known causes of noniatrogenic obstruction that do result in infertility.

Congenital absence of the vas deferens

Congenital absence of the vasa deferentia is a well-recognized cause of obstructive azoospermia and accounts for around 10% of all men with ductal obstruction (Jequier 1986). This lesion may also be seen in the domestic animal and is not that infrequently seen among bulls. In this species, unilateral absence of the vas deferens can also occur

It is genetically determined and is associated with the heterozygous presence of one of the gene anomalies (*CFTR* gene) causing cystic fibrosis (Dumur *et al.* 1990) that is carried on chromosome 7. Numerous studies have shown that populations of patients with congenital absence of the vasa deferentia carry mutations that have also been found in patients with cystic fibrosis. A small number of men with this problem also have lung disease and sinusitis, as do individuals with the homozygous condition of cystic fibrosis. There are, however, a large number of different mutations of this gene, all of which can be associated with congenital absence of the vasa deferentia. There is thus good reason to believe that men with congenital absence of the vasa deferentia and lung disease may carry an as yet unidentified mutation, perhaps on another chromosome. The most common mutation by far that is seen in this condition is Delta F508, which can be found in around 50% of all men with this condition. Other common mutations are G542X, R553X and W1282X (Patrizio & Zielenski 1996).

Congenital absence of the vas may involve the whole inguinal and scrotal vas, but in some men only sections of the duct may be missing. Absence of at least a portion of the epididymis is also very common (Fig. 6.10). As congenital absence of the vasa deferentia is due to a developmental abnormality of the wolffian duct, this lesion is also commonly associated with a concomitant absence or a hypoplasia of the seminal vesicles. However, this condition can also be associated with normal seminal vesicular morphology and function and in such patients the seminal fructose and ejaculatory volume will be normal.

Patients with this condition will therefore present with primary infertility. On examination, testicular size will be normal. As the outflow from the epididymis is obstructed and as the lower part of the epididymis is often absent, Bayle's sign will be positive, the distended caput epididymis being easily palpable. On examination of the spermatic cord, no vas is palpable. However, the vessels of the cord can be very easily be mistaken for the vas, and it is thus important to palpate this area very carefully to make sure that each vas deferens is truly absent.

On examination of the semen, azoospermia will be present as the seminal vesicles are frequently either absent or hypoplastic. As the seminal vesicles contribute to more than 40% of the total ejaculate, the seminal volume is frequently reduced; indeed, the seminal volume often totals less

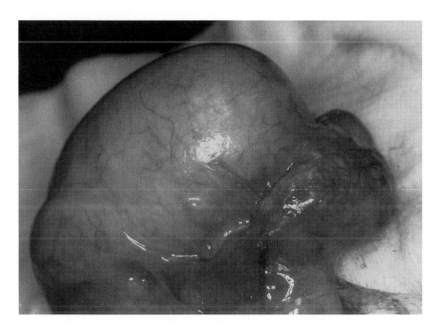

Fig. 6.10 A surgical photograph of the epididymis in a man with bilateral congenital absence of the vas deferentia. Note that the lower two-thirds of the epididymis is absent. This epididymal anomaly is a common finding among men with this condition.

than 1 mL. However, in the normal male, the prostatic contribution may occasionally exceed 1 or even 2 mL, and thus in a few of the men with this condition, and even when the seminal vesicles are totally absent, the seminal volume may be within the normal range. Because the seminal vesicles are often either hypoplastic or absent, the seminal fructose is usually markedly reduced or even absent (Amelar & Dubin 1974).

Infection as a cause of vasal obstruction

With the exception of vasectomy and of congenital absence of the vasa deferentia, vasal causes of obstructive azoospermia are relatively uncommon and make up less than 5% of the obstructive lesions in men with obstructive azoospermia.

All the infective agents that can cause obstruction of the epididymal duct are also capable of producing either strictures within the vas or of inducing a total occlusion of the lumen down its entire length. Occasionally the whole vas, including the muscle wall, may be obliterated, giving the initial impression that the vas is congenitally absent. However, at operation, a thin fibrous band of tissue at the site of the vas deferens may frequently be found. As the seminal vesicles are present in such patients, unlike those with congenital absence of the vas deferens, the ejaculatory volume is normal. Some infections, notably gonorrhoea, may also cause multiple stricture formation within the vasa, thus making the lesion impossible to treat surgically.

Surgical damage to the vas deferens

Surgical damage is not an infrequent cause of vasal obstruction. The most common site of such a lesion is in the groin and is the result of accidental damage to the vas during the operation of herniotomy in small children. During the dissection of the hernial sac in such patients, it is very easy either to cut, tie or surgically damage the vas, which in a very young child is very fine and rather fragile. A history of a herniotomy in childhood is thus relevant in a man presenting with signs of obstruction in an infertility clinic. Inadvertent ligation of the vas during a hernia repair in an adult does indeed occasionally occur, but it is much less common than that occurring in children. It must also be remembered that many of these vasal lesions may only occur unilaterally and such patients may therefore present in an infertility clinic not with azoospermia but with oligozoospermia and a high titre of antisperm antibodies (see below).

Cystic fibrosis

Cystic fibrosis is a genetically determined disease caused by the homozygous presence of two abnormal genes. In the male it is almost always associated with total obliteration of the vas deferentia and obstructive azoospermia. In this disorder the exocrine secretions are excessively viscid and thus the ducts of exocrine glands such as the pancreas, the biliary system, the bronchioles become damaged. The secretions that emanate from the testes and the epididymal ducts also appear to be very thick, and for this reason they occlude and then obliterate the vasa deferentia (Holsclaw 1969). These patients also demonstrate, at least in early childhood, an abnormally high salt content in the sweat. Patients with cystic fibrosis suffer from severe bronchiectasis and from pancreatic enzyme deficiency. Many individuals with cystic fibrosis die early in life, but with the advent of good antibiotic therapy many men with this disease are now surviving well into adult life. The great majority of the adult males with this disease are sterile because of the vasal obstruction and the obstructive azoospermia that such a lesion will produce. As almost all of the vas in these patients is occluded down its entire length, surgical treatment will be of no avail.

Clinical findings and investigation of vasal obstruction

On clinical examination of men with vasal obstruction, testis size will be normal as, in the absence of a second pathology, spermatogenesis will be unimpaired. In congenital absence of the vas deferens or among patients in whom the vas has been obliterated, it will not be possible to palpate the vas in the posterior part of the spermatic cord. The epididymis, however, will be distended. In men with congenital absence of the vas, the distal portions of the epididymis are often absent and so only a distended caput may be present, resulting in Bayle's sign being positive. In other types of vasal obstruction, the whole of the epididymis may be distended. In a patient with a stricture in the scrotal or inguinal portion of the vas, it may be possible to discern an increase in size of the vas itself proximal to the site of the suspected obstruction.

Vasography is of value in siting the point of obstruction. However, it must be remembered that the injection of contrast medium may itself cause vasal damage, especially if the obstruction remains unrelieved. It is thus important to perform vasography only during the course of a remedial operation where the intention is to resolve the obstruction.

The treatment of vasal obstruction

The first line of treatment of vasal obstruction is usually surgical and involves, where possible, the excision of the obstruction and a re-anastomosis of the vas. Such a procedure will only apply to a vasal stricture proximal to the deep ring of the inguinal canal and of no more than 3 cm in length. Usually if the stricture is longer than 5 cm, its excision and the subsequent anastomosis of the vas becomes technically very difficult. Strictures of 8 cm or more are probably best considered to be surgically irremediable.

The vasovasostomy operation

The position of the incision will depend on the suspected site of the obstruction. Where this is uncertain, a vasogram is first carried out. If the obstruction is in the scrotal vas, a midline incision is usually performed. If the obstruction is in the inguinal portion of the vas, then the inguinal canal is opened and this part of the cord may be examined. It is best to use some form of magnification for these procedures such as a loupe with at least ×4 magnification, or, if it is available, an operating microscope.

The vas is first isolated by blunt dissection and the site of the obstruction identified. The vas is then grasped some 2 cm on either side of the obstruction with Babcock forceps. It is important not to strip the vas of its coverings as this may induce vasal ischaemia and interfere with the healing of the vasovasal anastomosis.

Using a sharp knife, the obstructive lesion in the vas is now excised. At this point, it is important to ensure that (a) sperm are present in the fluid that exudes from the proximal cut end of the vas and (b) the vas, distal to the obstruction, is patent. Thus, a sterile microscope slide is now placed on the proximal cut end of the vas and the fluid examined microscopically for the presence of spermatozoa. Saline can now also be injected down the distal cut end of the vas to ensure distal patency. Should there be any doubt as to the presence of a normal vas deferens distal to the obstruction, then an intraoperative vasogram should be carried out.

The anastomosis of the vas is simple and can be performed using one layer of sutures (Fig. 6.11). Some surgeons advocate the use of three layers

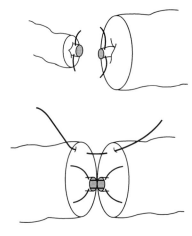

Fig. 6.11 A schematic representation of a vasovasostomy carried out for a stricture in the vas deferens. This is the same procedure that is used in vasectomy reversal. It is best carried out using some form of magnification.

but there is little evidence that this improves results. The sutures used can be absorbable or nonabsorbable. Suitable sutures include 6/0 polyglycolic acid or nylon. A second layer of sutures to the serosa of the vas can ensure a stable anastomosis without too much leakage of sperm around the anastomosis. The wound is then closed in the usual way with, as usual, very great care to ensure haemostasis.

Postoperatively these patients may have to remain in hospital for at least 24 h until the risk of haemorrhage is over and the postoperative discomfort is reduced. It is important that ejaculation is banned for a minimum of 10 days, as at ejaculation the vas contracts very strongly and there is thus a risk that ejaculation will cause a disruption of the vasovasal suture line.

A semen sample is taken some 4–6 weeks later to determine the presence of sperm in the ejaculate. If, however, azoospermia persists, it is worth waiting another 2–3 months as sometimes sperm will reappear in the ejaculate.

Ejaculatory duct obstruction

Ejaculatory duct obstruction is an uncommon cause of obstructive azoospermia and makes up only some 2% of all cases of ductal obstruction that present in an infertility clinic (Jequier 1986).

This type of obstruction may involve only the distal ends of the ejaculatory ducts or it may include the whole duct system, extending up to and including the terminal portions of the vasa deferentia. As with other types of obstruction, ejaculatory duct obstruction may be partial or complete and thus may give rise to semen that is either oligozoospermic or azoospermic (Carson 1984).

Causes of ejaculatory duct obstruction

Obstruction of the ejaculatory ducts may be congenital or acquired and there are several known causes of this problem.

Congenital atresia of the ejaculatory ducts

In this type of obstruction, the obstruction frequently involves the whole length of the ducts making it a difficult lesion to treat. This malformation is frequently associated with malformed distal vasa deferentia, which can produce a long stricture extending from the ejaculatory ducts up the vasa deferentia, often to the point where they arch over the ureters. Such a long stricture is thus not amenable to surgery.

Acquired ejaculatory duct obstruction

This may be found in patients who have undergone a variety of different forms of urethral surgery, in particular the excision of posterior urethral valves, transurethral resection of the prostate, and it may also be seen in men who have undergone prolonged urethral catheterization. The ejaculatory ducts may also be blocked in older men by both chronic prostatitis and benign prostatic hyperplasia. Occasionally the ejaculatory ducts can become blocked following a gonococcal infection.

It must also be remembered that, in the past, ejaculatory duct obstruction may also have been complicated by a concomitant epididymitis or epididymo-orchitis. Thus, these patients may have more than one site of ductal obstruction and, if sperm production has been compromised by such an infection, there may also be a second reason for their infertility.

Müllerian duct cysts

These are probably one of the most common causes of ejaculatory duct obstruction and are now one of the more common causes of haematospermia. These cysts form in the site of the prostatic utricle, which is one of two vestiges of the müllerian duct in the male, the other being the appendix testis within the tunica vaginalis. For reasons that are unknown, this small pit, which lies medial to and somewhat below the ejaculatory ducts on the verumontanum, deepens and begins to enlarge posteriorly and laterally (Fig. 6.12). The ejaculatory ducts then become compressed and their orifices turn inwards towards the cavity of the utricle causing the initially open pit on the verumontanum to form a cavity into which the ejaculatory ducts now open (Fig. 6.13). Thus, at ejaculation the secretions of the seminal vesicles and the testes are discharged not into the posterior urethra but into the newly formed cyst formed by the enlargement of the

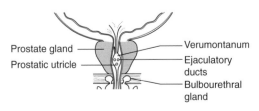

Fig. 6.12 The site of the prostatic utricle. This remnant of müllerian tissue may expand to form a müllerian duct cyst that can be a cause of ejaculatory duct obstruction.

Prostate gland —
Prostatic utricle —
— Verumontanum
— Ejaculatory ducts
— Bulbourethral gland

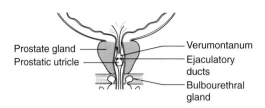

Prostate gland
Prostatic utricle

Verumontanum
Ejaculatory ducts
Bulbourethral gland

Fig. 6.13 A schematic representation of a müllerian duct cyst within the prostatic urethra.

prostatic utricle. This cystic prostatic utricle is now known as a müllerian duct cyst.

The cavity of a normal prostatic utricle is lined for the most part by transitional epithelium, but at the back of this small area can frequently be found a small area of endometrium-like epithelium which enlarges as the prostatic utricle grows to form a müllerian duct cyst. As the müllerian duct cyst is formed and ejaculation increases the pressure in this cyst, this endometrial tissue may bleed. Thus, on opening the cyst, it is almost the rule to find that it contains considerable amounts of altered blood.

Müllerian duct cysts as they form may obstruct only one ejaculatory duct and thus the patient may present in an infertility clinic with oligozoospermia and/or haematospermia.

The clinical presentation of ejaculatory duct obstruction

The main clinical feature of ejaculatory duct obstruction is a reduction in semen volume. Patients may indeed notice this and the low semen volume may be their major symptom on presentation at the clinic, and this symptomatology may precede an awareness of their infertility. However, patients who present with congenital ejaculatory duct obstruction may not realize that their semen volume is in fact abnormally low. Men with müllerian duct obstruction may, at least in the initial stages of the cyst formation when the obstruction is not complete, present with intermittent haematospermia.

On clinical examination and in the absence of a second pathology, the testes will be of normal size. However, in long-standing ejaculatory duct obstruction, it may be possible to detect distension of both epididymides. On rectal examination, it may or may not be possible to detect distension of the seminal vesicles but these, even when distended, are very soft and such abnormalities can easily be missed. In the presence of a large müllerian duct cyst (a cyst measuring more than 2 cm is considered to be large), it may be possible to detect such a swelling on digital rectal examination lying at the apex of the median lobe between the two lateral lobes of the prostate. If the cyst is small, it frequently remains undetectable even to a practised examiner of the prostate.

In ejaculatory duct obstruction the secretions of the seminal vesicles and the testes may be excluded from the ejaculate, thus reducing its volume to less than half. If the obstruction is complete and bilateral, this reduction in ejaculatory volume will be associated with azoospermia and an absence of fructose in the semen. The pH of the semen may also be con-

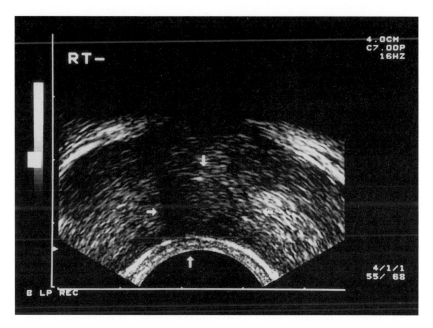

Fig. 6.14 A transrectal ultrasound showing the presence of a müllerian duct cyst within the prostate. This man presented with azoospermia and a low volume ejaculate. The cyst was around 2.5 cm in diameter. The somewhat hyperechoic appearance of this cyst is caused by the presence of blood contained within it.

siderably reduced. As a result of the exclusion of the seminal vesicular secretion by an obstruction of the ejaculatory ducts, the semen may also show a reduced ability to clot.

The most important investigation of ejaculatory duct obstruction involves the use of transrectal ultrasonography (Fig. 6.14). Transrectal ultrasound examination will outline the seminal vesicles, which will be distended in ejaculatory duct obstruction (Fig. 6.15). The ultrasound examination will also detect abnormalities of the prostate and will define the ampullae of the vasa deferentia. It will also demonstrate the patency or otherwise of the ejaculatory ducts themselves.

Antegrade vasography is also very useful to confirm such an obstructive lesion (Fig. 6.16) but, because of the small risk of ductal damage by the contrast media, it is best used during remedial surgery.

The treatment of ejaculatory duct obstruction

All surgery used in the alleviation of obstruction involving the ejaculatory ducts and the distal ends of the vas must be carried out by the transurethral route; surgery that is carried out behind the bladder runs a serious risk of causing impotence. Thus, transabdominal surgery in this area must be limited to the treatment of cancer and other life-threatening problems.

In men with congenital strictures of the ejaculatory duct, which are often associated with a concomitant atresia of the distal end of the vasa

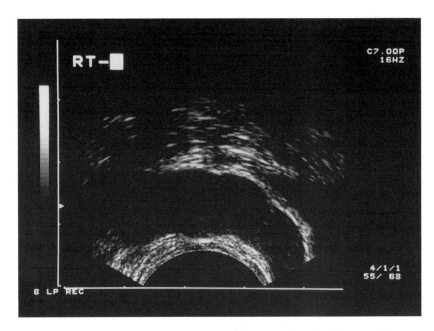

Fig. 6.15 A transrectal ultrasound at the level of the seminal vesicles showing their massive distension in a man with ejaculatory duct obstruction caused by the presence of a müllerian duct cyst.

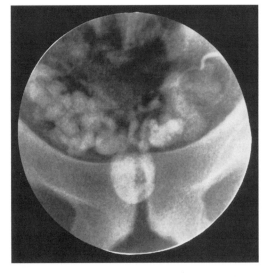

Fig. 6.16 A vasogram performed in a man undergoing surgery for a müllerian duct cyst. Note that the contrast injected into one vas enters the cyst and then passes up into the vas and the seminal vesicle of the opposite side.

deferentia, the length of the stricture is often too long to be amenable to surgery. Men with infertility due to this lesion are best treated by vasal flushing and IVF.

The acquired strictures, however, are much more amenable to surgery. Simple transurethral resection of the ducts is often sufficient to open a short stricture, but care must be taken not to resect too deeply in this area as this can damage the bladder neck mechanism. Transurethral resection can, however, be a very successful treatment of this problem and the subsequent pregnancy rates are high (Carson 1984). Patency of the ducts can be demonstrated by means of vasography or more simply by the injection of methylene blue down the vasa deferentia. This manoeuvre will also provide evidence of patency to the transurethral resectionist.

Very small lengths of obstruction in the ejaculatory ducts can be relieved by simple cannulation using the transurethral route. For this purpose, a no. 4 ureteric catheter is inserted into the orifices of the duct and contrast is then injected to demonstrate patency. Using a series of ureteric catheters, it is even possible to dilate the ducts in an attempt to prevent recurrence of the stricture.

The opening of a müllerian duct cyst, however, is more complex. It is best to have two operators to complete this operation (Low & Jequier, unpublished). The first procedure is to carry out vasography as this will demonstrate the size as well as the presence of the cyst. On hemisecting the vas to carry out the vasogram, it is very common to find copious quantities of old blood that exudes from its lumen. Having defined the cyst and determined that there is no other pathology present in this area, it is now useful to inject methylene blue down the vas to distend the cyst and make it visible to the second operator. The cyst can now be identified visually by an area of swelling and slight blue colour on the verumontanum.

Using a very small knife down the urethroscope, an incision is made longitudinally over the swelling until the old blood and the methylene blue escape into the urethra. A smaller transverse incision is now made and the cyst opened by excising the corners between these two incisions (Fig. 6.17). The cyst area can now be washed out and inspected. Postoperatively a catheter is left in overnight and, after its removal the following day, the patient can be discharged.

Postoperative complications following these procedures are few but a urinary tract infection and a postsurgical epididymitis can occur.

However, there are some problems that can specifically follow the opening of a müllerian duct cyst. After the incision of such a cyst, it does not appear to collapse; indeed, it may stay the same size for many months and thus can act as a small reservoir for urine (Fig. 6.18). The patient may thus complain of a postmicturition dribble or even of the contamination of the ejaculate with urine. This latter phenomenon can on occasions cause loss of

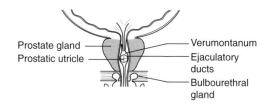

Prostate gland — Verumontanum
Prostatic utricle — Ejaculatory ducts
— Bulbourethral gland

Fig. 6.17 The incisions that are made transurethrally to drain a müllerian duct cyst. Great care must be taken to avoid damage to the ejaculatory ducts and also to the bladder neck that lies immediately above the site of the cyst.

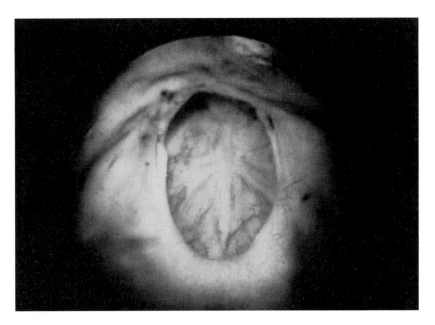

Fig. 6.18 A photograph, taken cystoscopically, of a müllerian duct cyst that had been opened more than 2 years previously. The position of the ejaculatory ducts at 10 and 2 o'clock can easily be seen. Note that the cyst does not collapse but maintains its size almost indefinitely. Thus, early drainage of these cysts is important in order to minimize their expansion. The persistence of these cavities can result in postoperative symptoms.

motility of sperm and could also cause persistence of infertility. The distortion of the ejaculatory ducts caused by the expansion of the müllerian duct cyst can also cause emission to take place into the opened cyst rather than into the urethra, thus giving rise to either a total loss of the ejaculate or a reduction in its force.

Partial or incomplete obstruction of the excurrent ducts

It must be remembered that obstruction of any part of the duct system may be partial or incomplete and can thus present with oligozoospermia rather than azoospermia (Jequier *et al.* 1983). It appears that many of the male patients with incomplete obstructive lesions will eventually progress to complete obstruction. However, the length of time taken for the lesion to progress to azoospermia may vary considerably and can range from several months to many years.

On clinical examination these men have normal-sized testes and their hormonal profile will, in the absence of a second pathology, also be normal. The diagnosis of partial obstruction is impossible to make without resorting to scrotal exploration. Even when lesions are found in the epididymis, the best method of management is unclear. Whether antibiotics are ever of value is dubious. At present, the best method of management of the infertility caused by this problem is the use of assisted conception.

Unilateral obstruction

Obstructive lesions of the excurrent ducts of the testes may occur unilaterally, and this is another way in which obstruction may present with oligozoospermia (Hendry *et al.* 1982). Such patients usually present with a low sperm count and the problem is also characterized by the presence of antisperm antibodies of the immunoglobulin G (IgG) group, which are found to involve predominantly the head region of the sperm. Thus, the infertility may indeed be caused by low sperm numbers but may equally be caused by the presence of antisperm antibodies that may impede fertilization.

Conclusion

It is thus clear from the discussion above that there are many causes of obstruction in men with infertility and there are also many ways in which this problem will present. It is important that the site of the obstruction is accurately identified as only then can a rational treatment be applied to this condition. The site of an obstruction can only be pin-pointed by a good clinical evaluation that includes careful history taking and a skilled clinical examination.

References

Amelar, R.D. & Hotchkiss, R.S. (1963) Congenital aplasia of the epididymes and vasa deferentia: effects on semen. *Fertility and Sterility* **14**, 44–48.

Averback, P. & Wight, D.G. (1979) Seminiferous tubule hypercurvature. A newly recognised common syndrome of human male infertility. *Lancet* **i**, 181–183.

Bayle, H. (1952) Azoospermia of excretory origin. *Proceedings of the Society for the Study of Fertility* **4**, 30–38.

Berger, R.E. (1994) Infection of the male reproductive tract. *Current Therapy in Endocrinology and Metabolism* **5**, 305–309.

Carson, C.C. (1984) Transurethral resection for ejaculatory duct stenosis and oligospermia. *Fertility and Sterility* **41**, 482–484.

Dumur, V., Gervais, R., Rigot, J.M. *et al.* (1990) Abnormal distribution of CF Delta F508 allele in azoospermic men with congenital aplasia of epididymis and vas deferens. *Lancet* **336**, 512.

El-Shiemy, S., El- Hefnawi, H., Abdel-Fattati, A., El-Okbi, M. & Farid, M. (1976) Testicular and epididymal involvement in leprosy patients with special reference to gynaecomastia. *International Journal of Dermatology* **15**, 52–58.

Ferrie, B.G. & Rundle, J.S.H. (1983) Tuberculous epididymo-orchitis—a review of 20 cases. *British Journal of Urology* **55**, 437–439.

Grant, J.B.F., Costello, C.B., Sequiera, P.J.L. & Blacklock, N.J. (1987) the role of *Chlamydia trachomatis* in epididymitis. *British Journal of Urology* **60**, 355–359.

Guerin, J.-F., Cyza, J.-C., Perrin, P. & Rollet, J. (1981) Les obstructions congenitales ou aquises d l'epididyme humain: étude de la mobilité des spermatoides en amont de l'obstruction. *Bulletin de l'Association Des Anatomistes,* **65**, 297–306.

Hamm, B. & Kelami, A. (1982) Experimental studies on the functional capacity of the alloplastic spermatocele (Kelami–Affeld prosthesis). *Urologia Internationalis* **37**, 314–323.

Handelsman, D., Conway, A.J., Boylan, A.J. & Turtle, J.R. (1984) Young's syndrome: obstructive azoospermia and chronic sino-pulmonary infections. *New England Journal of Medicine* **310**, 3–9.

Hassan, K.E. & Chui, M.A. (1985) Acute suppurative epididymitis in an intra-abdominal testis. *Urology* **57**, 244–245.

Heath, A.L., Mann, D.W.K. & Eckstein, H.B. (1984) Epididymal abnormalities associated with maldescent of the testes. *Journal of Paediatric Surgery* **19**, 47–49.

Hendry, W.F., Knight, R.K., Whitfield, H.N. *et al.* (1978) Obstructive azoospermia: respiratory function tests, electron microscopy and the results of surgery. *British Journal of Urology* **50**, 598–604.

Hendry, W.F., Parslow, J.M. & Stedronska, J. (1983) Exploratory scrototomy in 168 azoospermic males. *British Journal of Urology* **55**, 785–791.

Hendry, W.F., Parslow, J.M., Stedronska, J. & Wallace, D.M. (1982) Diagnosis of unilateral testicular obstruction in subfertile males. *British Journal of Urology* **54**, 774–779.

Hodges, R.D. & Hanley, H.G. (1966) Epididymovasostomy: a micro-dissection of two cases. *British Journal of Urology* **38**, 534–541.

Holsclaw, D.S. (1969) Cystic fibrosis and fertility. *British Medical Journal* **i**, 356.

Jequier, A.M. (1986) Obstructive azoospermia: a study of 102 patients. *Clinical Reproduction and Fertility* **3**, 21–36.

Jequier, A.M. (1991) Edward Martin (1859–1938). The founding father of modern clinical andrology. *International Journal of Andrology* **14**, 1–10.

Jequier, A.M., Crich, J.P. & Holmes, S.C. (1983) Incomplete obstruction of the male genital tract: a cause of oligozoospermia. *British Journal of Urology* **55**, 545–546.

Kelami, A. (1978) 'Infrapubic' approach in operative andrology. *Urology* **12**, 580–581.

Martin, E., Benton Carnett, J., Levy, J.V. & Pennington, M.E. (1902) The surgical treatment of sterility due to obstruction at the epididymis together with a study of the morphology of human sperm. *Therapeutics Gazette* **March,** 1–14.

Middlekauf, H.R., Fang, M.A. & Hahn, B.H. (1987) Polyarteritis nodosa of the epididymis in a patient with Whipple's disease. *Journal of Rheumatology* **14**, 1193–1195.

Nistal, M., Paniagua, R. & Picazo, M.L. (1983) Testicular and epididymal involvement in Fabry's disease. *Journal of Pathology* **141**, 113–124.

Nistal, M., Santamaria, L., Regadera, J. & Paniagua, R. (1988) Diverticula of human seminiferous tubules in the normal and pathologic testis. *Journal of Andrology* **9**, 55–61.

Pareek, S.S. & Tandon, R.C. (1985) Epididymal lesions in tuberculoid leprosy. *British Medical Journal* **291**, 313.

Patrizio, P. & Zielenski, J. (1996) Congenital absence of the vas deferens: a mild form of cystic fibrosis. *Molecular Medicine Today* **2**, 24–31.

Phadke, A.M., Samant, N.R. & Deval, S.D. (1973) Smallpox as an aetiological factor in male infertility. *Fertility and Sterility* **24**, 802–804.

Schoysman, R. (1981) Epididymal causes of male infertility: pathogenesis and management. In: *Pathology and Pathophysiology of the Epididymis* (eds C. Pollak & A. Klavert), pp. 102–113. Karger, Basle, Switzerland.

Silber, S.J. (1984) Microsurgery for vasectomy reversal and vasoepididymostomy. *Urology* **23**, 505–524.

Teichtahl, H., Temple Smith, P.D., Johnson, J.L., Southwick, G.J. & de Kretser, D.M. (1987) Obstructive azoospermia and chronic sinopulmonary disease in identical twins. *Fertility and Sterility* **47**, 879–881.

Wagenknecht, L.V. (1982) Obstruction in the male reproductive tract. In: *Treatment of Male Infertility* (eds J. Bain, W. B. Schill & L. Scjwarsteom), pp. 221–248. Springer-Verlag, Berlin.

Winnaker, J.T., Becker, K.L., Katz, S. & Mathews, M.J. (1967) Recurrent epididymitis in sarcoidosis: report of a patient treated with corticosteroids. *Annals of Internal Medicine* **66**, 743–748.

Wollin, M., Marshall, F.F., Fink, M.P., Malhotra, R. & Diamond, D.A. (1987) Aberrant epididymal tissue: a significant entity. *Journal of Urology* **138**, 1247–1250.

Young, D. (1970) Surgical treatment of male infertility. *Journal of Reproduction and Fertility* **23**, 541–542.

7: Primary Testicular Disease: a Common Cause of Male Infertility

Of all the many causes of infertility in the male, primary testicular disease is probably the most common (Jequier & Holmes 1993). For this reason it requires some attention and some understanding.

Unlike the situation of reduced gametogenesis in the female, most disorders of sperm production are the result of local damage to the testes themselves and are only rarely related to a disturbance of pituitary function. Thus, as its name implies, primary testicular disease is a primary disorder of the testes and is not secondary to any malfunction of the pituitary or the hypothalamus.

Primary testicular disease causes a disruption of the spermatogenic failure of varying severity and, as a consequence, there is a reduction in or a total obliteration of sperm production. This condition can also result in altered function of the Leydig cells and a fall in testosterone production. Depending on the degree of disruption of the process of sperm production and the distribution of the lesions within each testis, primary testicular disease will present in the clinic as either oligozoospermia, or in more severe cases, as azoospermia.

One of the reasons why the testis is so susceptible to damage may relate to its position, but it must also be remembered that the testicular blood flow is relatively low in relation to its metabolic needs. As a consequence the venous blood that leaves the testis through the pampiniform plexus is less well oxygenated than that from most other tissues in the body. The oxygen tension in the ram testis has been calculated to be only somewhere between 10 and 25 mmHg, and thus any interference with the tenuous oxygen supply to the testis is likely to result in hypoxic damage to the seminiferous epithelium. Likewise, any increase in demand for oxygen by the testis, such as that induced by an increase in temperature, could also result in ischaemic damage. This situation is worsened by the marked sensitivity of the testicular blood flow to vasoactive agents.

Although primary testicular disease is one of the most common causes of infertility in the male (Jequier & Holmes 1993), its aetiology is poorly understood and in some 65% of patients with this condition no cause can be ascertained (Table 7.1). This is a worrying aspect of this condition because, if its cause is not known, no means of prevention are available. However, there are a few known causes of this condition which, when present, can be elicited in a clinical history.

It must also be remembered that primary testicular disease is an untreatable condition: there are no therapies that improve the sperm count

Table 7.1 Some of the more common causes of primary testicular disease. Note that no cause can be identified in some two-thirds of the patients with this disorder

Suspected aetiology	%
Unknown	66
Testicular maldescent	20
Torsion	2
Trauma	5
Klinefelter's syndrome	5
Mumps orchitis	1
Chemotherapy	1

Jequier & Holmes (1993).

and there is no medication that will reverse this condition. The treatment of the infertility that this disorder may cause, relies entirely on the manipulation of the existing sperm in an ejaculate, whether that be by techniques such as intrauterine insemination or by the application of some form of assisted conception.

Another important feature of this disorder is the progressive demise of the sperm count and also of sperm function; therefore men with severe oligozoospermia caused by primary testicular disease may one day become azoospermic. Thus, if this condition is diagnosed and there is any sign of a continuing deterioration of semen quality then cryopreservation of one or two samples of semen from this patient may avoid the necessity, at a later date, of the retrieval of spermatozoa from the testis.

Causes of primary testicular disease

Although in the majority of men with this condition its aetiology may be unknown, there are causes of this condition that can be identified from the history.

Testicular maldescent

This is the most common of the identifiable causes of primary testicular disease and if it has occurred bilaterally may severely impair sperm production. A history of testicular maldescent is present in around 20% of men with primary testicular disease (Jequier & Holmes 1986) and may be present in around 9.5% of infertile men presenting at the clinic (Mieusset *et al.* 1995).

The exact cause of testicular maldescent in the human is not known. In the majority of children with this disorder, no other genital abnormalities are found, suggesting that this anomaly is not, in general, associated with any major hormonal disturbance. Nevertheless, there are hormonal abnormalities such as hypogonadotrophic hypogonadism with which maldescent is common and complete androgen resistance where it is the rule. Descent

113

of the testes can also be blocked by anatomical lesions such as 'prune belly syndrome'. The presence of posterior urethral valves where a full bladder will also impede testicular descent.

It has also been suggested that genitofemoral nerve may play an important part in the normal descent of the testes as transection of this nerve in neonatal rats inhibits the migration of the gubernaculum and thus interferes with testicular descent (Hutson & Beasley 1987). Transection of the cord may impede descent of the male gonads (Hutson *et al.* 1988), and thus maldescent of the testes is frequently seen in men with spina bifida. The substance known as calcitonin gene-related peptide (CGRP) is a neurotransmitter in the genitofemoral nerve and this substance may also influence testicular maldescent (Hutson & Beasley 1987).

Müllerian inhibitory substance (MIS) may also play a role in testicular maldescent. Persistence of the müllerian duct in the male is associated with cryptorchidism but its role in this condition has been difficult to define.

It is not known for sure whether the infertility that is associated with testicular maldescent is caused by a testicular degeneration that is secondary to the maldescent or whether the spermatogenic failure relates to the primary lesion that has initiated the maldescent. It is clear, however, that experimental cryptorchidism in the rat induces irreversible sterility (Kort *et al.* 1991) and that early orchidopexy in the human helps to preserve fertility (Quinn *et al.* 1991). It must also be remembered that the infertility associated with testicular maldescent may also relate to the presence of antisperm antibodies (Urry *et al.* 1994).

How testicular maldescent might damage sperm production is unclear. However, it is likely to be caused by the increased temperature that is present within the abdominal cavity: testicular temperature in the scrotum is around 35 °C whereas the intra-abdominal temperature is 37–38 °C. It is known that warming the testes impairs sperm production and that rendering the testes cryptorchid will also induce failure of spermatogenesis.

The infertility associated with testicular maldescent may also be complicated by abnormalities of the excurrent ducts. There is an association between deletions of sections of the epididymal ducts and of the vasa deferentia resulting in a superimposed obstructive problem (Terrone *et al.* 1996). Ectopic tissue may also be found in relation to a maldescended testes such as renal, splenic or even adrenal tissue (Mininberg & Dattwyler 1973). Such tissue may initially be mistaken for a testicular malignancy. It is also not uncommon for the excurrent ducts of the testis, especially the epididymal duct, to become damaged during orchidopexy resulting in a secondary obstructive lesion. Maldescended testes are also prone to undergo torsion, and as torsion itself can result in damage to the spermatogenic epithelium, such an accident may worsen the problem of infertility.

Most patients with this disorder know of its presence and will give a history of this problem. Some men will have undergone at least an attempt at orchidopexy at some time in their lives, and this procedure is usually carried out just prior to puberty. However, as early orchidopexy may be more effective in preventing infertility than is an operation closer to puberty, children today often undergo this procedure at 18–24 months of age.

It is, however, important to differentiate a true maldescended testis from the ectopic testis. In the latter situation, the testes descend normally but then take an aberrant route out of the scrotum to end up in different positions on the front of the superior pubic rami. Thus, maldescended testes remain in the line of descent whereas ectopic testis come to lie outside this pathway. Testes in these ectopic sites are very susceptible to trauma and, as trauma is a very important cause of primary testicular disease, ectopic testes may also show evidence of damage to sperm production.

Testes that are maldescended are usually reduced in size and may show a reduction in sensation. If these testes are palpable, they should be examined carefully for any possible presence of a tumour. If the damage to the spermatogenic epithelium is major and has occurred bilaterally, then the serum FSH will be raised. Likewise, if the damage to the testes is severe enough to interfere with Leydig cell function, then the LH may also be raised and the testosterone level may be below that of normal.

Impalpable cryptorchid testes are best sited using the laparoscope but their position can also be identified by arteriography. The most common position for a maldescended testis is just above the deep inguinal ring.

Testes that remain cryptorchid are dangerous as they can be the site of testicular tumours. Tumours may occur in some 3% of maldescended testes. However, the removal of bilaterally maldescended testes will deprive the patient of his main source of testosterone. However, a unilaterally cryptorchid testis that is too high for orchidopexy is best removed. Tumours that do develop in an intra-abdominal testis tend to present late and thus may frequently undergo widespread dissemination before their presence is detected.

If the testis is easily palpable, the patient should be instructed in its regular palpation in order to detect any development of a tumour. If the testis is within the inguinal ring or close to it, it may be possible to carry out an orchidopexy even in an adult as this will preserve natural testosterone production and avoid the use of replacement therapy.

The operation of autotransplantation of maldescended testes has also been described. In this procedure, a high paranephric testis is excised and placed within the scrotum. The testicular vessels are then microsurgically anastomosed to the inferior epigastric vessels (Wacksman *et al.* 1982) in an attempt to maintain natural testosterone production. However this operation does not succeed very often and has now largely been abandoned.

In children who present at or around puberty with inadequate testicular descent, especially if there is evidence of hypo-androgenization, may respond to a course of treatment with human chorionic gonadotrophin. However, this type of therapy is little used now as most cases of testicular maldescent are today treated surgically at a much earlier age. Treatment by orchidopexy when the child is less than 10 years of age may reduce the subsequent occurrence of testicular tumours (Lee 1995).

Torsion

Torsion of the testis often results in failure of the production of sperm by that testis and in a reduction or even in the total obliteration of the spermatogenic epithelium. It commonly occurs in children and is especially common in children with a maldescended testis. Testicular torsion may be unilateral or bilateral and is frequently associated with testicular maldescent. When a testis undergoes torsion, the venous return and then the arterial input are cut off. As a consequence, the testis, whose normal blood supply is precarious, will become ischaemic and the damage to the spermatogenic epithelium that may result from this ischaemia is frequently irreversible. If the torsion is associated with maldescent, the spermatogenic epithelium may have been abnormal even before the onset of the ischaemia caused by the torsion. Thus, the prognosis for fertility following torsion will be, for the most part, very poor.

Testicular torsion presents acutely with a sudden onset of testicular pain. In children this disorder can also present with pain referred to the renal area, and torsion can thus be mistaken for renal colic or an acute pyelonephritis. The diagnosis can often be confirmed by using colour Doppler ultrasound, which will demonstrate a lack of blood flow through the testis which has undergone torsion (Yazbeck & Patriquin 1994).

On examination, however, the testis is often acutely tender and may be a little enlarged. Where a torsion is suspected, a scrotal exploration must be carried out and the diagnosis confirmed or excluded. The testes undergo torsion in a lateral direction around the spermatic cord and may have undergone more than one turn. The testis must be examined and its viability assessed. A torted testis is a dusky blue in colour, and if the torsion is long standing, it may in fact already show evidence of gangrene. If, on untwisting the torsion, there is no colour change nor is there evidence of a returning blood supply, then the testis should be removed. A testicular biopsy and frozen section can also sometimes be helpful diagnostically in this situation. In any long-standing torsion, the spermatogenic potential of the testis is almost always lost.

There has been considerable controversy as to whether torsion of one testis causes spermatogenic damage in the contralateral gonad and this question has never been satisfactorily answered. As many torted testes are already maldescended, it could be the possible delay in descent that causes this change in the opposite testis. Torsion may also generate antisperm antibodies and this could contribute to an abnormal sperm count postoperatively. More recently, it has been suggested that torsion may also induce apoptosis in the opposite testis (Hadziselimovic *et al.* 1997).

In some patients with infertility, a retractile testis or a testis that is easily elevated into the inguinal canal may be present. Such a retractile testis is

116

normal in a young child but cannot be deemed to be normal in a adult. A retractile testis may simply represent a testis that is severely reduced in size but its movement to an intra-abdominal position can only damage its potential for sperm production. It is thus suggested by some authors that such retractile testes should be held in the scrotum surgically (Jarrett *et al.* 1992). In this procedure a pouch is fashioned in the dartos muscle and the testis is stitched into position within this pouch.

Trauma

Injury to the testis is an important cause of primary testicular disease. It may even be sustained in early life as it is known that nearly 10% of children have suffered from significant genital injury prior to puberty (Finkelhor & Wolak 1995). It has even been suggested that testicular damage may occur during a breech delivery of a male infant (Lips *et al.* 1979).

Testicular trauma can also be sustained in sports activities, fights and falls and may also form part of an array of multiple injuries, particularly those that are the result of motor vehicle accidents. Injury may cause oedema or induce the presence of an intratesticular haematoma. In either situation, the intratesticular pressure will rise. As the fibrous tunica albuginea is poorly distensible, any increase in intratesticular pressure can result in a reduction in blood flow to the testis. The consequent ischaemia if prolonged will thus result in a reduction in the activity of the spermatogenic epithelium from which it may not recover. Indeed, ischaemia may be the underlying problem in many men with primary testicular disease as several of the histological features of this disorder may be present in the experimental testis that has been rendered ischaemic (Markey *et al.* 1995).

Trauma may also damage the epididymal duct and so there may also be an obstructive lesion that is superimposed upon the primary testicular disease. A history of trauma is thus important among patients with this problem, but it is often difficult to relate the traumatic incident to any subsequent reduction in the sperm count.

It must also be remembered that one common form of trauma is the testicular biopsy. There is no doubt that needle biopsy may result in a high incidence of intratesticular haematomata (Schlegel & Su 1997), and indeed the damage done to the testis can sometimes be sufficient to reduce its secretion of testosterone (Manning *et al.* 1998).

Orchitis

Orchitis occurs as the result of some form of infection that can be either bacterial or viral. These infections will be discussed individually and in more detail in Chapter 14. Orchitis may also be secondary to an epididymitis when it is known as epididymo-orchitis. Any inflammatory condition of the testis will result in intratesticular oedema and, because of the lack of distensibility of the tunica albuginea, this oedema will reduce the blood

117

flow through the testis. As a consequence, ischaemic damage to the spermatogenic epithelium can occur which can be irreversible. The most common bacterial agents that cause epididymo-orchitis include chlamydia and the coliform group of organisms.

An acute epididymo-orchitis will present as a sudden onset of pain in the scrotum and this usually occurs bilaterally. Such a problem may also be associated with the presence of a urinary tract infection. The testis and epididymis are acutely tender and the gonads are often swollen. The scrotum may also be reddened. It can be quite difficult to distinguish an acute epididymo-orchitis from testicular torsion and if there is any doubt, a careful ultrasound examination and Doppler imaging of the testicular arterial blood flow will usually distinguish the two (Paltiel *et al.* 1998). If such imaging is not available and doubt about the diagnosis persists, then scrotal exploration must be performed.

The most famous cause of orchitis as an agent of infertility is the viral disease of mumps (Jameson 1981). However, mumps only causes infertility when it induces an orchitis that is bilateral. As mumps orchitis only occurs in postpubertal males, mumps that occurs in childhood has no implications for future fertility. In adults, a mumps orchitis only occurs in some 25% of men with the clinical disease. The severity of the mumps orchitis does vary greatly between individuals, and there are many men with a history of bilateral orchitis who are able to maintain a normal sperm production postinfection. Thus, in men with a history of mumps orchitis, infertility is not the rule.

More exotic infections may also involve the testis and these may form granulomatous lesions; examples of these include the lesions produced by *Mycobacterium tuberculosis*, *M. leprae* and even by bilharzia. Very rarely, one may see a testicular gumma that is the result of a chronic syphilitic infection.

Chromosomal anomalies

Chromosomal anomalies may also cause infertility. The best known of these disorders involve the sex chromosomes, although autosomal anomalies have great relevance to fertility as well.

Klinefelter's syndrome

This condition was first described by Harry F. Klinefelter and two very distinguished colleagues from Boston, Massachusetts, in 1942 (Klinefelter *et al.* 1942). Klinefelter's syndrome is the most common sex chromosomal abnormality seen in an infertility clinic. It may represent around 3–4% of all infertile men with a karyotypic abnormality who attend an infertility clinic (Pandiyan & Jequier 1996). In this condition, the white cell karyotype shows the presence of a 47,XXY configuration. However, this condition can exist as a mosaic, an example of which would be 47,XXY/46,XY.

Interestingly, this disorder can also be seen in the domestic cat, the horse, the sheep and in cattle: the male tortoiseshell cat has a triploid sex chromosome pattern and, like men with Klinefelter's syndrome, it is frequently sterile (Long *et al.* 1981). Testicular histology in these animals is also remarkably similar to that in the human with Klinefelter's syndrome.

The phenotype associated with this anomaly varies greatly between individuals. However, most patients with this condition are hypo-androgenized, having poor beard growth and scanty body hair. Libido may be reduced and sexual function may also not be normal. Gynaecomastia may also be present. Testicular size is always reduced and the serum levels of the gonadotrophins are raised. Serum testosterone is either in the lower range of normal or is reduced. In later life, this reduction in testosterone production may predispose the patient to osteoporosis.

This karyotypic anomaly is always associated with a fairly severe abnormality of the semen analysis and signs of primary testicular disease. The vast majority of patients with this disorder are in fact azoospermic, but very occasionally men with Klinefelter's syndrome may be oligozoospermic and a case of natural paternity has been reported.

The testicular histology is characterized by almost total atrophy of the seminiferous tubules that are replaced by sheets of Leydig cells. However, one may see, in testicular biopsies from these patients, the occasional tubule in which spermatogenic activity is taking place.

Today it is now possible to collect sperm from these biopsies and, using the techniques of IVF and ICSI, pregnancies from these patients have now been achieved (Bourne *et al.* 1997). It is of interest that the offspring produced from testicular sperm taken from men with Klinefelter's syndrome seem to show no evidence of any abnormality in their sex chromosome complement. It is thus likely that only sperm with a haploid sex chromatin are capable of normal fertilization.

Noonan's syndrome

This is a much rarer karyotypic abnormality involving the sex chromosomes and is the male equivalent of Turner's syndrome in an individual with a male phenotype. Chromosomal analysis shows an apparent 45,XO configuration but a portion of the Y chromosome is present within the karyotype to provide the patient with his male phenotype.

Men with this condition are very obviously hypo-androgenized and the diagnosis has almost always been made before the patient arrives in an infertility clinic. There are obvious abnormalities of the genital tract (Elsawi *et al.* 1994). Puberty has almost always been delayed. The testes are often maldesended and testicular size is very reduced. The serum testosterone is low in the presence of raised gonadotrophin levels. Histology of the testis shows atrophy of the seminiferous tubules, although occasionally sperm can be present in the ejaculate.

There is no treatment of the infertility associated with this condition apart from the application of assisted conception to those men with sperm in their ejaculate or within a testicular biopsy.

Autosomal abnormalities

A wide variety of autosomal anomalies have been described in association with abnormalities in the seminal fluid in men with infertility. However, it is often difficult to be sure that the autosomal abnormality is indeed the cause of the abnormal sperm count. It is possible for almost identical autosomal abnormalities to be found in both infertile and the fertile man. Nevertheless, autosomal abnormalities are found much more commonly amongst infertile men than those with normal semen analyses.

Translocations of parts of the autosomal chromosomes are commonly found among infertile men, and it is possible that these anomalies give rise to chromosomally unbalanced haploid spermatozoa that can cause developmental problems in the embryo. Such autosomal translocations also have the potential of producing a trisomy in any resultant conception. Chromosomal abnormalities in the infertile male is thus of great relevance, not only to the patient himself but to his partner. In this situation, the outcome in terms of the offspring must also be considered.

Testis size in men with autosomal abnormalites can be normal or reduced depending upon the severity of the related (or unrelated) primary testicular disease. Similarly, the serum gonadotrophins can also be normal or raised.

The routine use of white cell karyotypic analyses in the evaluation of the infertile male has been much argued in the past, its cost being a major disincentive to its use in this context. Although this analysis is of little value in many of the other causes of infertility in the male, it is indeed of value in the diagnosis of the causation of primary testicular disease and should be carried out in all men with who appear clinically to have this condition.

Deletions on the long arm of the Y chromosome

Recently, deletions involving Region 9 on the long arm of the Y chromosome have been described in relation to both azoospermia and oligozoospermia. However, no phenotype has been ascribed to infertile men with this disorder, and to date the only way to diagnose this anomaly is by the identification of these genetic lesions using the polymerase chain reaction. These disorders are discussed in more detail in Chapter 16, which relates to genetics and infertility.

Chemotherapeutic agents and X-irradiation therapy

The use of both anticancer therapy and X-irradiation in the treatment of malignancy is a not uncommon cause of infertility. The use of these agents in the management of disorders such as Hodgkin's disease, which so frequently occurs in young people, is indeed a cause of primary testicular disease. Sadly, there is little one can do to protect the fertility of young men undergoing this form of therapy, which, owing to the nature of their disease, must take precedence over their future fertility. It is, however, important in young adults to conserve samples of semen prior to any chemotherapy or radiotherapy. However, such a collection of semen would be impossible in a child.

It is also very difficult to predict the long-term effect of these antimitotics on the spermatogenic epithelium and in many instances either partial or total recovery does indeed occur. However, when the number of drugs that are used is increased, as in triple or quadruple therapy, recovery is much less likely to occur.

Severe damage to the spermatogenic epithelium can also be induced by X-irradiation (Rowley *et al.* 1974) and only a relatively small dose is sufficient to damage spermatogenesis permanently. Irradiation of the groin area following the removal of a testicular cancer or even the scatter from the irradiation of the upper abdomen may also be sufficient to damage sperm production. In many patients, the effects upon the testes produced by irradiation is frequently irreversible. Patients who undergo total body irradiation and marrow transplantation are also almost always infertile at the completion of their treatment.

The clinical features of primary testicular disease

Men with this disorder present at the infertility clinic with either azoospermia or oligozoospermia (Jequier & Holmes 1993). The abnormality found in the semen of men with this condition will depend upon: (a) the nature of the histological change; (b) the severity of the lesions; (c) the distribution of the lesions within the testes; and (d) the presence or absence of a second pathology. The damage to the testes that has caused the primary testicular disease may affect only the spermatogenic epithelium. However, in more severe damage to the testis, Leydig cell function may also be compromised. Thus, in some patients only the production of sperm is damaged, whereas in other patients testosterone production is also reduced (Table 7.2).

In general, patients with this problem have no disturbance in sexual function and are usually normally androgenized. However, when the damage to the spermatogenic epithelium is severe and Leydig cell function

Table 7.2 Some of the clinical features associated with primary testicular disease

Oligozoospermia or azoospermia
Reduced testis size
Loss of testicular sensation
Raised serum FSH level
Abnormal LH and testosterone levels
Abnormal testicular histology

is also damaged, loss of testosterone production may also result, causing a reduction in libido, alterations in sexual function and clinical evidence of hypo-androgenization. The Leydig cells are, interestingly, extremely resistant to damage of any sort, including the damage induced by ischaemia, and thus hypo-androgenization only occurs very infrequently among most men with primary testicular disease. Indeed, the only group of patients with primary testicular disease who are commonly hypo-androgenized are those with anomalies of their sex chromosomes such as men with Klinefelter's and Noonan's syndromes.

Any damage to the spermatogenic epithelium can result in a reduction in the width of the epithelium and a consequent narrowing of the seminiferous tubule. If these changes are widespread, then the size of the testis as a whole will be reduced. The more severe the damage to the seminiferous tubular epithelium, the more likely it will be that the testis volume will fall. Testis size will be reduced in around 70% of men with this disorder (Jequier & Holmes 1993).

However, in some men, particularly those with the histological change in the seminiferous tubules that is known as germinal aplasia, testis volume can remain normal (*vide infra*). Thus, it must be remembered that not all men with primary testicular disease will have a reduction in the size of their testes.

Testis volume is best estimated using the orchimeter invented by Prader (Prader 1966). The plastic or wooden ovoids that make up this orchiometer are made in volumes varying from 5 to 25 mL. Testis size is compared with these ovoids and an estimate is made of the volume of each testis.

In primary testicular disease, there can also be some loss of testicular sensation. This physical sign can be demonstrated by applying a very *gentle* squeeze to each testis. In some patients with primary testicular disease, a loss of sensation is obvious but this is certainly not the case in all men with this disorder.

One aspect of this condition that is not given enough attention is that this may be a progressive disorder. Thus, men with severe oligozoospermia may, 1 year later, find themselves to be azoospermic. Although today one can frequently find spermatozoa for use in IVF and ICSI in these patients, storing samples of even very abnormal semen will avoid the necessity of testicular biopsy and the testicular harvesting of sperm at a later date.

Serum FSH, LH and testosterone in men with primary testicular disease

Elevated serum FSH levels indicate a reduced inhibin secretion by the Sertoli cells. Thus, a raised FSH level in serum is indicative of the severity of abnormal Sertoli cell function and is a common occurrence among patients with primary testicular disease (Bergmann *et al.* 1994). The serum FSH level is thus nearly always raised in azoospermic men with primary testicular disease but may be raised in about one-third of men whose primary testicular disease only renders them oligozoospermic (Fig. 7.1).

Serum LH levels may also be raised in men with this condition and almost certainly indicates a disturbance in Leydig cell function. Serum LH levels are elevated in around one-third of the azoospermic men with this

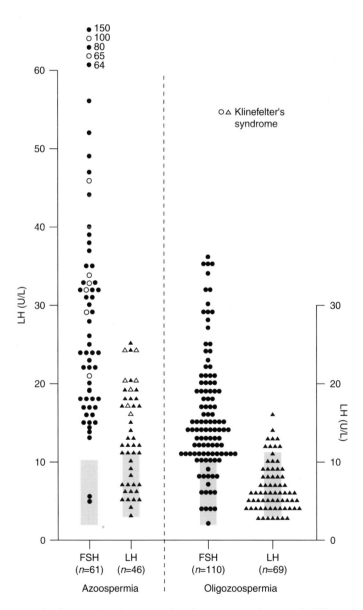

Fig. 7.1 Levels of FSH and LH in serum taken from a group of men with different forms of primary testicular disease. Note that even in men who are azoospermic, the serum FSH levels can occasionally be normal. However, the serum FSH level is normal in some one-third of men who are only oligozoospermic as a result of primary testicular disease. (Reproduced by kind permission of the *British Journal of Urology.*)

condition but is raised in only 10% of oligozoospermic men with primary testicular disease. However, it must be remembered that primary testicular disease may be a progressive disorder, and therefore if the serum LH is already raised, there is the possibility that hypogonadism can eventually occur at a later date and give rise to a distressing degree of sexual dysfunction. Thus, patients with primary testicular disease and a raised serum LH level should be warned of this possibility and reassured that its treatment, when required, will be simple and very effective.

Serum testosterone levels are usually only abnormal when there is clear clinical evidence of hypo-androgenization and often a history of sexual dysfunction (Fig. 7.2). However, occasionally, reduced serum testosterone may be present in men with this condition who give no such history and who are clinically eugonadal.

Thus, the serum levels of FSH, LH and testosterone should be measured in all patients with this condition.

It is also useful, especially if there is any doubt about the diagnosis and in particular where there is a history of sexual dysfunction, to check that these men are not suffering from hyperprolactinaemia or some other endocrine disorder. This problem can be simply excluded by measuring the serum prolactin.

Semen quality in men with primary testicular disease

Semen quality varies greatly in men with this condition and no specific change can be related to the presence of primary testicular disease. Although patients with primary testicular disease show varying degrees of asthenozoospermia and teratozoospermia together with oligozoospermia in their semen samples and many aspects of sperm function are often abnormal, there are no changes in semen quality that are specific to this

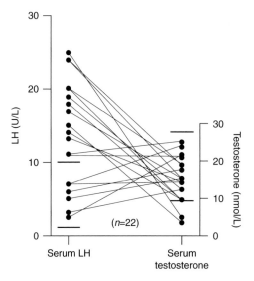

Fig. 7.2 Levels of LH and testosterone in serum taken from a group of men with primary testicular disease. Note that the serum testosterone is frequently within the normal range even when the serum LH is raised. (Reproduced by kind permission of the *British Journal of Urology*.)

particular cause of male infertility. Thus, as is the case with many disorders resulting in infertility in the male, the diagnosis cannot be made from a semen analysis.

Testicular histology in men with primary testicular disease

The histological changes that may be seen in men with primary testicular disease are varied and can be very focal in their distribution through the testis (Silber *et al.* 1997). Indeed, one can sometimes see different changes in seminiferous tubular histology within one field of a testicular biopsy. This variable distribution of changes within a single testicular biopsy make its interpretation very difficult. It must thus be remembered that in a testicular biopsy, we are only examining a very small portion of the total testicular content of spermatogenic epithelium. The semen analysis represents the output of sperm from not only the whole testis from whence the biopsy came but also the output from the testis on the opposite side. As the great feature of the histological changes that are seen in this condition is their focality, normal biopsies can be obtained from men with very low sperm counts. It is common to find that the appearance of the testicular biopsy may be at odds with the findings of a semen analysis. The diagnostic capabilities of a testicular biopsy can thus be very limited.

The histological changes that can be found among the seminiferous tubules in men with primary testicular disease can be divided into five major categories.

Normal testicular tissue

Because of the focal distribution of lesions within the testis in this disorder, biopsies that are histologically normal are not infrequently seen in men with clinically obvious primary testicular disease. Such a phenomenon may be seen in as many as 15% of all men with primary testicular disease that undergo a testicular biopsy (Jequier, unpublished). Such a result is clearly not helpful diagnostically but does indicate that sperm are present within the testis.

Maturational arrest

This is a common finding among men with this disorder and indicates the presence of an arrest of maturation in those tubules. For reasons that are not clear, the arrest usually occurs during spermatogenesis at the secondary spermatocyte stage (Fig. 7.3).

Thickening of the tubular basement membrane

This is a common finding in men with primary testicular failure (Fig. 7.4). A marked hypertrophy of the myoid cells that make up the basement

125

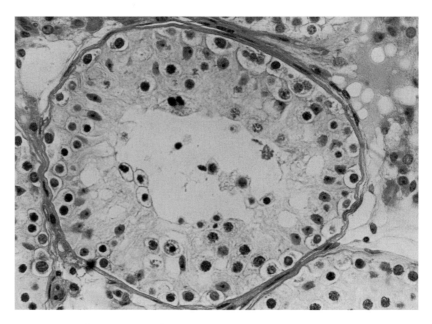

Fig. 7.3 A histological section of a seminiferous tubule showing maturational arrest. In this section there is no maturation of the sperm precursors beyond the spermatocyte stage.

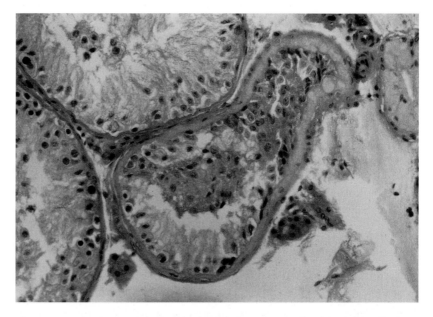

Fig. 7.4 A section from a testicular biopsy taken from an infertile, oligozoospermic man that shows marked thickening of the seminiferous tubular basement membrane. This change is frequently seen in testicular biopsies from men with disordered spermatogenesis.

membrane occurs and its mode of induction is unclear. It is also possible that this morphological change may interfere with the transfer of testosterone from the Leydig cells and thus enhance the reduction in sperm production, or may even be a cause of infertility in itself.

Germinal aplasia

This histological changes also occur both focally and as a generalized change in men with primary testicular disease. The tubules contain only Sertoli cells (Fig. 7.5). These Sertoli cells can appear to be normal on light microscopy, but electron microscopic examination of these cells often reveals fairly gross abnormalities. Where the Sertoli cells are normal in size and the condition is generalized throughout the testis, then testis size can also be normal. If inhibin production by these Sertoli cells remains adequate, then the serum FSH level can also be normal, making the diagnosis of this condition difficult (see below).

Tubular atrophy

In this histological change, some tubules show atrophy and contain no cellular tissue at all while others may show ghost-like outlines of past Sertoli cells (Fig. 7.6). Hyalinization of the tubules can also be seen in these biopsies.

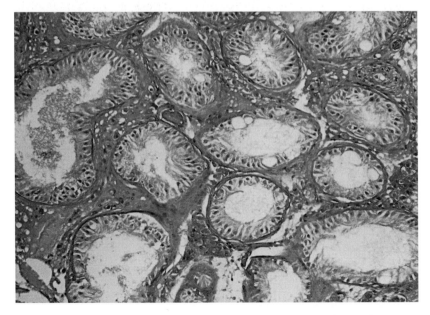

Fig. 7.5 A section from a testicular biopsy showing germinal aplasia. This condition is also known as Sertoli cell only syndrome. In this biopsy, the tubules are of reasonably normal size and only Sertoli cells are visible in each of the tubules.

127

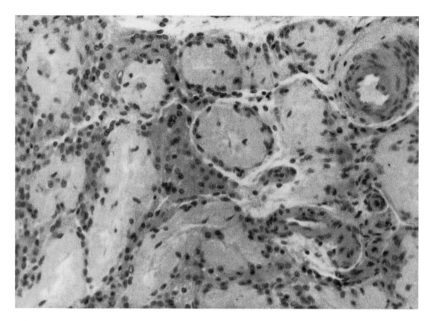

Fig. 7.6 A testicular biopsy showing almost total atrophy and hyalinization of the seminiferous tubules. No Sertoli cells can be seen in any of these tubules.

Testicular microlithiasis

In this condition, multiple small areas of calcification are present in the testis. This calcification can exist in two forms. The first involves amorphous calcific debris and the second consists of calcium laminates that are seen in the testicular tissue. This disorder can be diagnosed on an X-ray of these testes and of course is also seen on testicular biopsy. The exact implications of these anomalies is unclear, but microlithiasis is more likely to be seen in maldescended testes and its presence may indicate an increased risk of malignant change (Renshaw 1998). Laminated calcification may indicate an increased aggressiveness of a tumour. Microlithiasis can, however, be seen in normal testes.

Germinal aplasia and focal tubular atrophy and some difficulties in diagnosis in men with primary testicular disease

There are three types of primary testicular disease that deserve special mention for they can be diagnostically very confusing. The first of these disorders is generalized germinal aplasia and the second is a condition best described as focal tubular atrophy.

Generalized germinal aplasia

In this condition, all the tubules contain only the Sertoli cells. In around 30% of men with this condition, the diameter of the tubules is normal

(Jequier *et al.* 1984) and, in such a patient, testicular size will also be normal. Likewise, if Sertoli cell function and the inhibin production is adequate, then the serum FSH level will also be normal. Such patients can thus easily be mistakenly diagnosed as having obstructive azoospermia and not primary testicular disease. The true diagnosis can thus only be made from a testicular biopsy.

Focal tubular atrophy

In this interesting condition, the testes show the presence of a mixture of tubules showing many different types of histological change ranging from total tubular atrophy to tubules that appear to be completely normal and which show full maturation of spermatogonia into spermatozoa (Fig. 7.7). Patients with this form of infertility present with a reduced sperm count, but often motility and morphology may be normal. Even though the sperm count can be quite low in this condition, sperm function is frequently normal and thus many men with these histological changes may not even be infertile.

Depending upon the proportion of tubules that are atrophied, testis size, however, will often be quite markedly reduced. Despite the reduction in testis size, the serum FSH level is frequently normal. Such patients are

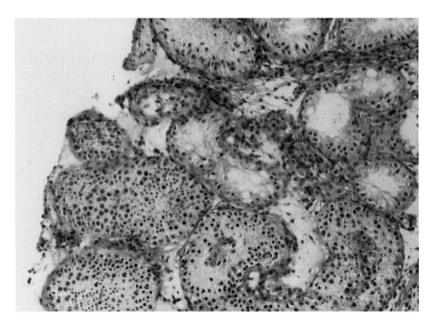

Fig. 7.7 This testicular biopsy contains seminiferous tubules that show a variety of different histological abnormalities even though they are all contained within one field. At the top of the section are tubules showing germinal aplasia while others show either maturational arrest or the presence of normal spermatogenesis. This illustration demonstrates the focality of the changes that may occur in the testis in men with primary testicular disease.

clearly diagnostically confusing and it is thus important that clinicians are aware of this diagnostic problem among men with primary testicular disease. As sperm function is normal, patients with this condition are usually only infertile if sperm numbers are severely reduced.

Carcinoma *in situ* of the testis in men with primary testicular disease

Testicular maldescent is associated with a marked increase in the incidence of testicular cancer (Giwercman 1992). Indeed between the ages of 16 and 30 years, the incidence of testicular malignancy is as high as 1 in 30. In around 5% of infertile men with a history of testicular maldescent, carcinoma *in situ* will be found on a testicular biopsy. The presence of this change almost guarantees the onset of testicular cancer at a later date. It is therefore important that the presence of this condition is identified in men with primary testicular disease, and for this reason it has been suggested that all men with a history of testicular maldescent should undergo a testicular biopsy.

If present in a testicular biopsy, this condition is best treated by low-dose irradiation of the testes (Giwercman *et al.* 1994). However, it must be remembered that this will destroy all the germ cells within the testes and render the patient azoospermic. It is thus important if possible to store sperm prior to treatment as these sperm can then be used to generate pregnancies after the treatment has been completed. As these patients have been cryptorchid in the past, the sperm count may be low even prior to treatment, and thus it may be necessary to consider the use of IVF and ICSI in the management of the infertility among patients with this condition.

Testicular biopsy and its place in the management of primary testicular disease

Testicular biopsy and its role in the diagnosis of male infertility has been a subject of considerable controversy for many years. Testicular biopsy has two major places in the management of primary testicular disease, one in diagnosis and another in the treatment of the associated infertility.

Testicular biopsy can be useful diagnostically, especially in confirming the diagnosis of primary testicular disease where the testes are normal in size and where the serum FSH is within the range of normal. However, as primary testicular disease is often focal, it is possible to obtain normal biopsies in men with this condition. Thus, testicular biopsy is not a very reliable method of diagnosis. In general, however, the testicular biopsy does for the most part aid diagnosis considerably and is indeed an aid in differentiating primary testicular disease from other causes of infertility in the male.

Testicular biopsy is also very useful for treatment. Sperm can be found in a testicular biopsy in around 60% of azoospermic men with primary testicular disease. Using the technique of IVF and ICSI, pregnancies can now be reliably generated from many azoospermic men with primary testicular disease, even where not a single sperm can be found in the ejaculate. Although often no more than a few sperm can be isolated from a testicular biopsy, usually sufficient numbers are obtained to generate several embryos and complete treatment using IVF.

Thus testicular biopsy has an important part to play in both the diagnosis of infertility and its treatment.

The performance of a testicular biopsy

Testicular biopsies can be carried out in several ways. They can be performed using simple aspiration needles, prostatic biopsy guns or using the more traditional method of open biopsy. As the testis is a very sensitive organ, good analgesia is always required.

The testis can be rendered analgesic using local regional or general anaesthesia. Local anaesthesia is achieved by the use of a cord block where around 20 mL of bupivacaine is injected around the scrotal portion of the spermatic cord. This type of analgesia is used for the needle aspiration of the testicular tissue. A spinal anaesthetic is also a useful technique and can be used for either a needle aspiration or for an open biopsy. General anaesthesia is usually reserved for men undergoing an open biopsy.

Needle biopsy

The advantage of a needle biopsy is that it is simple and diagnostic. However, it is blind and may be associated with the formation of a haematoma within the testis itself. It also has the disadvantage that, because the testis and its excurrent ducts are not visualized, any associated pathology may pass unnoticed.

The scrotum is firstly shaved and then scrupulously cleaned using antiseptic solution, preferably an iodine-based compound such as the povidone–iodine preparations. The biopsy needle used can be a Menghini needle or other biopsy needles that have been designed specifically for taking testicular biopsies.

The testis is then held firmly between the finger and thumb and the surface of the testis at a distance from the epididymis is identified. A needle biopsy is then taken from about 1–2 cm into the testis itself. Firm pressure is then placed on the biopsy site to minimize any bleeding.

Other instruments that have been used to obtain a testicular biopsy are guns such as the 'BIP' gun, which has been in use for many years as an instrument for obtaining prostatic biopsies. It is the author's view that this needle is too big for use in testicular biopsy and the risk of intratesticular bleeding may be high. Just because the patient does not complain of any major testicular pain, it does not mean that a testicular haematoma is not present.

Open biopsy

An open biopsy is often carried out in men where a view of the epididymis is required for diagnosis. The author uses this approach for therapeutic biopsies as this technique allows the clinician to obtain a larger biopsy and thus may provide enough sperm for cryopreservation.

This procedure is usually carried out using general anaesthesia. After scrupulous cleaning of the scrotum and the surrounding area, an incision is made in the scrotum. The dartos is incised and the tunica albuginea opened to expose the testis. The epididymis can now be visualized.

A site on the surface of the testis is identified which is not traversed by blood vessels and a small incision is now made in the tunica albuginea. The underlying seminiferous tubules now bulge out through the incision and are cut off using a very sharp knife or fine, sharp scissors while making sure that the tubules are not crushed in the process. The biopsy is now placed in fixative if histology is needed or placed in medium if the biopsy is to be used to obtain spermatozoa for IVF and ICSI. If the purpose of the biopsy is to obtain a sample for histology as well as to collect sperm, then two biopsies can be taken. In some patients sperm may not be obtainable from this biopsy in which case the incision is closed and a further biopsy must be taken from either another site or from the opposite testis.

The incision is closed using a fine polydiaxonone (PDS, Ethicon Ltd) or polyglactin (Vicryl, Ethicon Ltd) suture. Very careful attention to haemostasis is essential. The tunica vaginalis is closed and very careful haemostasis of the connective tissue containing the dartos muscle must now be achieved. Most of the postoperative bleeding that occurs after testicular biopsy or after any form of scrotal exploration comes from this area. The skin may be closed with sutures of the surgeon's choice, although the author favours the use of a fine subcuticular suture of polyglactin (Vicryl, Ethicon Ltd).

The fixation and staining of testicular biopsies

Testicular biopsies should *never* be fixed in formalin. In the testis, formalin destroys cellular detail and disrupts the spermatogenic epithelium. Only special fixatives such as Bouin's, Zenker's or Stieve's fixatives can be used for the fixation of biopsies from the testis. If the biopsy is to be examined electron microscopically, the standard glutaraldehyde fixative can also be used. A biopsy placed in Bouins's solution must be transferred to a solution of 70% alcohol after 24 h or the biopsy will fragment.

Staining of the biopsy can be carried out using the usual laboratory stains such as haematoxylin and eosin. A modification of the Gomori trichrome stain makes particularly striking sections of testicular biopsies, which is useful for black and white reproduction in journal publications.

The treatment of primary testicular disease

There is no known treatment for primary testicular disease. Sperm counts from men with this condition can frequently be improved by removing other factors that may be worsening the problem, an example of which may be the presence of a varicocele. There is otherwise no known way of increasing the sperm count nor of altering any abnormal morphology, although a number of regimens such as courses of vitamins C and E and even gonadotrophin therapy have been tried. However, it may be possible to enhance sperm movement *in vitro* at least temporarily using stimulants such as pentoxyfilline.

Thus, in order to counsel the patients properly concerning the rationale for their treatment, correct diagnosis is important and that can only be achieved in primary testicular disease from careful clinical examination evaluation.

It must be remembered, however, that not all primary testicular disease, especially if it is not severe, may need treatment: just because the semen analysis may be abnormal, it does not necessarily mean that this is the cause of the infertility.

Today it is possible to overcome much of the infertility caused by this condition by the application of reproductive technology. Using techniques such as IVF, and in particular what are known as the 'microassisted' techniques of fertilization such as ICSI, it is possible to generate pregnancies from only a few sperm obtained either from an ejaculate or from a testicular biopsy.

The alternative treatment of the infertility caused by primary testicular disease is of course the use of donated sperm. Most patients, however, prefer to use their own sperm and the use of gamete donation is becoming less and less frequent.

References

Bergmann, M., Behre, H.M. & Nieschlag, E. (1994) Serum FSH and testicular morphology in male infertility. *Clinical Endocrinology* **40**, 133–136.

Bourne, H., Stern, K., Clarke, G., Pertile, M. & Baker, H.W. (1997) Delivery of normal twins following the intracytoplasmic injection of sperm from a patient with 437,XXY Klinefelter's syndrome. *Human Reproduction* **12**, 2447–2450.

Elsawi, M.M., Pryor, J.P., Klufio, G., Barnes, C. & Patton, M. (1994) Genital tract function in men with Noonan syndrome. *Journal of Medical Genetics* **31**, 468–470.

Finkelhor, D. & Wolak, J. (1995) Nonsexual assaults to the genitalia in the youth population. *Journal of the American Medical Association* **274**, 1692–1697.

Giwercman, A. (1992) Carcinoma-in-situ of the testis. Screening and management. *Scandinavian Journal of Urology and Nephrology Supplementum* **148**, 1–47.

Giwercman, A., von der Maase, H., Rorth, M. & Skakkebaek, N.E. (1994) Current concepts of radiation treatment of carcinoma in situ of the testis. *World Journal of Urology* **12**, 125–130.

Hadziselimovic, F., Geneto, R. & Emmons, L.R. (1997) Increased apoptosis in the contralateral testis in patients with testicular torsion. *Lancet* **350**, 118.

Hutson, J.M. & Beasley, S.W. (1987) The mechanism of testicular descent. *Australian Paediatric Journal* **23**, 215–216.

Hutson, J.M., Beasley, S.W. & Bryan, A.D. (1988) Cryptorchidism in spina bifida and spinal cord transection: a clue to the mechanism of transinguinal descent of the testis. *Journal of Paediatric Surgery* **23**, 275–277.

Jameson, R.M. (1981) Clinical aspects of infections associated with male infertility: a review. *Journal of the Royal Society of Medicine* **74**, 371–373.

Jarrett, T.W., Mininberg, D.T. & Golstein, M. (1992) Infertility in patients with retractile testes. *Journal of Urology* **147**, 397A.

Jequier, A.M., Ansell, I.D. & Bullimore, N.J. (1984) Germinal aplasia: how it may mimic obstructive azoospermia. *British Journal of Urology* **56**, 537–539.

Jequier, A.M. & Holmes, S.C. (1993) Primary testicular disease presenting as azoospermia or oligozoospermia in an infertility clinic. *British Journal of Urology* **7**, 731–735.

Klinefelter, H.F., Reifenstein, E.C. & Albright, F. (1942) Syndrome characterised by gynaecomastia, aspermatogenesis without A-Leydigism, and increased secretion of follicle-stimulating hormone. *Journal of Clinical Endocrinology* **II,** 615–627.

Kort, W.J., Hekking-Weijma, I. & Vermeij, M. (1991) Temporary intraabdominal cryptorchidism in the weanling rat leads to irreversible azoospermia. *Journal of Surgical Research* **51**, 138–142.

Lee, P.A. (1995) Consequence of cryptorchidism: relationship to etiology and treatment. *Current Problems in Pediatrics* **25**, 232–236.

Lips, U., Francke, C. & Prader, A. (1979) Testicular function in adolescence after breech delivery. *Helvetica Paediatrica Acta* **34**, 437–442.

Long, S.E., Gruffyd-Jones, T. & David, M. (1981) Male tortoiseshell cats: an examination of testicular histology and chromosome complement. *Research in Veterinary Science* **30**, 274–280.

Manning, M., Junemann, K.-P. & Aitken, P. (1998) Decrease in testosterone blood concentrations after testicular sperm extraction for intracytoplasmic sperm injection in azoospermic men. *Lancet* **352**, 37.

Markey, C.M., Jequier, A.M., Meyer, G.T. & Martin, G.B. (1995) Relationship between testicular morphology and sperm production following ischaemia in the ram. *Reproduction Fertility and Development* **7**, 119–128.

Mieusset, R., Bijan, L., Massat, G., Mansat, A. & Pontonnier, F. (1995) Clinical and biological characteristics of infertile men with a history of cryptorchidism. *Human Reproduction* **10**, 613–619.

Mininberg, D.T. & Dattwyler, B. (1973) Ectopic adrenal tumor presenting as torsion of the spermatic cord in a new born infant. *Journal of Urology* **13**, 2037–1038.

Paltiel, H.J., Connolly, L.P., Atala, A., Paltiel, A.D., Zurakowski, D. & Treves, S.T. (1998) Acute scrotal symptoms in boys with an indeterminate clinical presentation: comparison of color Doppler and scintigraphy. *Radiology* **207**, 223–231.

Pandiyan, N. & Jequier, A.M. (1996) Mitotic chromosomal anomalies among 1210 infertile men. *Human Reproduction* **11**, 2604–2608.

Prader, A. (1966) Testicular size assessment and clinical importance. *Triangle* **7**, 240–243.

Quinn, F.M.J., Crockard, A.D. & Brown, S. (1991) Reversal of degenerative changes in the scrotal testis after orchidopexy in experimental unilateral cryptorchidism. *Journal of Paediatric Surgery* **26**, 451–454.

Renshaw, A.A. (1998) Testicular calcifications: incidence, histology and proposed pathological criteria for testicular microlithiasis. *Journal of Urology* **160**, 1625–1628.

Rowley, M.J., Leach, D.R., Warner, G.A. & Heller, C.G. (1974) Effect of graded doses of ionising radiation on the human testis. *Radiation Research* **59**, 665–678.

Schlegel, P.N. & Su, L.-M. (1997) Physiological consequences of testicular sperm aspiration. *Human Reproduction* **12**, 1688–1692.

Silber, S.J., Nagy, Z., Devroey, P., Tournaye, H. & Van Steirteghem, A.C. (1997) Distribution of spermatogenesis in the testicles of azoospermic men: the presence or absence of spermatids in the testes of men with germinal failure. *Human Reproduction* **12**, 2422–2428.

Terrone, C., Ceratti, G., Bonazzi, A., Rocca Rossetti, S. & Bianchi, M. (1996) Obstructive azoospermia and malformations of the seminal tract. *Archivio Italiano Di Urologia, Andrologia* **68**, 353–357.

Urry, R.L., Carrell, D.T., Starr, N.T., Snow, B.W. & Middleton, R.G. (1994) The incidence of antisperm antibodies in infertility patients with a history of cryptorchidism. *Journal of Urology* **151**, 381–383.

Wacksman, J., Dinner, M. & Nandler, M. (1982) Results of testicular autotransplantation using microvascular techniques: experience with 8 intra-abdominal testes. *Journal of Urology* **128**, 1319–1321.

Yazbeck, S. & Patriquin, H.B. (1994) Accuracy of Doppler sonography in the evaluation of acute conditions of the scrotum in children. *Journal of Pediatric Surgery* **29**, 1270–1272.

8: Varicocele and its Role in Male Infertility

The condition called varicocele has been known to medicine for around 2000 years. It was described by the nineteenth-century surgeon Ambroise Pare as a 'compact pack of vessels filled with melancholic blood'. The role of varicocele as a cause of infertility was first suggested by Macomber and Saunders in 1929 but the demonstration that its ligation increased the sperm count and resolved infertility was first demonstrated clinically by Tulloch in one patient in 1955 (Tulloch 1955).

Varicocele is caused by a dilatation of the venous drainage of the testis. This venous distension is usually caused by a pathological dilatation of the pampiniform plexus and/or a dilatation of the cremasteric venous system.

The role of varicocele in the causation of infertility in the male has been a contentious issue for many years as this condition is frequently found in normally fertile men. The arguments began in 1979 when Nilssen and colleagues (Nilsson *et al.* 1979) reported that they could not demonstrate any therapeutic effect on fertility in men undergoing ligation of a varicocele. Likewise, in 1985, Baker and colleagues (Baker *et al.* 1985) also demonstrated that varicocele ligation produced no changes in sperm count among a large group of infertile males.

These findings were countered by a large study in which it was reported that in adolescents with a varicocele, unilateral ligation increased testicular size over that of the opposite or control side. In 1995, a German group demonstrated that varicocele ligation did not increase the pregnancy rate more than simple counselling and concluded that varicocele tie had little part to play in the treatment of infertility (Nieschlag *et al.* 1995).

However, it has recently been reported that obvious improvements in semen quality occurred after varicocele ligation in men who had previously undergone an orchidectomy but who also had a contralateral varicocele (Hendry 1992). It is also known that varicocele size may relate to a reduction in testicular size and to reduced sperm numbers in the ejaculate (Sigman & Jarow 1997). The response to ligation is also greater when the varicocele is large rather than when it is small (Steckel *et al.* 1993). However, improvement in the sperm count has been seen following repair even among men with a subclinical varicocele (Jarow *et al.* 1996). Varicocele is also associated with abnormal testicular histology and a reduced biopsy score, both of which appear to improve after ligation.

There is also some evidence that there may be defective mitochondrial oxidative phosphorylation in a varicocele-bearing testis (Hsu *et al.* 1995) which, because of the generation of reactive oxygen species (Zalata *et al.* 1995), is therefore likely to result in defective sperm function, poor fertilization rates and infertility. Indeed it is known that fertilization rates within an IVF programme may also improve after ligation of a varicocele (Ashkenazi *et al.* 1989). There is also evidence that the presence of a varicocele causes a progressive deterioration in semen quality (Chehval & Purcell 1992), but these changes could relate to the presence of a second pathology and not to the presence of the varicocele alone. More powerful evidence that varicocele is indeed a cause of infertility is the improvement that occurs after varicocele ligation where the ipsilateral testis is atrophic (Hendry 1992).

It has also been suggested that varicocele may only cause infertility in the presence of a second pathology in the so-called 'cofactor' theory (Peng *et al.* 1990). One of the cofactors cited is nicotine and this theory suggests that the effect of cigarette smoking on testicular function may enhance the infertility effect of a varicocele. Such a theory would also indicate that the response to ligation may be dependent upon the severity of a possible second pathology. If the second pathology is very severe or very mild, little response will be seen after ligation.

Because of all of these contrasting reports, it is not surprising that the argument over varicocele as a cause of infertility continues to cause disagreement. However, it would appear that there is indeed a place for varicocele ligation in the management of male infertility, even though it is still very difficult for the clinician to predict success or failure of this procedure in an individual infertile male patient (Hargreave 1995). It must also be remembered that if varicocele ligation was indeed having an effect that involved only a small percentage of patients, such changes could, individually, go unnoticed within a much larger group of infertile males. The studies quoted above, however, do not conclusively show that varicocele never causes infertility or that it necessarily always causes infertility. That varicocele does at times cause infertility is strongly supported by the most recent and much larger study carried out by the World Health Organization (World Health Organization 1985).

All these factors do indeed indicate that varicocele can indeed be a cause of testicular and/or epididymal dysfunction. The fact that varicocele has been associated with azoospermia, a problem that has been promptly resolved by varicocele ligation, makes it very difficult to postulate that this condition is never a cause of infertility.

The incidence of varicocele

Varicoceles may be found in around 9–15% of all adolescent males and in about the same percentage of fertile adult males who present for vasectomy (Handelsman *et al.* 1984). A varicocele may be unilateral or bilateral. A left-sided varicocele is much more common than is a varicocele on the right. A varicocele may be found in around 20–35% of men who present with infertility (Comhaire 1986). If indeed varicocele does contribute to the problem of infertility in the male, then its occurrence is likely to be a common phenomenon.

The anatomy of a varicocele

The blood supply to the testis is made up of three main systems. These three systems are composed of the internal spermatic artery, the artery of the vas deferens and the cremasteric artery.

The internal spermatic vessels

The internal spermatic arteries are derived from the aorta and arise just below the renal arteries. They pass downwards and laterally on the psoas major retroperitoneally, crossing in front of the ureter and the external iliac artery and passing through the deep inguinal ring to enter the spermatic cord and the scrotum. At the upper and posterior aspect of the upper pole of each testis, the artery divides into two branches that enter the testis on its medial and lateral surfaces (Fig. 8.1).

The internal spermatic veins exit the testes on their posterior border to form the pampiniform plexus, a major component of the spermatic cord.

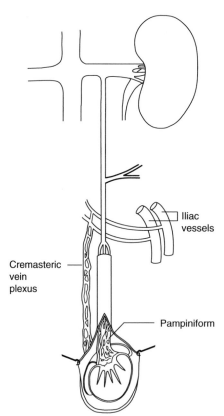

Iliac
vessels

Cremasteric
vein
plexus

Pampiniform

Fig. 8.1 The venous anatomy of a varicocele.

These join together to form three or four veins within the inguinal canal and emerge through the deep inguinal ring as two veins which ascend retroperitoneally lateral to the arteries in front of the psoas major. On the left side, these veins join to form a single vessel that enters the renal vein at a right angle. On the right side, the vessels also join to become a single vessel that enters the inferior vena cava just below the right renal vein. However, it must be remembered that there is a great variation in the venous anatomy of the spermatic veins especially on the left side (Comhaire *et al.* 1981a).

The deferential vessels

The deferential artery on each side arises from the superior vesical artery and accompanies each vas deferens to the testis. It provides blood flow to the vas deferens and also a small blood supply to the testis itself by forming numerous anastomotic connections with the internal spermatic artery.

The cremasteric system

The cremasteric artery arises from the inferior epigastric artery on each side and enters the spermatic cord at or close to the deep inguinal ring. It supplies the cremaster muscle and the coverings of the spermatic cord. It anastomoses with the internal spermatic artery, and thus provides some blood supply to each testis. It is accompanied by the cremasteric vein, which drains into the inferior epigastric vein of that side. Because of the anastomoses that exist between the cremasteric veins and the pampiniform plexus, the cremasteric veins can also form varicosities that may make up a significant part of a varicocele.

The intratesticular varicocele

This is a rare form of varicocele and it is probable that only five cases have ever been described (Mehta & Dogra 1998). In this condition the varicocele is contained within the testis and can only be diagnosed by means of testicular ultrasound (Ozcan *et al.* 1997), when serpiginous dilated veins can be seen within the testis.

These varices may present clinically with either infertility or testicular pain. Testicular size appears to be normal in these patients. Reversal of the venous blood flow may be seen on Doppler imaging during a Valsalva manoeuvre. It must also be remembered that these lesions can be mistaken for testicular cysts, abscesses or tumours. Dilatation of the rete testis may also resemble an intratesticular varicocele.

The formation of a varicocele

A varicocele is the result of the retrograde reflux of blood down the internal spermatic vein causing dilatation of the pampiniform plexus. Reflux must be present in the venous system before any venous dilatation can be called a varicocele. However, quite how a varicocele forms remains unclear. It was at one time believed that varicocele was caused by the absence of valves in the internal spermatic vein, but it is now known that valves may be absent in the internal spermatic vein in men without varicocele (Wishahi 1991).

Left-sided varicoceles are 10 times more common than those on the right side, but varicoceles can present bilaterally in around 5% of patients. This high incidence of left-sided varicocele is likely to be caused by the right-angled 'T' junction between the left internal spermatic vein and the left renal vein, as such a junction allows reflux from the renal vein down into the internal spermatic vein. Such pressure will gradually cause a dilatation of the internal spermatic vein down its whole length and will then involve the pampiniform plexus.

There are, however, other means by which the formation of a varicocele could be enhanced if not induced. On the left side, a loaded, distended colon may impede the venous return from the testis and so induce distension of the internal spermatic vein. On the right side, venous distension and the impedance of the venous return may also be enhanced by a 'nutcracker' effect that may be applied to the internal spermatic vein by the posterior abdominal wall and the branches of the superior mesenteric artery.

In the large majority of varicoceles, the major part of the venous dilatation occurs in the pampiniform plexus proximal to the formation of the single internal spermatic vein. However, this venous distension may be augmented by a concomitant dilatation of the cremasteric venous system within the inguinal canal. When the dilatation involves the pampiniform plexus alone, the lesion is known as a grade I varicocele, but, if the cremasteric venous system also forms part of the varicocele, it is known as a grade II varicocele. Occasionally, varicosities can form in the cremasteric venous system alone, but these lesions rarely give rise to varicoceles of any size and are not likely to be of great significance clinically.

Possible causes of testicular and epididymal dysfunction in infertile men with varicocele

Several hypotheses have been put forward to explain the suggested relationship between varicocele and infertility. However, it must be remembered that a varicocele may have a variable effect on fertility depending on the individual in whom it occurs and the presence of the many cofactors that might enhance testicular or epididymal dysfunction. There are, however, a number of factors that may play an important role in inducing the infertility that can be associated with the presence of a varicocele.

An increase in testicular temperature

That the dilated vessels of a varicocele cause an increase in the intrascrotal temperature has been the most popular theory to date in the attempt to explain effects of a varicocele on fertility (Tessler & Kahn 1966).

Although there is no doubt that increased testicular temperature has a deleterious effect on sperm production both in man and in experimental animals, the evidence for changes in temperature as the cause of infertility in varicocele is disputed; some clinicians report that no differences in scrotal temperature have been found (Lund & Nielsen 1996) while others have demonstrated a reduction in temperature after varicocele ligation (Wright *et al.* 1997). However, it has also been postulated that the presence of the dilatations in the pampiniform plexus in varicocele may disturb heat between the venous system and the artery. This may result in a slight increase in the temperature of the arterial blood and hence of the temperature of the testis itself. These changes may, however, be dependent upon other pathological changes that may have occurred in the testis, and which are unrelated to the presence of the varicocele (Turner *et al.* 1996).

Despite these data, some authors have claimed that scrotal cooling will improve fertility and semen quality in infertile men with varicocele (Zorgniotti & Macleod 1973).

Impedance of the arterial input

Among patients with large varicoceles, it is possible that the weight of the blood in a varicocele could impede the arterial input into the testis and thus cause infertility by a simple ischaemic change. Using technetium pertechetate perfusion studies, such impedance of the arterial input in men with varicocele has indeed been demonstrated in the past (Comhaire *et al.* 1983). These authors also demonstrated that in men whose semen did not show an improved quality after varicocele ligation, no increase in the arterial blood flow could be demonstrated. However, more recently, using colour Doppler ultrasonography, such a reduction in testicular blood flow has been disputed (Ross *et al.* 1994).

The effect of catecholamines

Significant increases in the concentration of catecholamines have been demonstrated in the testicular blood of men with varicocele, and it has been suggested that this may be the result of blood from the adrenal vein refluxing down the dilated internal spermatic vein from the renal vein (Comhaire & Vermeulen 1974). There may also be a countercurrent exchange of noradrenaline (norepinephrine) between the dilated pampiniform plexus and the testicular artery, which itself could explain a reduction in arterial blood flow that occurs in men with varicocele. Long-term exposure to such vasoconstrictors could also cause endothelial hyperplasia and a permanent reduction in testicular blood flow.

Changes in hormonal levels

Changes in levels of both the gonadotrophins and testosterone have been demonstrated in men with varicocele. Although changes in FSH and LH levels may alter in men with varicocele, these hormones may also change in other causes of infertility that are not associated with varicocele.

In men with varicocele, a minor degree of Leydig cell resistance has been reported and the Leydig cell reserve also seems to be depleted (Ando *et al.* 1984). However, it also appears that the serum testosterone levels may increase significantly following varicocele repair.

The cofactor theory

This theory postulates that before a varicocele can cause a deterioration in semen quality and result in infertility, it must interact with another factor (Peng *et al.* 1990). It is suggested for example that if a varicocele is present together with another toxic factor such as nicotine, a varicocele may then be able to suppress sperm production, and there is indeed some evidence to support such a theory. It is thus possible that the presence of a second pathology may also enhance an otherwise minor effect of the varicocele itself. It is, however, going to be very difficult to separate the effects of each of these factors from one other. Such interactions are, however, likely to be important in the eventual understanding of the mechanism of action of a varicocele and the way in which it induces infertility.

Varicocele as a cause of partial obstruction

It has also been suggested that the dilatations of the pampiniform plexus may cause an incomplete obstruction of the efferent ductules with which it would be in close proximity (Nistal *et al.* 1988). Such patients may thus present with oligozoospermia.

The semen analysis in varicocele

It must be remembered that semen analysis will be normal in the majority of men with a varicocele. The seminal volume, the pH of the ejaculate and its liquefaction are normal.

It was suggested some years ago by Macleod (1965) that varicocele was associated with an increased number of tapered heads among the sperm in the ejaculate, producing the so-called 'stress pattern'. It is now known, however, that there is in fact no pattern of change that can be associated with this possible cause of infertility. Thus, in men with varicocele the changes that may be found in their semen are now thought by many to be nonspecific and, even in the presence of a large varicocele, the semen analysis can be normal (Lemcke *et al.* 1997). The diagnosis of a varicocele thus really cannot be determined from the examination of a sample of semen.

The semen from men with infertility related to varicocele may contain an excess of peroxidase-negative round cells which represent germinal cells that have sloughed into the lumen of the seminiferous tubules and entered the ejaculate. The presence of these immature cells in semen may indicate a disturbance in sperm production by the seminiferous epithelium.

Testicular histology in varicocele

All the changes that may be seen in relation to all the different causes of infertility may be seen on the examination of a testicular biopsy taken from a man with infertility and a varicocele. Testicular histology may vary from a mild impairment of sperm production to testicular atrophy. The more severe the changes in the testicular histology, the less likely will the patient respond to varicocele ligation (Foresta *et al.* 1984). The maturation of the spermatogenic cells is defective and changes may also be seen in the Sertoli cells, which frequently show vacuolation (Cameron *et al.* 1980). It is likely that many of these changes represent a second pathology and are not just the result of the varicocele. The Leydig cells usually remain histologically normal. The histological changes, however, tend to be more severe in the testis on the side of the varicocele than in the contralateral testis.

Endocrine changes in varicocele

Despite their normal appearance, a varicocele is said to interfere with the function of the Leydig cells. The serum testosterone may be at or even below the lower limits of the normal range (Ando *et al.* 1984) and may rise to normal levels after ligation. Despite this reduction in serum testosterone, the serum LH is usually normal.

The serum FSH may be raised if sperm production is severely compromised. However, it is always possible that some of these histological and endocrine changes may occur as the result of a second pathology rather than being the direct effect of the varicocele.

Clinical presentation of a varicocele

Many varicoceles will go unnoticed by the patient but, especially when they are large, they may give rise to an ache in the scrotum. When a varicocele is extremely large, the patient may notice a swelling around the testicle.

Varicoceles are usually described in relation to their size. They may be reported as large, moderate or small, although there are other clinicians who use the terms grade I, grade II and grade III to describe their dimensions. It must be remembered that in some clinics, the terms grade I and grade II are simply subdivisions created at surgery and relate only to the presence or absence of a cremasteric input to the dilated venous plexus. There are also subclinical varicoceles, which are clinically undetectable and which need technical aids such as radiology for their demonstration. It is now believed that subclinical varicoceles do not induce infertility.

Clinical varicoceles are detected by palpation of the scrotum in the standing position. The venous distension is accentuated by asking the patient to perform the Valsalva manoeuvre, during which the examining clinician can feel the increasing distension of the dilated plexus. The distension will also completely disappear when the patient lies down. Palpation of the testes may reveal them to be small, and this change in size is usually asymmetric, the testis on the side of the varicocele often being smaller than the testis on the opposite side.

Other methods of demonstrating the presence of a varicocele

The diagnosis of a varicocele can be confirmed in a number of different ways and these techniques can also be used to demonstrate the presence of a subclinical varicocele.

Doppler echography

These techniques, which can be used in the clinic, enable one to demonstrate the size and direction of flow of blood within the pampiniform plexus and is a simple and effective way to demonstrate the presence of a varicocele (Fig. 8.2). As the internal spermatic artery is situated within the pampiniform plexus, its presence on the Doppler display indicates the correct position of the probe. After siting the artery, the patient, who is lying in the supine position, is asked to carry out a Valsalva manoeuvre when the reversal of flow in the venous plexus can be demonstrated. Often at this point, especially among patients with large varicoceles, the arterial flow is masked by this venous reflux.

The blood flow in and out of the testis can also be imaged using colour flow and power Doppler imaging of the testes (Dubinsky *et al.* 1998) and this can be useful in an attempting to quantify, at least approximately, the blood flow in the testis. This facet of ultrasonography can also be valuable in the diagnosis of torsion of the testis, where the blood flow will be at or close to nil.

Retrograde venography

This method of demonstrating a varicocele provides the clinician with a very detailed picture of this venous anomaly; however, it is a very invasive procedure that probably should never be carried out for diagnostic pur-

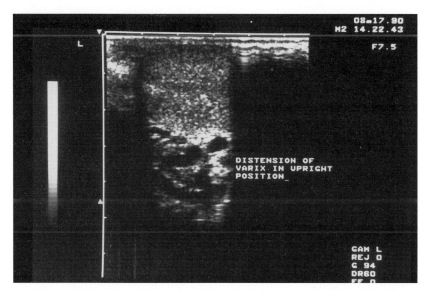

DISTENSION OF
VARIX IN UPRIGHT
POSITION_

Fig. 8.2 An ultrasound image of the scrotum showing the presence of a varicocele. Note its close relationship with the epididymis.

poses alone but only when it forms part of the therapeutic process of embolization of a varicocele (Comhaire *et al*. 1981b). Under radiological screening and under local anaesthesia, a Seldinger catheter is inserted into the right femoral vein and advanced via the inferior vena cava, from where it can be directed into the left renal vein and then into the internal spermatic vein. After injection of contrast medium up the catheter at appropriate sites and with the patient carrying out the Valsalva manoeuvre, the exact extent of the varicocele on either side can be demonstrated and the reflux down the internal spermatic vein can be confirmed.

Venous scintigraphy

In this technique, the presence of a radioisotope within the venous system allows the demonstration of the pooling of blood within the pampiniform plexus (Comhaire *et al*. 1981b). This type of investigation is also useful for the study of the arterial perfusion of the testis in patients with many conditions other than varicocele that cause infertility.

A 15-mCi dose of the isotope technetium-99 pertechnetate is injected intravenously and the activity over the scrotal region is imaged using a static scanner. The pooling of blood caused by a varicocele in either hemiscrotum is easily demonstrated.

The selection of patients for treatment of varicocele

Not all patients with varicocele need treatment. Some men present with

145

this condition complaining of testicular ache and this symptom is indeed frequently relieved by ligation. If an infertile patient presents with oligozoospermia, slightly reduced testicular size and a normal serum FSH level, then response to ligation in terms of an improved semen analysis can be expected. If, however, the varicocele is associated with azoospermia, very reduced testicular size and a raised serum FSH level, any response to ligation in terms of fertility will be unlikely.

The clinical management of a varicocele

The treatment of a varicocele must involve the obliteration of the reflux of blood down the internal spermatic vein and therefore must involve the obstruction or the ligation of this vessel. This result can be accomplished in a number of different ways.

Surgical ligation

In the past, and using macrosurgery and not microsurgery, the pampiniform plexus was ligated within the scrotum. However, the high incidence of haematoma using this approach and also the possibility of damage to the spermatic artery close to the testis with its attendant risk of testicular atrophy have made this surgical approach very unpopular. As a consequence this operation has now been abandoned. There are today four approaches to varicocele ligation.

The inguinal operation

In this technique, the dilated veins of the pampiniform are ligated within the inguinal canal.

A 5-cm incision is made over the inguinal canal to expose the aponeurosis that forms the anterior wall of the canal (Fig. 8.3). The aponeurosis is incised over the canal, taking care not to damage the ilioinguinal nerve that lies on the anterior surface of the cord. The cord is then elevated up out of the wound. The thin covering of the cord is incised and the veins are then very carefully dissected out of the cord. At this point the internal spermatic artery lies posteriorly and is thus reasonably safe from damage. The veins in the cord are identified, dissected out, cut and ligated, usually with catgut. Prior to closure, the cremasteric vein can be inspected and, if this is clearly dilated, it can also be ligated and cut.

The cord is then replaced back into the canal and the wound is closed taking care not to compress the cord within the canal when closing the aponeurosis. The aponeurosis is best closed using polyglactin (Vicryl, Ethicon Ltd). Most patients who have undergone this procedure can go home on the same day.

High ligation operation

This approach was popularized by Palomo (1949) and later by Ivanissavich (1960). In this operation, the vessels are ligated above the inguinal ring (Fig. 8.3).

A transverse incision is made just above and lateral to the anterior superior iliac spine. The fibres of the underlying muscles are split to expose the peritoneum. The peritoneum is now retracted medially to expose the spermatic vein on its undersurface. At this point the spermatic vein is some distance from both the internal spermatic artery and the vas deferens, which are thus safe from injury.

Interestingly, damage to the spermatic artery at this point appears to make little difference to testicular function, doubtless because of the extensive anastomoses that exist between the spermatic and the cremasteric arterial systems both in the inguinal canal and within the cord. Indeed, ligation of the artery at this point has been suggested as a means of reducing the blood flow through the testes and hence reducing the venous return. At this point the internal spermatic vein has usually been reduced to a single vessel, which is now clamped, cut and tied.

The single disadvantage of this technique is that one cannot inspect and, if necessary, ligate any part of the varicocele that involves the cremasteric vein. However, it appears to be a satisfactory way in which to repair a varicocele (Magdar *et al.* 1995).

Laparoscopic ligation

This operation is now a very popular way in which to carry out a varicocele ligation (Winfield & Donovan 1992).

In this technique, the vein is identified laparoscopically at a point above the deep inguinal ring. The peritoneum on the anterior abdominal wall is

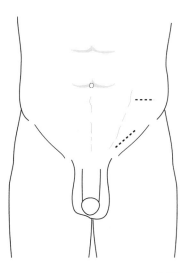

Fig. 8.3 A diagrammatic illustration of the sites of the common incisions used in the surgical approach to varicocele ligation. These are marked with dotted lines.

147

first incised. The vessel that lies beneath it is then clamped and its lumen is usually obliterated by bipolar diathermy. Alternatively, the vein can be occluded using some form of haemostatic clip. However, care must be taken not to damage the vas deferens as it curves around the medial edge of the deep inguinal ring where it lies close to the spermatic veins.

The main disadvantage of this method is that it takes much longer to complete than the other two surgical approaches and the surgeon cannot identify or treat any concomitant dilation of the cremasteric venous system. Like the other techniques described above, laparoscopic varicocele ligation is carried out on a 'day case' basis and is a safe and efficient way in which to ligate a varicocele (Tan *et al.* 1995).

Subinguinal microsurgical ligation

This technique involves the microsurgical ligation of each of the dilated veins in the spermatic cord and this is carried out through a 2-cm incision in the scrotum. It may be carried out under either local or general anaesthesia. After opening the inguinal canal, all dilated vessels within the pampiniform plexus are sought in the cremasteric fascia and ligated. The cord is now exposed and elevated out through the wound and dilated posterior cremasteric vessels are now clamped with haemostatic clips and ligated. The dilated veins within the spermatic cord are now isolated in groups and carefully identified before being clamped and ligated. Care is taken to make sure that the spermatic artery is not included in the procedure of ligation. During the course of this operation, the vasal veins are also identified and ligated. The wound may then be closed in the usual way.

This procedure therefore conserves the testicular arterial supply and preserves the lymphatic drainage of the testis. This latter advantage may reduce the incidence of hydrocele postoperatively. It is also likely to minimize the incidence of scrotal haematoma. Because of the accurate identification of even the smallest dilated vein within the spermatic cord, the recurrence rate of the varicocele is said to be substantially reduced and the pregnancy rate following the use of this technique may also be increased.

Percutaneous treatment of varicocele

The percutaneous approach to the treatment of varicocele has become a much used and a very useful way of managing this condition (Ferguson *et al.* 1995). The internal spermatic vein is approached via either the jugular vein or more commonly from the right femoral vein and the inferior vena cava (Fig. 8.4).

These procedures are best carried out under general anaesthesia. A standard Seldinger needle is used to introduce a no. 9 French vascular catheter into the femoral vein. A no. 7 French catheter is now introduced through the sheath and guided radiologically into the internal spermatic vein. Reflux

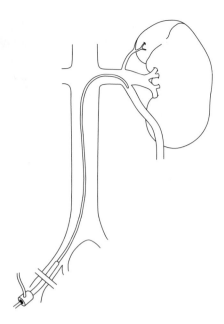

Fig. 8.4 The percutaneous approach to the left internal spermatic vein used for the injection of sclerosing and other agents that are used to occlude the internal spermatic vein in men with varicocele.

can now be demonstrated on X-ray by asking the anaesthetist to maintain the patient in inspiration for a few seconds. A variety of different methods of occlusion of the internal spermatic vein can now be employed.

Solid devices

A wide variety of devices have been designed to occlude the internal spermatic vein in the treatment of varicocele. These include stainless steel coils, Dacron plugs and detachable mini-balloons that are made of silicone. Such devices inserted into the internal spermatic vein cause the formation of a thrombus and thus occlude the vein. They are introduced by means of an intravenous catheter, the size of the occlusive device being chosen to produce a snug fit into the internal spermatic vein. All these devices are relatively easy to insert but tend to be reasonably expensive to purchase.

The insertion is carried out under radiological control. A standard Seldinger catheter is used to introduce a no. 9 French gauge vascular catheter into the femoral vein. A no. 7 French gauge catheter is now inserted into the no. 9 catheter and advanced into the inferior vena cava and from there into the internal spermatic vein on either the left or the right side. The reflux can now be demonstrated using contrast and by asking the patient to carry out a Valsalva manoeuvre. The device is then introduced into the internal spermatic vein using a wire to advance the device out of the catheter.

Sclerosing agents

Agents that induce thrombosis can also be used in the treatment of varicocele. These are also introduced by means of a radiologically controlled catheterization of the internal spermatic vein. The most commonly used agent in this technique is a substance that is a mixture of sodium morrhate and benzyl alcohol. Other substances used in this way include sodium tetradecyl sulphate and absolute alcohol. The sclerosant is introduced into the vein while the spermatic cord is compressed to prevent the spread of the sclerosant down the vein and into the testis. Sclerosants are able to occlude the internal spermatic vein in around 90% of all patients so treated. They also have the advantage that, unlike the devices that may be inserted into the vein, they do not embolize or migrate. However, atrophy of the testis has been described in relation to this use of sclerosants (Wegner *et al*. 1996).

Fibrin plugs

Plugs of fibrin may also be used to occlude the internal spermatic vein. These are also introduced by means of an intravenous catheter. These are a useful means of occluding the internal spermatic vein and have the advantage of being relatively cheap.

Complications of varicocele surgery

There are several well-known complications of varicocele surgery.

Hydrocele formation

The commonest complication of varicocele surgery is the development of a hydrocele which may be seen in around 7–9% of all cases (Goldstein *et al*. 1992; Mellinger 1995). Hydroceles are usually only seen after surgical treatment and are never seen after percutaneous occlusion. Their presence may relate to the interference in the lymphatic drainage of the testis that may occur during a varicocele operation. These hydroceles are not usually large and rarely need any treatment.

Testicular atrophy

Testicular atrophy should never be seen after varicocele surgery and indeed never occurs after any of the percutaneous methods of treatment. Whenever surgery for varicocele is carried out in the groin area the internal spermatic artery should be sought and preserved.

Vasal damage

Vasal damage has also been reported after laparoscopic varicocele ligation, but this problem can be avoided if careful identification of all the structures around the deep inguinal ring is made prior to diathermy.

As can happen in any operation, the formation of a haematoma can occur. However, this is uncommon in varicocele surgery. The complication of the percutaneous route really only involves the formation of a haematoma at the site of the puncture of the femoral vein.

There is little doubt today that at least some varicoceles are indeed a cause of infertility and that their ligation will improve semen quality in some patients. The aetiology of varicocele and the means by which it causes infertility remains obscure. The identification of those infertile men who will benefit from varicocele ligation continues to be a problem.

The problem of the recurrent varicocele

A varicocele may recur after surgery. This is almost never caused by recanalization of the vein even after percutaneous therapy but is a result of either an inadequate ligation of all of the vessels involved in the production of the varicocele or the subsequent development of reflux into a smaller collateral vein.

The varicocele in the child and adolescent

It is not uncommon for a varicocele to present and even become symptomatic in an adolescent. Its presence can cause embarrassment in the changing rooms at school and even in a child can cause pain or a dull ache in the testicle.

There appears to be little doubt that in a child, a varicocele may impair the natural increase in testicular size that occurs at puberty (Rivilla & Casillas 1997) and that repair of the varicocele returns that growth to normal (Kass & Reitelman 1995). Most paediatric surgeons now feel that where a varicocele in an adolescent or in a child appears to be reducing the size of a testis either unilaterally or bilaterally, then ligation or embolization of the internal spermatic vein is indicated.

References

Ando, S., Giachetto, C., Beraldi, E. *et al.* (1984) The influence of age on Leydig cell function in patients with varicocele. *International Journal of Andrology* **7**, 104–118.

Ashkenazi, J., Dicker, D., Feldberg, D., Shelef, M., Goldman, G.A. & Goldman, J. (1989) The impact of spermatic vein ligation on the male factor in *in vitro* fertilization–embryo transfer and its relation to testosterone levels before and after operation. *Fertility and Sterility* **51**, 471–474.

Baker, H.W.G., Burger, H.G., de Kretser, D.M., Hudson, B., Rennie, G.C. & Straffon, W.G.E. (1985) Testicular vein ligation and fertility in men with varicoceles. *British Medical Journal* **291**, 1678–1680.

Cameron, D.F., Snydle, F.E., Ross, M.H. & Drylie, D.M. (1980) Ultrastructural alterations in the adluminal testicular compartment in men with varicocele. *Fertility and Sterility* **33**, 526–533.

Chehval, M.J. & Purcell, M.H. (1992) Deterioration of semen parameters with time in men with untreated varicocele: evidence for progressice testicular damage. *Fertility and Sterility* **57**, 174–177.

Comhaire, F.H. (1986) Varicocele and its role in male infertility. In: *Oxford Reviews in Reproductive Biology*, Vol. 8 (ed. J.R. Clarke), pp. 165–213. Oxford University Press, Oxford.

Comhaire, F., Kunnen, M. & Nahoum, C. (1981a) Radiological anatomy of the internal spermatic vein (s) in 200 retrograde venograms. *International Journal of Andrology* **4**, 379–387.

Comhaire, F.H., Kunnen, M. & Vermeulen, L. (1983) Testicular arterial perfusion in varicocele: the role of rapid sequence scintigraphy with technetium in varicocele evaluation. *Journal of Urology* **130**, 923–926.

Comhaire, F., Simons, M., Kunnen, M. & Vermeulen, L. (1981b) Testicular arterial perfusion in varicocele: the role of rapid sequence scinitgraphy with technetium in varicocele evaluation. *Journal of Urology* **130**, 923–926.

Comhaire, F.H. & Vermeulen, A. (1974) Varicocele sterility: cortisol and catecholamines. *Fertility and Sterility* **25**, 88–95.

Dubinsky, T.J., Chen, P. & Maklad, N. (1998) Color-flow and power Doppler imaging of the testes. *World Journal of Urology* **16**, 35–40.

Ferguson, J.M., Gillespie, I.N., Chalmers, N., Elton, R. & Hargreave, T.B. (1995) Percutaneous varicocele embolization in the treatment of infertility. *British Journal of Radiology* **68**, 700–703.

Foresta, C., Ruzza, G., Rizzotti, A., Lembo, A., Valente, M.L. & Mastrogiacomo, I. (1984) Varicocele and infertility. Pre-operative prognostic elements. *Journal of Andrology* **5**, 135–147.

Goldstein, M., Gilbert, B.R., Dicker, A.P., Dwosh, J. & Gnecco, C. (1992) Microsurgical inguinal varicocelectomy with delivery of the testis: an artery and lymphatic sparing technique. *Journal of Urology* **148**, 1808–1811.

Handelsman, D.J., Conway, A.J., Boylan, L.M. & Turtle, J.R. (1984) Testicular function in potential sperm donors: normal ranges and the effects of smoking and varicocele. *International Journal of Andrology* **7**, 369–382.

Hargreave, T.B. (1995) Debate on the pros and cons of varicocele treatment in favour of varicocele treatment. *Human Reproduction* (**Suppl. 1**) (10), 151–157.

Hendry, W.F. (1992) Effects of left varicocele ligation in subfertile males with absent or atrophic testes. *Fertility and Sterility* **57**, 1342–1343.

Hsu, H.S., Wei, Y.H., Li, A.F., Chen, M.T. & Chang, L.S. (1995) Defective mitochondrial phophorylation in varicocele-bearing testicles. *Urology* **46**, 545–549.

Ivanissavich, O. (1960) Left varicocele due to reflux. Experience with 4709 operative cases in 42 years. *Journal of the International College of Surgeons* **34**, 742–745.

Jarow, J.P., Ogle, S.R. & Eskew, L.A. (1996) Seminal improvement following repair of ultrasound detected subclinical varicoceles. *Journal of Urology* **155**, 1287–1290.

Kass, E.J. & Reitelman, C. (1995) Adolescent varicocele. *Urologic Clinics of North America* **22**, 151–159.

Lemcke, B., Behre, H.M. & Nieschlag, E. (1997) Frequently subnormal semen profiles of normal volunteers recruited over 17 years. *International Journal of Andrology* **20**, 144–152.

Lund, L. & Nielsen, K.T. (1996) Varicocele testis and testicular temperature. *British Journal of Urology* **78**, 113–115.

Macleod, J. (1965) Seminal cytology in the presence of varicocele. *Fertility and Sterility* **16**, 735–757.

Magdar, I., Weissenberg, R., Lunenfeld, B., Karsik, A. & Goldwasser, B. (1995) Controlled trial of high spermatic vein ligation for varicocele in infertile men. *Fertility and Sterility* **63**, 120–124.

Mehta, A.L. & Dogra, V.S. (1998) Intratesticular varicocele. *Journal of Clinical Ultrasound* **26**, 49–51.

Mellinger, B.C. (1995) Varicocelectomy. *Techniques in Urology* **1**, 188–196.

Nieschlag, E., Hertle, L., Fischedick, A. & Behre, H.M. (1995) Treatment of varicocele:

counselling is as effective as occlusion of the vena spermatica. *Human Reproduction* **10**, 347–353.

Nilsson, S., Edvinson, A. & Nilsson, B. (1979) Improvement of semen and pregnancy rate afterligation and division of the internal spermatic vein; fact or fiction? *British Journal of Urology* **51**, 591–596.

Nistal, M., Paniagua, R., Regadera, J. & Santamaria, L. (1984) Obstruction of the tubuli recti and ductuli efferentes by dilated veins in the testes of men with varicocele and its possible role in causing atrophy of the seminiferous tubules. *International Journal of Andrology* **7**, 309–323.

Ozcan, H., Aytac, S., Yagci, C., Turkolmez, K., Kosar, A. & Erden, I. (1997) Color Doppler ultrasonographic findings in intratesticular varicocele. *Journal of Clinical Ultrasound* **25**, 325–329.

Palomo, A. (1949) Radical cure of varicocele by a new technique: preliminary report. *Journal of Urology* **61**, 604–607.

Peng, B.C.H., Tomashevsky, P. & Nagler, H.M. (1990) The co-factor effect: varicocele and infertility. *Fertility and Sterility* **54**, 145–148.

Rivilla, F. & Casillas, J.G. (1997) Testicular size following therapy for paediatric left varicocele. *Scandinavian Journal of Urology and Nephrology* **31**, 63–65.

Ross, J.A., Watson, N.E. & Jarow, J. (1994) the effect of varicoceles on testicular blood flow in man. *Urology* **44**, 535–530.

Sigman, M. & Jarow, J. (1997) Ipsilateral testicular hypotrophy is associated with decreased sperm counts in infertile men with varicoceles. *Journal of Urology* **158**, 605–607.

Steckel, J., Dicker, A.P. & Goldstein, M. (1993) Relationship between varicoele size and reponse to varicoelectomy. *Journal of Urology* **149**, 769–771.

Tan, S.M., Ng, F.C., Ravintharan, T., Lim, P.H. & Chang, H.C. (1995) Laparoscopic varicocelectomy: technique and results. *British Journal of Urology* **75**, 523–528.

Tessler, A.N. & Kahn, H.P. (1966) Varicocele and testicular temperature. *Fertility and Sterility* **17**, 201–203.

Tulloch, W.S. (1955) Varicocele in subfertility: results of treatment. *British Medical Journal* **2**, 536.

Turner, T.T., Caplis, L. & Miller, D.W. (1996) Testicular microvascular blood flow: alteration after Leydig cell eradication and ischaemia but not varicocele. *Journal of Andrology* **17**, 239–248.

Wegner, H.E., Meier, T. & Miller, K. (1996) Testicular necrosis after antegrade sclerotherapy of varicocele. *International Urology and Nephrology* **28**, 357–358.

Winfield, H.N. & Donovan, J.F. (1992) Laparoscopic varicocelectomy. *Seminars in Urology* **10**, 152–160.

Wishahi, M.M. (1991) Anatomy of the venous drainage of the human testis: testicular vein cast, microdissection and radiographic demonstration. a new anatomical concept. *European Urology* **20**, 154–160.

World Health Organization (1985) Comparision among different methods of diagnosis of varicocele. *Fertility and Sterility* **43**, 575–582.

Wright, E.J., Young, G.P. & Goldstein, M. (1997) Reduction in testicular temperature after varicocelectomy in infertile men. *Urology* **50**, 257–259.

Zalata, A., Hafez, T. & Comhaire, F. (1995) Evaluation of the role of reactive oxygen species in male infertility. *Human Reproduction* **10**, 1444–1451.

Zorgniotti, A.W. & Macleod, J. (1973) Studies in temperature, human semen quality and varicocele. *Fertility and Sterility* **24**, 854–863.

9: Endocrine Causes of Infertility in the Male

Endocrine disease is an uncommon cause of infertility in men: in only some 2% of patients with an abnormal semen analysis will a primary endocrine cause be found to be at the root of the problem. In the management of the infertile male, it is, however, important to understand how the common endocrinopathies may cause testicular and sexual dysfunction. Normal function of the gonads is dependent upon an adequate production of the trophic hormones by the anterior pituitary gland. Thus, normal activity of the gonads can be interrupted by reduced gonadotrophin secretion but may also be altered by abnormal gonadal responses to gonadotrophins as well as by the interaction of other nongonadal endocrine abnormalities on the hypothalamic–pituitary–gonadal axis.

In this section, the common endocrine disorders that may occur in men and their action on fertility will be discussed. The diagnosis of these conditions and the manner in which they may induce infertility will be described.

Pituitary tumours

There are a number of different tumours of the pituitary that can give rise to infertility in the male.

Acromegaly

Acromegaly is an uncommon disease with an incidence of only 2–4 per million of the population and is predominantly seen among women (Alexander *et al.* 1980) and in the middle aged. It is thus only rarely seen among men attending an infertility clinic. However, young men can occasionally suffer from this disorder and infertility and sexual dysfunction are common among such patients.

Causation of infertility in acromegaly

The disease of acromegaly is caused by the overproduction of growth hormone by the anterior pituitary gland and is usually associated with the growth of an acidophil adenoma of the pituitary. The serum prolactin may also be elevated in these patients (Franks *et al.* 1976) and thus galactorrhoea may also occur among these men. This rise in serum prolactin may be either caused by the concurrent production of prolactin by the growth

154

hormone secreting pituitary adenoma or because of hypothalamic dysfunction resulting from the suprasellar extension of that adenoma and the consequent reduction in dopamine production by the hypothalamus. Hyperprolactinaemia in men results in a reduction in the serum testosterone levels and also induces a relative LH deficiency. These two factors will result in hypo-androgenization and sexual dysfunction. An elevation of the serum prolactin is more commonly, but not exclusively, seen among acromegalic men who are impotent.

A further factor in acromegaly that may give rise to sexual dysfunction is the presence of diabetes mellitus. Growth hormone is a diabetogenic hormone and clinical diabetes may be present in some 10–20% of acromegalic patients (Nabarro 1987); indeed, some of these patients may even require insulin therapy. It is thus possible that the diabetes associated with acromegaly may at least contribute to the sexual dysfunction that is so often seen in male patients with this disorder.

Clinical presentation of acromegaly

Patients with acromegaly complain of general fatigue, of enlarged hands and feet and of coarsening of the skin. Vision may be disturbed and, because of an overgrowth of the facial bones, a variety of maxillary sinus and dental problems can also arise. Impotence and loss of libido occur in around one-third of men with this disease (Eastman *et al.* 1979; Nabarro 1987) and this is probably one of the major causes of infertility in these men.

Because of the reduction of the serum testosterone in men with acromegaly, sperm production and motility may be reduced. Thus, the infertility in men with acromegaly may be caused by an abnormal semen analysis as well as the presence of sexual dysfunction.

Treatment of acromegaly

The treatment of the infertility associated with acromegaly is clearly closely related to the treatment of the acromegaly itself. Pituitary adenomata may be removed surgically or reduced in size by radiotherapy, both of which will not only reduce growth hormone production but also that of prolactin (Tsuchiya *et al.* 1985). Treatment with dopamine agonists such as bromocriptine can also shrink tumour size and may normalize the levels of both growth hormone and prolactin in serum. Surprisingly, there are patients who, despite a return of the growth hormone levels to normal, remain impotent; likewise, there are some acromegalic men whose prolactin remains high but who retain normal sexual function and potency.

Thus, it would appear that there are a variety of factors present in men with this disorder that influence sexual function and the occurrence of hypogonadism in acromegaly.

Cushing's disease

In the condition known as Cushing's disease, the anterior pituitary gland secretes excessive quantities of adrenocorticotrophic hormone (ACTH) and in 75% of patients with this disorder a pituitary adenoma can be demonstrated (Cushing 1932). As a consequence of the high ACTH secretion, the adrenal gland produces excessive amounts of cortisol. It must also be remembered that hypercortisolism can also occur in primary adrenal hyperplasia or as the result of the administration of large doses of corticosteroids for a variety of different therapeutic reasons.

Cushing's disease is much less common in men than in women, the male–female ratio being only 1:8. This condition will thus only rarely be seen in men with infertility.

Causation of infertility in cushing's disease

In male patients with Cushing's disease, there is usually a reduction in both LH and testosterone levels in serum. The LH and FSH responses to gonadotrophin-releasing hormone are also blunted (Luton *et al.* 1977). As the result of these changes, these men show signs of hypogonadism.

There are in fact few reports concerning Cushing's disease and testicular function but in a small number of men who have been studied, oligozoospermia was frequently encountered. Testicular histology usually shows the presence of hypospermatogenesis. The seminiferous tubular basement membranes are often thickened and the Leydig cells are reduced in number (Gavrilove *et al.* 1974).

The infertility may also be enhanced by the presence of hyperprolactinaemia. Although concurrent secretion of prolactin and ACTH within a pituitary adenoma may occur in this disorder, hyperprolactinaemia in men with Cushing's disease would seem to be uncommon.

Clinical presentation of Cushing's disease

Patients with Cushing's disease may complain of muscle weakness, of increasing amounts of centrally distributed fat and also some patients with this disorder may suffer from psychiatric disturbances.

Sexual dysfunction is very common among men with Cushing's disease, and indeed this was even reported by Harvey Cushing in his original paper on this subject. Loss of libido and a reduction in potency occurs in more than half the men with this condition (Luton *et al.* 1977).

On clinical examination, these men are overweight and show obvious body striae over the abdomen and thighs. Hypertension is always present and may be severe.

Treatment of Cushing's disease

Surgical removal of the pituitary adenoma results in a prompt rise in serum levels of LH and testosterone. Secondary hypopituitarism seems to be uncommon following pituitary surgery for Cushing's disease. The ablation of the pituitary tumour can also be achieved using irradiation therapy. Consequent normalization of adrenal function will result in a rapid recovery in terms of both sexual function and semen quality.

However, infertility in these patients may be worsened by the preoperative use of aminoglutethimide, which blocks the conversion of cholesterol to pregnenolone, and which may further reduce testosterone secretion.

Where no adenoma of the pituitary exists, this condition must be treated medically, and for this purpose ketoconazole is used. This substance also blocks steroid synthesis. Therapy with ketoconazole has been shown to reduce serum levels of both free and bound testosterone and also causes a marked reduction in sperm numbers in semen (Pont *et al.* 1984). Thus, not only does Cushing's disease cause infertility but this may be worsened by the medical methods used to control the hypercortisolism.

Hyperprolactinaemia

Unlike its counterpart in women, hyperprolactinaemia is an uncommon disorder among men. Estimates of the incidence of hyperprolactinaemia vary greatly between clinics (Jequier *et al.* 1979) and may depend upon the definition of hyperprolactinaemia. One infertility clinic failed to identify a single case of hyperprolactinaemia from a very large number of men with abnormal semen analyses (Hargreave *et al.* 1981).

Because the presentation of hyperprolactinaemia in men tends to be more subtle than its counterpart in women, the condition can have been present for many years prior to diagnosis. Thus, pituitary tumours in hyperprolactinaemic men tend to be surprisingly large (Fig. 9.1). Suprasellar

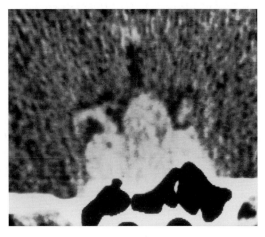

Fig. 9.1 A magnetic resonance image of a very large pituitary prolactinoma showing massive suprasellar extension. This tumour was found in a patient who presented with sexual dysfunction. The serum prolactin level was very raised. The insidious onset of hyperprolactinaemia in the male allows such tumours to grow to a great size before they are detected. (Published by kind permission of Dr Peter Pullan, PhD, FRACP.)

157

extension is also very common (Franks *et al.* 1978). Such large tumours often cause loss of the peripheral vision and they may even invade the cavernous sinuses producing various types of ophthalmoplegia.

Another cause of hyperprolactinaemia is a condition known as the empty sella syndrome. This disorder is cause by a herniation of the dura and the subarachnoid space into the sella turcica. It can also be the result of a degenerated pituitary adenoma.

Other causes of hyperprolactinaemia in men include ingestion of any of the many drugs that raise serum prolactin. Serum prolactin may also be elevated in conditions such as renal failure and hypothyroidism. It must not be forgotten that sexual dysfunction and a raised serum prolactin are also associated with the presence of other forms of pituitary disease such as acromegaly and Cushing's disease.

Causation of infertility in hyperprolactinaemia

The excess secretion of prolactin results in reduced secretion of LH and a decrease in the frequency of the LH pulses. There is thus an overall reduction of LH secretion resulting in a reduction in testosterone secretion. Serum testosterone levels are low and the testosterone responses to human chorionic gonadotrophin (hCG) are also impaired. Thus hyperprolactinaemia may present with a low sperm count and infertility (Merino *et al.* 1997), although interestingly hyperprolactinaemia appears to have little effect on sperm function (Okada *et al.* 1996).

Other causes of infertility may also be found among hyperprolactinaemic men: these include retrograde ejaculation (Ishikawa *et al.* 1993) and even epididymal obstruction (Jequier *et al.* 1979). Hyperprolactinaemia is also frequently seen in patients in renal failure (Lim 1994).

Clinical presentation of hyperprolactinaemia

Patients with hyperprolactinaemia usually present with a variety of forms of sexual dysfunction such as impotence, loss of libido and disorders of ejaculation (Franks *et al.* 1978). As any pituitary tumour may be large, these men can also present with headaches and loss of peripheral vision. Gynaecomastia and galactorrhoea may also be seen among these patients but this is uncommon because of both the absence of oestrogen stimulation of the breast and also the small amounts of breast tissue present in men.

The investigation of these men is similar to that used in women. The exclusion of thyroid disease and of the other associated causes of pituitary disease is very important. Because of the high incidence of pituitary tumours in these men, examination of the pituitary using either computerized tomography (CT) or magnetic resonance imaging (MRI) is essential.

158

Treatment of hyperprolactinaemia

The treatment of hyperprolactinaemia in men is essentially the same as that in women. Because of the large size of these pituitary tumours in men as well as the high incidence of both recurrence and postoperative hypogonadotrophic hypogonadism following surgery, hyperprolactinaemia in this group of patients is best treated medically. The dopamine agonist cabergoline (Dostinex, Pharmacia and Upjohn Ltd) is the first line of treatment and is given in doses ranging from 0.5 to 2 mg per week. The better-known drug bromocriptine can also be used for this purpose. Even very large tumours will respond well to this type of therapy, but treatment may need to be lifelong.

However, despite restoration of the serum prolactin to normal, the serum testosterone in some men may remain low and such individuals may require testosterone replacement therapy to normalize sexual function. Sexual dysfunction may also persist in these men even when the testosterone levels do return to normal, and it has been suggested that prolonged hyperprolactinaemia may induce a degree of androgen resistance.

In many hyperprolactinaemic patients, especially those receiving testosterone replacement, the hypospermatogenesis that is causing infertility will also require treatment using gonadotrophins as endogenous LH secretion will be suppressed by the testosterone therapy. Thus, in severely hyperprolactinaemic men, a return to normal cannot be guaranteed either in terms of sexual function nor fertility.

Gonadotrophin-secreting pituitary tumours

The anterior pituitary gland contains gonadotrophin-producing cells known as gonadotrophs that secrete both LH and FSH. The secretions of the gonadotrophs are modulated by the secretions of the gonads. Just occasionally, however, gonadotroph adenomata can form within the anterior pituitary and produce excessive amounts of FSH and LH (Snyder 1987). Should this happen in an infertile man, it can lead to considerable diagnostic confusion (Table 9.1).

Gonadotroph cell adenomata were at one time thought to be a rarity but they are now reported to make up as much as 17% of all large pituitary tumours (Snyder 1985). How these tumours are initiated is unknown but they seem to be more common among men than women. The age range of patients with this disorder is wide, and a gonadotrophin-secreting adenoma has even been reported in a child with precocious puberty. However, they seem to occur predominantly in men over 40 years and are thus unlikely to present in an infertility clinic. Most of these tumours secrete FSH alone including both its α- and β-subunits but there can also be limited secretion of the β-subunit of LH. The serum LH and therefore the serum testosterone levels will be normal in these patients, as will the testosterone response to hCG.

159

Table 9.1 The differentiation of an FSH-secreting pituitary adenoma from secondary hypergonadotrophism due to primary testicular disease

	Gonadotroph adenoma	Primary testicular disease
Age	Usually > 40 years	Usually < 40 years
Testis size	Normal	Reduced
Fertility	Normal	Reduced
Sexual function	Usually normal	Usually normal
Serum FSH	Raised	Raised
Serum LH	Normal	Normal or raised
Testosterone	Normal	Normal or raised
FSH response	Enhanced	Normal or enhanced
Testosterone	Normal	Normal or impaired
FSH response to TRH	Enhanced	Normal
Testosterone response to hCG	Normal	Normal or impaired

Clinical presentation of gonadotrophin-secreting tumours

In the adult male, excess FSH secretion will produce few symptoms and thus patients with this lesion are frequently undetected until the tumour has reached a considerable size. Such tumours may thus present only when chiasmal compression and suprasellar extension has occurred and the intracranial pressure is elevated. Men with this tumour may appear to be clinically normal and fertility is usually unimpaired. However, major degrees of suprasellar extension in these men may result in a secondary hyperprolactinaemia.

Serum FSH levels will of course be elevated in men with primary testicular disease. Thus, care must be taken not to assume that high levels of FSH in serum always indicate the presence of testicular pathology, as very rarely they may indicate the presence of a gonadotrophin-secreting tumour of the pituitary. The important differences are that many with these tumours usually have normal sized testes and a normal semen analysis. One interesting feature of this condition is an enhancement in the release of FSH in response to a bolus dose of thyrotropin releasing hormone (TRH) and indeed this response may be of use diagnostically (Snyder 1993). The differences between a gonadotrophin-secreting adenoma and primary testicular disease are outlined in Table 9.1.

These tumours, as are all adenomata of the pituitary, are best imaged using either a CT scan of the pituitary or by MRI.

Causation of infertility in men with gonadotrophin-secreting pituitary tumours

The only way that these tumours can cause infertility is by inducing hyperprolactinaemia or perhaps by the concurrent presence of another pathology. For the most part these patients retain their fertility, and the only major problem among men with this condition is the confusion that the raised serum FSH levels can bring about.

Treatment of men with gonadotrophin-secreting tumours

Treatment of these tumours can be carried out by either transphenoidal surgery or irradiation of the pituitary fossa (Snyder 1993). However, it is known that a reduction in tumour size will occur following treatment with bromocryptine (Snyder 1985) and this is now the standard treatment for most prolactin-secreting pituitary adenomata.

Hypogonadotrophic hypogonadism

Lesions of either the hypothalamus or of the anterior pituitary will result in a loss of gonadotrophin secretion. Hypothalamic lesions will reduce or obliterate the production of gonadotrophin-releasing hormone (GnRH), while impaired pituitary function will in turn reduce or prevent a response in terms of gonadotrophin secretion. Loss of gonadotrophin production will thus result in reduced function of the gonad causing the condition known as hypogonadotrophic hypogonadism, in which both the pituitary as well as the gonadal secretions are impaired or even absent altogether.

Causes of hypogonadotrophic hypogonadism

There are very many causes of this condition that may involve either the hypothalamus or the pituitary—or indeed both at once.

Hypothalamic lesions and hypothalamic malfunction

Damage to the hypothalamus can be the result of a number of different lesions. Inflammatory changes as occur in meningitis and encephalitis can result in hypothalamic malfunction, as can the deposition of granulomatous lesions in this area, a more common example being sarcoidosis. Tumours of this regions such as the craniopharyngioma (a tumour of Rathke's pouch), optic gliomata and also meningiomata can also involve the hypothalamus and disrupt it functionally. Both surgery and radiotherapy in this area may also induce hypothalamic malfunction (Lam *et al.* 1986), and the hypothalamic area can also be temporarily or permanently damaged by trauma such as that occurring in a fracture of the base of the skull. A hamartoma of the hypothalamus is also known to be a cause of reproductive failure.

It must also be remembered that large pituitary adenomata that extend upwards out of the pituitary fossa may impinge on the hypothalamus and interfere with its function.

161

Pituitary malfunction

Hypopituitarism is most commonly caused by the presence of pituitary adenomata but pituitary function can also be impaired by infiltrative lesions such as sarcoidosis. Such a problem may also occur because of iron deposition within the anterior pituitary that is seen in patients with haemochromatosis. Autoimmune disorders may also disrupt pituitary function, as is seen in the condition of lymphocytic hypophysitis.

Vascular disturbance, such as may occur as the result of disseminated intravascular coagulation as well as the impairment of the blood supply to the pituitary by a carotid aneurysm, can also gravely disturb pituitary function and reduce gonadotrophin secretion.

Trauma to the pituitary or accidental stalk section, as can occur together with a serious base of skull fracture, may also interfere with pituitary function. Pituitary damage can also be the result of irradiation to the sella turcica.

There is a rare and less severe form of hypopituitarism where only LH secretion is affected. These individuals have normal FSH levels and spermatogenesis is near normal. However, in these men, the LH secretion, and thus the testosterone production is very low, and this condition is known as the fertile eunuch syndrome (McCullogh *et al.* 1953).

More rarely, an isolated FSH deficiency can also give rise to infertility (Stewart-Bentley & Wallack 1975).

Idiopathic hypogonadotrophic hypogonadism (IHH)

This disorder is a common cause of delayed puberty that extends over the age of 18 years and, as there is frequently a family history of this disorder, it is almost certainly genetically predetermined.

Patients with IHH have a variable body habitus, as there may not be a complete absence of gonadotrophin secretion in many of these patients. Some men with this condition are of short stature while others may be tall, and these differences relate to the amount of testosterone being produced by the testes. However, patients with hypogonadotrophic hypogonadism usually have scant or no secondary sexual hair and the testes are reduced in size. Testicular maldescent may also be present. Histology of the testes shows a range of features varying from the completely unstimulated prepuberal seminiferous tubules to those showing some spermatogenic differentiation, but which also show maturational arrest. The changes are of course dependent upon the amount of gonadotrophins that are being produced by the anterior pituitary.

Kallman's syndrome

This condition of severe hypogonadotrophic hypogonadism (Kallman *et al.* 1944) appears to be inherited either as an X-linked recessive trait or as a dominant condition with varying degrees of expression. Its presence results in a total absence of puberty and it is associated with a maldevelopment of some of the midline structures of the brain and these include the hypothalamus. However, patients with this condition are also frequently anosmic because of an aplasia of the olfactory nerves (Lieblich *et al.* 1987). They present with lack of secondary sexual development and fail to go through puberty.

Again the physical signs in these patients relate to the severity of the hypothalamic dysfunction, but usually severe hypogonadism is present.

Prader–Labhart–Willi syndrome

This condition is often known simply as the Prader–Willi syndrome (Prader *et al.* 1956), but is probably more fairly known as the Prader–Labhart–Willi syndrome. It is now known to have a genetic basis and appears to be caused by an absence of the paternal or maternal contribution to an area on the long arm of chromosome 15 in the 11–13 regions (LaSalle *et al.* 1998), as does its close relation the Angelman syndrome. Deletion of a portion of the long arm of chromosome 6 has also been reported in relation to the Prader–Willi syndrome (Butler *et al.* 1998).

The disorder consists of gross obesity, mental subnormality and hypogonadism. The obesity is now thought to relate to a resistance to leptin (Isotani *et al.* 1997). The presence of the Prader–Willi syndrome is frequently suspected in early life, as this condition may cause neonatal hypotonia.

The degree of hypogonadism in this condition is very variable, but there is always some disruption of pubertal development. These patients have no beard growth and the distribution of the sexual hair is always female. The penis remains infantile and the testes are markedly reduced in size.

Histology of the testes shows an absence of spermatogonia and scanty number of Leydig cells (Katcher *et al.* 1977). The serum levels of FSH and LH are generally very low and there is a subnormal response to GnRH and hCG stimulation. There is also a reduced gonadotrophic response to stimulation with clomifene and these factors indicate the presence of a hypothalamic lesion (Tolis *et al.* 1974; Jeffcoate *et al.* 1980).

Haemochromatosis

Men with this condition are frequently infertile (Tweed & Roland 1998): indeed hypogonadism may be present in as many as 75% of patients with this disorder. Haemochromatosis is a disorder of iron metabolism and iron binding. Whether this is a primary disease or is related to large-scale breakdown of red blood cells, excessive quantities of iron are laid down in the tissues. Patients suffering haemochromatosis develop considerable iron deposition in the pancreas, and thus diabetes frequently accompanies this disease. Thus, all the vascular and neurological complications of diabetes may be seen in patients with haemochromatosis and disorders of potency and ejaculation that relate to diabetes may occur in the male patients with this disorder.

In most men with this disease, infertility is caused by gonadotrophin deficiency. Large amounts of iron are deposited in the cells of the anterior pituitary (Peillon & Racadot 1969), resulting in a reduced or even absent production of both FSH and LH. The situation may be worsened by the presence of both erectile and ejaculatory problems. However, it must be remembered that anterior pituitary function may sometimes be normal in these patients, and in this situation the patient's infertility will be a result of a separate lesion.

Male patients with haemochromatosis usually present in an infertility clinic with impotence, loss of libido, and on examination are frequently grossly hypo-androgenized. There is a general lack of body hair and poor beard growth. The testes are often reduced in size but this will be dependant upon the degree of reduction in gonadotrophin production. Apart from the physical signs that accompany haemochromatosis and the marked bronzed pigmentation of the skin that is so characteristic of this condition, no other physical signs are usually present.

The serum levels of FSH and LH are low and the serum testosterone levels are concomitantly reduced (Stocks & Powell 1972). Testicular histology in hypogonadotrophic men with haemochromatosis will show a gross reduction in sperm production and there will be a marked reduction in the number of germ cells. The Leydig cells are often very reduced in number (Peillon & Racadot 1969). It is of interest that iron deposition does not seem to occur in the testes.

Improvement in testicular function, together with sexual function, can be brought about by depletion of the tissue of their deposits of iron. This can be achieved by vigorous and repeated phlebotomy; indeed, removal of blood has been shown to resolve the infertility in a male patient with haemochromatosis within 3–4 months (Siemons & Mahler 1987). However, as the major part of a patient's infertility is caused by pituitary insufficiency, it is also possible to treat these men with gonadotrophins.

Anabolic steroid abuse

The abuse of steroids by athletes, weightlifters and individuals involved in sports that require a large muscle bulk is becoming an increasingly common cause of hypogonadotrophic hypogonadism and infertility. Suppression of gonadotrophin secretion by these agents can be very profound and may persist for several years (Jarow & Lipshultz 1990). As the acquisition of these drugs has often been through illegal channels, some patients will, at least initially, deny their use, and this can at times lead to diagnostic difficulties.

These men present with acute hypogonadism with both impotence and azoospermia. As the onset of this type of hypogonadism is rapid, these

164

patients may arrive in the clinic with few clinical signs of testosterone deficiency, for these clinical signs may not have had time to become manifest. Such patients will also complain of loss of libido and, of course, of infertility.

The serum levels of FSH and LH are frequently unmeasurable and the serum testosterone will be very low, often in the range seen in the normal female. The semen analysis is always abnormal.

The treatment of the infertility in these men is by means of gonadotrophin therapy.

The reproductive endocrine changes that can occur in male patients with uraemia

In many male patients in renal failure, and particularly those undergoing dialysis, testosterone production is reduced and spermatogenesis may be impaired (Lim 1994). These changes usually correlate with a small rise in LH while FSH tends to remain within the normal range. Zinc deficiency may also occur in men with renal failure but whether this plays any part in the patient's infertility is not known. However, therapy with zinc compounds may improve gonadal function in some patients with renal disease (Mahajan *et al.* 1982).

The serum prolactin may also be raised in these patients and this may contribute to the reduction in testosterone secretion. Thus, the administration of dopamine agonists may also raise the serum testosterone level and improve sexual function in these men

Thus, such men may present with infertility and an abnormal sperm count. More importantly, patients in end-stage renal failure and an abnormal sperm count may occasionally present for the first time to an infertility clinic. Such men may also complain of impotence and loss of libido, but this may not necessarily correlate with the reduction in testosterone production. There may also be an element of Leydig cell resistance in these men as blunted responses to hCG in these men (Holdsworth *et al.* 1977).

The testicular histology among men with uraemia seems to be very variable and may range from a total absence of germ cells to a mild maturational arrest. It must be remembered, however, that part of any effect upon the testicular histology may relate to any cytotoxic therapy that may have been given to the patient rather than the effect of the uraemia itself.

The treatment of any infertility associated with renal failure is difficult, and probably is best treated by assisted conception as it is difficult to raise the sperm count in these patients. Simple loss of libido is often most easily managed by testosterone therapy but it must be remembered that testosterone will often reduce the sperm count to the point of azoospermia.

Liver disease

Severe liver disease, especially that seen in relation to alcoholic cirrhosis, can also be a cause of infertility. Hepatocellular damage results in poor metabolism of the sex hormones and the accumulation of oestrogen in the circulation. These changes gives rise to the well-known 'spider naevi', which are characteristic of liver disease in the male. In this situation, gonadotrophin secretion is reduced and spermatogenesis is suppressed. Liver disease can thus be a cause of hypogonadotrophic hypogonadism. Alcohol also has a direct effect on the testis and so excess consumption can affect fertility without there being any major damage to liver function.

The treatment of hypogonadotrophic hypogonadism

There are three objectives in the treatment of hypogonadotrophic hypogonadism. These involve: (i) the induction of the secondary sex characteristics for those patients that have not undergone a normal puberty; (ii) the maintenance or restoration of normal sexual function; and (iii) the induction or return of fertility. These aims can be achieved by using androgen therapy, treatment with gonadotrophins or, in men with hypothalamic lesions, by the use of gonadotrophin-releasing hormone.

Androgen therapy

Androgen therapy is a useful means of restoring sexual function but it will not, in these circumstances, treat the patient's infertility. Androgen therapy has the advantage that it is much cheaper than gonadotrophin therapy and it can be used to manage hypogonadotrophic hypogonadism when fertility is not desired or required. It is also useful for the induction of puberty.

Natural testosterone when taken by mouth is absorbed and rapidly degraded by the liver so that only small amounts of the hormone are left to enter the systemic system. Androgen therapy must therefore consist of chemically modified androgens that are only slowly metabolized by the liver or by the use of natural testosterone that must be administered by alternative routes.

In order to prevent rapid metabolism by the liver, many of the oral androgen preparations have been modified by 17-α alkylation and/or by the modification of their ring structure. Those androgens that are administered systemically have been esterified so that their absorption into fat is enhanced and their release into the circulation is considerably slowed.

Testosterone replacement therapy can be carried out in a number of different ways. Injection of the long-acting esters of testosterone in doses of 100–250 mg, given as an intramuscular injection every 3–4 weeks, will provide a steady level of androgen replacement and will bring the serum testosterone levels into the range of normal in the majority of patients. In younger patients who have not been through puberty, it is best to begin treatment with smaller doses of androgen that can be increased as puberty progresses.

There are two main sources of intramuscular androgen replacement. One is a preparation of testosterone enanthate manufactured in doses of

100 and 200 mg (Primoteston, Schering Pharmaceuticals). The second preparation of this type is a mixture of testosterone esters that include testosterone propionate, phenylpropionate, isocaproate and decanoate (Sustenon, Organon Pharmaceuticals) and this preparation is available in doses of 100 and 250 mg.

Natural testosterone can also be given as a cystalline preparation in the form of a pellet (Testosterone Implant, Organon Pharmaceuticals) which is available in doses of 100 and 200 mg. These are inserted using a special introducer in doses of 100–600 mg every 3–6 months. Although this preparation will free the patient from the chore of monthly injections, this type of therapy tends to be more expensive for the patient.

Oral preparations for androgen replacement are also available. The testosterone ester, testosterone undecanoate (Andriol, Organon Pharmaceuticals), given in doses of 120–160 mg per day in divided doses, is a useful preparation and has the advantage that any return of endogenous gonadotrophin secretion will not be suppressed. Another preparation is the modified androgen mesterolone (Proviron, Schering Pharmaceuticals), which is administered in doses of 50–75 mg per day. The older preparation of oral testosterone, namely methyl testosterone, is little used today. For any therapy that is long term (and all therapy of hypogonadotrophic hypogonadism will need to be long term), it is best to avoid the alkylated oral preparations as these can occasionally, after prolonged use, induce liver damage. The short-term use of these preparations, however, usually produces no problems.

More recently, preparations of testosterone have come onto the market that deliver testosterone transdermally and are prepared as either a patch or a cream. These preparations may also prove very useful in the management of this form of hypogonadism.

Gonadotrophin therapy

The application of gonadotrophins to hypogonadotrophic hypogonadism involves the use of both gonadotrophins.

For the initiation of puberty and the generation of the secondary sex characteristics, testosterone, and thus LH, is needed. However, for the initiation of spermatogenesis, FSH is essential; but for the production of mature sperm, testosterone, and therefore LH, is required. As there is no commercial preparation of LH, the much longer-acting preparation of hCG is always used in place of LH.

Among patients who have not gone through puberty, treatment can be commenced using small doses of androgen replacement. However, the advantage of treatment with gonadotrophins is that initiation of spermatogenesis will take place at the same time as the development of the secondary sex characteristics. Thus, for the initiation of spermatogenesis, FSH is needed, while for the changes associated with puberty, LH or its equivalent in hCG is required.

167

Most commercial preparations of gonadotrophins are now manufactured using the recombinant technology and the urinary preparations are now largely being phased out. These preparations are sold in 75- or 150-IU ampoules (Gonal F, Serono) or in 50- and 100-IU ampoules (Puregon, NV Organon). The commercial preparations of hCG are today still all based on urinary extracts and are marketed as Profasi (Serono) and Pregnyl (NV Organon). The hCG preparations are available in ampoules containing 1000, 2000 or 5000 IU.

Treatment of the prepubertal adult

Among patients with hypogonadotrophic hypogonadism who show few signs of puberty, a combined therapeutic regime consisting of FSH and hCG is recommended. A number of different treatment protocols have been described. However, the most commonly used regimen consists of:

1   hCG 2000 IU three times per week i.m. for 6 weeks as this will elevate the serum testosterone to normal male levels.

2   At the end of 6 weeks, a dose of FSH of 37.5 IU (i.e. half an ampoule) added to the hCG also three times per week (Spratt *et al.* 1986).

During this protocol and if fertility is desired, the semen should be examined on a monthly basis to assess the fertility potential of the patient. Careful evaluation of the female partner is essential so that the chances of pregnancy are maximized as gonadotrophin therapy is expensive and should be kept to a minimum. This combined therapy may need to be continued for 3–6 months before fertility is achieved. If there is no response in terms of testis size or fertility after 3 months the dose of FSH and hCG should be doubled. In patients who are resistant to treatment, especially those who are found to have very small testes at the initial examination and who have shown no signs of pubertal changes, therapy may have to be continued for as long as 1–2 years. If the patient is also cryptorchid, then the prognosis for fertility is poor even if the treatment induces testicular descent.

Treatment of the postpubertal adult

Among patients whose hypogonadism is incomplete, or in whom the hypogonadotrophic hypogonadism has been induced in adulthood, then only hCG will be required to restore both their androgenization and their fertility. The usual treatment is simply hCG 2000 IU given intramuscularly three times per week.

The major problem with this treatment is its cost. It is important that as much potentially fertile semen as possible is cryopreserved so that more than one pregnancy can be generated from a single course of therapy. Increasing resistance to hCG is a well-recognized complication of too frequent hCG injections, which can induce receptor 'down-regulation', but this problem can be prevented by adequate spacing of therapy (Glass &

Vigersky 1980). A further possible complication of gonadotrophin treatment is the formation of antibodies that can block the action of hCG, but in practice these are rarely of much significance clinically; indeed, this resistance is easily overcome by increasing the dose of hCG (Sokol *et al.* 1981).

Gonadotrophin-releasing hormone therapy

This type of therapy has been used in men with hypothalamic lesions, but of course such treatment will not be of any value among patients with pituitary disease. However, in most patients this lesion is a hypothalamic one and thus can be treated with gonadotrophin-releasing hormone (Nachtigall *et al.* 1997). This agent is commercially available in ampoules containing 100 or 500 µg of the releasing hormone (Gonadorelin, Ayerst Laboratories).

Gonadotrophin-releasing hormone is administered in a pulsatile manner either subcutaneously or intravenously using an electronically driven pump (Fig. 9.2). The pulses are best administered some 90 min apart and the dose of releasing hormone should be around 25 ng/kg body weight. This regime provides a dose of around 1–2 µg per pulse. However, in many patients with a very profound suppression of hypothalamic function, doses as high as 300 ng/kg body weight may have to be used (Spratt *et al.* 1986).

Using this treatment, there should be an unequivocal rise in both gonadotrophin and testosterone levels in serum at the end of 7 days of

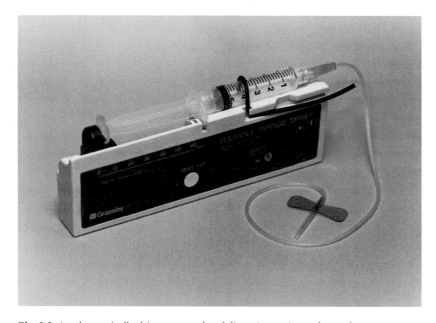

Fig. 9.2 An electronically driven pump that delivers intermittent doses of gonadotrophin-releasing hormone either subcutaneously or intravenously. The size of the pump and the difficulties involved in trying to hide it under clothes made this type of therapy unpopular among patients.

treatment. However, it may take 2–3 months before sperm will appear in the semen in an azoospermic man and as long to see changes in semen quality in an infertile patient with oligozoospermia. Semen should be examined monthly following 3 months of this treatment. When the semen is of good quality, samples should be cryopreserved for use in insemination.

Like gonadotrophin therapy, treatment with releasing hormone is expensive. Many patients object to the presence of the pump, which may become visible, especially under summer clothes, and which also impedes activities such as swimming and many other outdoor recreations. As with gonadotrophin therapy, fertility is not assured, especially among patients with very small testes and profound hypogonadism.

It is also possible to develop antibodies to the releasing hormone administered in this way, but this problem can be overcome simply by increasing the dose. However, a single case of anaphylactic reaction has been described in one woman undergoing this therapy (MacLeod *et al.* 1987).

Thyroid disease

The current literature concerning the fertility status of men with thyroid disease is sparse, but it would appear that thyroid disease does indeed have a deleterious effect on male reproductive performance. Thyroid disease is predominantly found in women and thus it will only occasionally found among male patients in an infertility clinic.

Hypothyroidism

Hypothyroidism can cause male infertility in several ways. Firstly sexual dysfunction may be present in as many as 80% of male patients with severe primary myxoedema (Griboff 1962). Loss of libido and a reduction in potency are common features of reduced thyroid function. It is also known that hyperprolactinaemia is a frequent complication of myxoedema in women (Thomas *et al.* 1987), but whether this occurs in men and contributes to the sexual dysfunction in this condition is not known.

Experimentally, congenital hypothyroidism is associated with a reduced sperm production and this abnormality is reversed by treatment with thyroxine (Matsumishi *et al.* 1986). It would thus appear that young male patients with thyroid hypofunction are at risk of both testicular malfunction and sexual difficulties. This form of thyroid disease may also affect semen quality (Buitrago & Diez 1987). Treatment of the hypothyroidism should resolve both the hypothyroidism and any associated infertility.

Hyperthyroidism

It has been demonstrated in the past that moderately large doses of thyroid extract cause a reduction in spermatogenic activity in peripubertal animals

170

(Maqsood 1954). However, there is little evidence that thyrotoxicosis *per se* is a cause of infertility in the human male. Nevertheless, hyperthyroidism causes weight loss, which, if profound, may cause varying degrees of hypogonadotrophic hypogonadism. There is also some evidence that excessive production of thyroxin may sensitize the pituitary gonadotrophs to the action of gonadotrophin-releasing hormone, as in such patients the response to a bolus dose of gonadotrophin-releasing hormone is enhanced; but despite this the serum levels of gonadotrophins and testosterone remain unchanged by treatment (Rojdmark *et al.* 1988). Thus, thyrotoxicosis could be an indirect rather than a direct cause of male infertility. As with myxoedema, treatment of the excessive thyroid activity should resolve any associated fertility problem.

Diabetes mellitus

Diabetes is one of the most common endocrine diseases and will indeed frequently present in an infertility clinic. The most common way in which diabetes presents in an infertility clinic is by the way in which it interferes with normal sexual function (Sexton & Jarow 1997). Both neurological and vascular factors are likely to be the cause of erectile failure in diabetics, while an autonomic neuropathy is almost certainly the cause of the ejaculatory disturbance in these patients (Dunsmuir & Holmes 1996).

Causes of infertility in diabetes mellitus

Impotence is a very common complication of diabetes and occurs in 50% of all diabetics (McCullogh *et al.* 1980). Nocturnal penile tumescence in the impotent diabetic is reduced or absent (Murray *et al.* 1987), demonstrating the presence of an organic lesion. Disorders of ejaculation may also be present in diabetic males, and around one-third of all men presenting in an infertility clinic with retrograde ejaculation will have diabetes mellitus (Jequier, unpublished). Not infrequently, retrograde ejaculation will progress in diabetics to ejaculatory failure.

The serum testosterone in men with diabetic impotence may be reduced, and the possible role of hypo-androgenization in this group of men with erectile failure is emphasized by the fact that testosterone replacement therapy may alleviate impotence in a proportion of these patients (Murray *et al.* 1987).

The effect of diabetes on spermatogenic activity is much more difficult to assess. Testicular biopsies from impotent diabetic patients show a wide range of changes that vary from a minimal reduction in spermatogenesis to the presence of totally hyalinized and nonfunctional seminiferous tubule (Cameron *et al.* 1985). The Sertoli cell tight junctions are often also abnormal and ultrastructural abnormalities in the Sertoli cell cytoplasm can often be demonstrated. Even the Leydig cells may be abnormal and can show the presence of large lipoid droplets and pathological vacuoles. It is thus clear that diabetic male patients do have significant testicular pathology that can not only account for their infertility but also for at least part of their sexual dysfunction.

Treatment of infertility caused by diabetes mellitus

Treatment of the infertile diabetic will depend upon the severity of the testicular lesion and upon the severity of the sexual dysfunction. If the testes are reduced in size and the serum FSH raised, primary testicular disease is present and significant damage to sperm production will have occurred. There will thus be little that can be done to improve semen quality.

It must be remembered also that diabetic patients can develop disorders of sperm maturation at any time. Thus, if a diabetic patient is able to produce a good fertile ejaculate it may be wise to cryopreserve some semen for insemination in the future, should primary testicular disease or ejaculatory failure suddenly supervene.

If the patient has erectile failure, a wide variety of means of correcting this disorder are available for this problem, and retrograde ejaculation and ejaculatory failure are best treated in the manner described in Chapter 8.

Overall, diabetes is commonly seen in an infertility clinic and the reproductive failure that it so commonly causes needs very careful clinical evaluation and precise diagnosis.

Congenital adrenal hyperplasia

Congenital adrenal hyperplasia is a complex, genetically determined disease, in which there is an absence or a deficiency of the enzymes necessary for the production of the steroid precursors of cortisol.

As a consequence of the enzyme defect, the secretion of cortisol is very reduced or absent and therefore the pituitary secretion of ACTH is considerably enhanced. As ACTH acts to convert cholesterol to pregnenelone, this excess ACTH activity together with all the steroidogenesis that takes place 'upstream' from the site of action of the absent or deficient enzymes is markedly increased. In response to the action of the ACTH, the size of the adrenal glands is also greatly increased (Table 9.2).

The extra ACTH drive increases pregnenelone production and will result in greatly increased levels of testosterone as well as of the other androgens in the serum.

When this enzyme is totally absent, no aldosterone or cortisol will be produced. Gross salt depletion will result and such an obvious abnormality will be diagnosed at birth. Thus male patients who present at an infertility clinic with congenital adrenal hyperplasia will usually be men in whom the condition has already been diagnosed or treated or they will have a partial or incomplete enzyme deficiency. In a partial enzyme deficiency, the cortisol and aldosterone production will be sufficiently high to prevent any major salt loss that would otherwise jeopardize health.

Table 9.2 Steroid production by the adrenal gland and the common sites of enzyme deficiency that may be seen among patients with congenital adrenal hyperplasia

Cholesterol
　I
Pregnenolone　　　　　17-OH pregnenolone　　　DHEA
　II　　　17 hydroxylase　　II　　　　　　　II
Progesterone　　　　　　17-OH Progesterone
Androstenedione
　III　　　21 hydroxylase　　III　　　　　　IV
Desoxycorticosterone　　17-Desoxycorticosterone
Testosterone
　IV　　　　　　　　　　IV　　　　　　　IX
Corticosterone　　　　　　Cortisol
Dihydrotestosterone
　V
Aldosterone

In women, the excess testosterone production will cause obvious virilization but in men the increase in testosterone secretion will cause no problems apart from infertility. Thus, it is only the nonsalt-losing congenital adrenal hyperplasia in men that will be diagnosed in an infertility clinic.

The cause of infertility in congenital adrenal hyperplasia

The infertility seen among men with congenital adrenal hyperplasia is solely caused by the excess testosterone production (Wischusen *et al.* 1981). There is frequently, however, a history of precocious puberty in these men (Bornaccorsi *et al.* 1987). As the result of the high serum testosterone and other androgens, pituitary LH secretion is decreased and the pulsatile nature of its release may be depressed (Redfar *et al.* 1977). Leydig cell activity is therefore reduced and the amount of testosterone crossing the seminiferous tubular basement membrane is thus depressed. Spermatogenesis is therefore usually seriously impaired.

Clinical presentation of congenital adrenal hyperplasia

On clinical examination these men are usually normally androgenized but the testes are markedly reduced in size. The semen is often severely oligozoospermic or may even be azoospermic.

Testicular biopsies taken from men with infertility and congenital adrenal hyperplasia show spermatogenic arrest and even hyalinization of the seminiferous tubules together with a marked reduction in the number of Leydig cells (Bornaccorsi *et al.* 1987).

Some patients, for reasons that are unclear, may remain fertile despite very high levels of testosterone in the serum (Urban *et al.* 1978).

An uncommon complication of congenital adrenal hyperplasia is the development of gross testicular enlargement in association with massive

Leydig cell hyperplasia (Dahl & Bahn 1962). In these patients aberrant adrenal tissue can sometimes be found close to the testis, which itself undergoes hyperplasia.

Treatment of the infertility caused by congenital adrenal hyperplasia

Corticosteroid therapy, in particular treatment with dexamethasone, will reduce testosterone levels and return the Leydig hypoplasia to normal (Augarten *et al.* 1991). As a consequence, LH secretion will increase, intratesticular testosterone concentrations will rise and fertility may return to normal. However, it must be remembered that this condition can be associated with permanent damage to the seminiferous tubules and thus not all patients will respond to treatment in terms of their fertility. The gross enlargement of the testes that is sometimes also associated with this condition will also respond to corticosteroid therapy.

Androgen resistance

Resistance to the action of androgens is a genetically determined defect. The androgen receptor gene has also now been identified. Depending upon its severity, androgen resistance can produce a wide spectrum of phenotypic and endocrine abnormalities.

Resistance to the action of the androgens is caused by abnormalities in the androgen receptors that are present in normally androgen-sensitive tissues. In its most profound form, a patient who is karyotypically male may thus show no evidence of androgen activity and thus will be phenotypically female, the clinical condition of 'total androgen insensitivity' also known as 'testicular feminization'. However, as ovarian tissue and müllerian stimulating hormone are both necessary for the development of the müllerian duct system, these patients are without fallopian tubes, uterus or the upper two-thirds of the vagina. Among patients with an androgen receptor abnormality, androgen receptors in the pituitary and hypothalamus will also not be functional and thus the secretion of LH will be greatly increased, as will the production of testosterone by the ovary. Thus, the clinical features of a patient with androgen receptor abnormalities is that they appear hypogonadal but both the LH as well as the testosterone levels in serum are increased (Griffin & Wilson 1980).

It is of course possible that the resistance to androgen is incomplete. This phenomenon will result in a phenotype that is clearly male but whose genitalia may show a variety of abnormalities, and it is this group of patients that may present in an infertility clinic (Morrow *et al.* 1987). The male patients with partial or incomplete androgen insensitivity who may present in an infertility clinic may be divided into three categories.

Type I androgen insensitivity (at one time known as Reifenstein's syndrome)

This condition was originally described by Reifenstein in 1947, when its cause was unknown (Reifenstein 1947). In 1974, Wilson and colleagues demonstrated that it was caused by an abnormality of the androgen receptor (Wilson *et al.* 1974). It is now known more simply as type I androgen insensitivity. Patients with this condition are always infertile.

Cause of infertility in Type I androgen resistance

Testosterone is essential for spermatogenesis as well as for the normal function of the accessory glands and also for sperm transport within the genital tract. As none of these functions will be normal, infertility is the rule and the semen in these patients is frequently azoospermic.

Clinical presentation of Type I androgen deficiency

Patients with this condition have a fairly severe form of androgen resistance but nevertheless have an unambiguously male phenotype. However, hypo-androgenization is very evident, beard growth is poor and the sexual hair tends to be in a female distribution. Genital abnormalities that may be present include hypospadias, bifid scrotum and cryptorchidism. As androgens are being secreted in excess, some are converted to oestrogen and thus gynaecomastia is common among these patients. The penis and the prostate are small and the testes are markedly reduced in size.

The association between hypo-androgenization, gynaecomastia and very small testes makes this condition phenotypically very similar to that seen in patients with Klinefelter's disease; indeed, even the histological picture of atrophied seminiferous tubules and large numbers of Leydig cells makes for confusion. However, in Type I androgen insensitivity, the serum testosterone is high and the karyotype normal while in Klinefelter's disease the testosterone is low and the karyotype is abnormal (Table 9.3).

Patients with Type I androgen insensitivity therefore demonstrate the apparent paradox of clinical androgen deficiency in the presence of high levels of both LH and testosterone. One useful way for the clinician to determine the possible presence of androgen receptor abnormalities is to

Table 9.3 The clinical differentiation of androgen receptor abnormalities from Klinefelter's syndrome

	Androgen receptor abnormalities	Klinefelter's syndrome
Karyotype	46, XY	47, XXY
LH	Raised	Raised
Testosterone	Raised	Low

calculate the androgen receptor index. (Aiman & Griffin 1982). This index is derived from the sum of the values of the serum LH and the serum testosterone. An androgen resistance index (where the serum testosterone is measured in nmol/L) of greater than 250 is generally believed to be indicative of an insensitivity to androgen.

Type II androgen insensitivity (previously known as Rosewater's syndrome)

This condition was first described by Rosewater and colleagues in 1965, when again its cause was unknown (Rosewater *et al.* 1965). It is now known to be caused by androgen insensitivity but which is much less severe that that seen in the Type I disorder.

Clinical presentation of Type II androgen deficiency

Among patients with this condition again the penis and prostate are small but the testes are usually of normal size. Hypogonadism may be seen, but it is of much less severity than that seen in men with the Type I form of androgen insensitivity. Minor abnormalities of the genitalia such as glandular hypospadias may be present. Semen analysis usually shows the presence of oligozoospermia, but not all men with this condition are infertile. Testicular histology may show varying degrees of maturational arrest.

Treatment of this condition will have to involve some form of assisted reproduction as there are no ways of improving the semen quality. It has, however, been reported that treatment with FSH may increase sperm numbers in the semen. It must, however, be remembered that these distressing conditions are genetically predetermined.

Idiopathic oligozoospermia

In recent years it has been pointed out that some men who are clinically normal but who have oligozoospermia may in fact have a minor degree of androgen resistance, as elevated testosterone levels were noted in a group of oligozoospermic men. The presence of elevated levels of LH as well as testosterone together with a raised androgen resistance index was also described among a group of oligozoospermic men (Aiman & Griffin 1982). The role of mild androgen insensitivity in the general overview of infertility in the male remains unclear, but it would appear at least to play a role in its aetiology. However, recent studies suggest that this is a much less common cause of male infertility than was previously supposed (Tincello *et al.* 1997).

Endocrine disease is an infrequent but nevertheless important and often highly treatable cause of infertility in the male. However, for both diagnostic and therapeutic success in this area of infertility, careful history taking together with a careful clinical examination and general evaluation of each patient are all very important.

References

Aiman, J. & Griffin, J.E. (1982) The frequency of androgen receptor deficiency in infertile men. *Journal of Clinical Endocrinology and Metabolism* **54**, 725–732.

Alexander, L., Appleton, D., Hall, R., Ross, W.M. & Wilkinson, R. (1980) Epidemiology of acromegaly in the Newcastle region. *Clinical Endocrinology* **12**, 71–79.

Augarten, A., Weissenberg, R., Pariente, C. & Sack, J. (1991) Reversible male infertility in late onset congenital adrenal hyperplasia. *Journal of Clinical Investigation* **14**, 237–240.

Bornaccorsi, A.C., Adler, I. & Figueirdo, J.G. (1987) Male infertility due to congenital adrenal hyperplasia: testicular biopsy findings, hormonal evaluation and therapeutic results in three patients. *Fertility and Sterility* **40**, 809–814.

Buitrago, J.M. & Diez, L.C. (1987) Serum hormones and seminal parameters in males with thyroid disease. *Andrologia* **19**, 37–41.

Butler, M.G., Moore, J., Moraweicki, A. & Nicolson, M. (1998) Comparision of leptin protein levels in Prader–Willi syndrome and control individuals. *American Journal of Medical Genetics* **75**, 7–12.

Cameron, D.F., Murray, F.T. & Drylie, D.D. (1985) Interstitial compartment pathology and spermatogenic disruption in testes from impotent diabetic men. *Anatomical Record* **213**, 53–62.

Cushing, H. (1932) The basophil adenomas of the pituitary body and their clinical manifestations. *Bulletin of Johns Hopkins Hospital* **50**, 137–195.

Dahl, E.V. & Bahn, R.C. (1962) Aberrant adrenal cortical tissue near the testees in human infants. *Fertility and Sterility* **40**, 809–814.

Dunsmuir, W.D. & Holmes, S.A. (1996) The aetiology and management of erectile, ejaculatory, and fertility problems in men with diabetes mellitus. *Diabetic Medicine* **13**, 700–708.

Eastman, R.C., Gordon, P. & Roth, J. (1979) Conventional supervoltage irradiation is an effective treatment for acromegaly. *Journal of Endocrinology and Metabolism* **48**, 931–940.

Franks, S., Jacobs, H.S. & Nabarro, J.D.N.N. (1976) Prolactin concentrations in patients with acromegaly: clinical significance and response to surgery. *Clinical Endocrinology* **5**, 63–69.

Franks, S., Jacobs, H.S., Martin, N. & Nabarro, J.D. (1978) Hyperprolactinaemia and impotence. *Clinical Endocrinology* **14**, 277–287.

Gavrilove, J.L., Nicolis, C.L. & Sohval, A.R. (1974) The testis in Cushing's syndrome. *Journal of Urology* **112**, 95–99.

Glass, A.R. & Vigersky, R.A. (1980) Resensitisation of testosterone production in men with human chorionic gonadotropin-induced desensitisation. *Journal of Clinical Endocrinology and Metabolism* **51**, 1395–1400.

Griboff, S.I. (1962) Semen analysis in myxoedema. *Fertility and Sterility* **13**, 436–443.

Griffin, J.E. & Wilson, J.D. (1980) The syndromes of androgen resistance. *New England Journal of Medicine* **302**, 198–209.

Hargreave, T.B., Richmond, J.D., Liakatis, J., Elton, R.A. & Brown, N.S. (1981) Searching for the infertile man with hyperprolactinaemia. *Fertility and Sterility* **36**, 630–632.

Holdsworth, S., Atkins, R.C. & De Kretser, D.M. (1977) The pituitary–testicular axis in men with chronic renal failure. *New England Journal of Medicine* **296**, 1245–1249.

Ishikawa, H., Kaneko, S., Ohashi, M., Nakagawa, K. & Hata, M. (1993) Retrograde ejaculation accompanying hyperprolactinaemia. *Archives of Andrology* **30**, 153–155.

Isotani, H., Kameoka, K. & Furakawa, K. (1997) Dialy profile of serum leptin in Prader–Willi syndrome complicated by diabetes mellitus—a case report. *Hormone and Metabolic Research* **29**, 611–612.

Jarow, J.P. & Lipshultz, L.I. (1990) Anabolic steroid-induced hypogonadotrophic hypogonadism. *American Journal of Sports Medicine* **18**, 429–431.

Jeffcoate, W.J., Laurence, B.M., Edwards, C.R.W. & Besser, G.M. (1980) Endocrine function in the Prader–Willi syndrome. *Clinical Endocrinology* **12**, 81–89.

Jequier, A.M., Crich, J.P. & Ansell, I.D. (1979) Clinical findings and testicular histology in three hyperprolactinaemic men. *Fertility and Sterility* **31**, 525–530.

Kallmann, F.J., Choenfeld, W.A. & Barrera, S.E. (1944) The genetic aspects of primary eunuchoidism. *American Journal of Mental Deficiency* **48**, 203–236.

Katcher, M.L., Bargman, G.J., Gilbert, E.F. & Opitz, J.M. (1977) Absence of spermatogonia in the Prader–Willi syndrome. *European Journal of Paediatrics* **124**, 257–260.

Lam, K.S.L., Wang, C., Yeung, R.T.T. *et al.* (1986) Hypothalamic hypopituitarism following cranial irradiation for nasopharyngeal carcinoma. *Clinical Endocrinology* **24**, 643–651.

LaSalle, J.M., Ritchie, R.J., Glatt, H. & Lalande, M. (1998) Clonal heterogeneity at alleleic methylation sites diagnostic for Prader–Willi and Angelman syndromes. *Proceedings of the National Academy of Sciences of the USA* **95**, 1675–1680.

Lieblich, J.M., Rogol, A.D., White, B.J. & Sussman, G.L. (1987) Syndrome of anosmia with hypogonadotrophic hypogonadism (Kallman's syndrome): clinical and laboratory studies in 23 cases. *American Journal of Medicine* **73**, 506–519.

Lim, V.S. (1994) Reproductive endocrinology in uraemia. *Baillière's Clinical Obstetrics and Gynaecology* **8**, 469–480.

Luton, J.-P., Thieblot, P., Valcke, J.-C., Mahoudeau, J.A. & Bricaire, H. (1977) Reversible gonadotrophin deficiency in male Cushing's disease. *Journal of Clinical Endocrinology and Metabolism* **45**, 488–495.

MacLeod, T.L., Eisen, A. & Sussman, G.L. (1987) Anaphylactic reaction to LHRH. *Fertility and Sterility* **48**, 500–502.

Mahajan, S.K., Abbasi, A.A., Prasad, A.S., Rabbani, P., Briggs, W.A. & McDonald, F.D. (1982) Affect of oral zinc therapy on gonadal function in hemodialysis patients. A double blind study. *Annals of Internal Medicine* **97**, 357–361.

Maqsood, M. (1954) Role of the thyroid on maturity and fertility in the male. *Fertility and Sterility* **5**, 382–401.

Matsumishi, M.T., Kuroda, K., Shirai, M., Ando, K. & Sugisaki, T. (1986) Spermatogenesis in Snell dwarf, little and congenitally hypothyroid mice. *International Journal of Fertility* **9**, 289–295.

McCullogh, E.P., Beck, J.C. & Schaffenburg, C.A. (1953) A syndrome of eunuchoidism with spermatogenesis, normal urinary FSH and low or normal ICSH ('fertile eunuchs'). *Journal of Clinical Endocrinology and Metabolism* **13**, 489–509.

McCullogh, D.K., Campbell, I.W., Wu, F.C., Prescott, R.J. & Clarke, B.E. (1980) The prevalence of diabetic impotence. *Diabetologia* **18**, 279–283.

Merino, G., Carranza-Lira, S., Martinez-Chequer, J.C., Barahona, E., Moran, C. & Bermudez, J.A. (1997) Hyperprolactinaemia in men with asthenozoospermia, oligozoospermia or azoospermia. *Archives of Andrology* **38**, 201–206.

Morrow, A.F., Gyorki, S., Warne, G.L. *et al.* (1987) Variable androgen levels in infertile men. *Journal of Clinical Endocrinology and Metabolism* **64**, 1115–1121.

Murray, F.T., Wyss, H.U., Thomas, R.G., Spevack, M. & Glaros, A.G. (1987) Gonadal dysfunction in diabetic men with organic impotence. *Journal of Clinical Endocrinology and Metabolism* **65**, 127–135.

Nabarro, J.D.N.N. (1987) Acromegaly. *Clinical Endocrinology* **26**, 481–512.

Nachtigall, L.B., Boepple, P.A., Pralong, F.P. & Crowley, W.F. (1997) Adult-onset idiopathic hypogonadotrophic hypogonadism—a treatable form of male infertility. *New England Journal of Medicine* **336**, 410–415.

Okada, H., Iwamoto, T., Fujioka, H., Shirakawa, T., Tatsumi, N., Kanzaki, M., Minayoshi, K., Ohya, K., Fujisawa, M., Arakawa, S., Kamidono, S. & Ishigami, J. (1996) Hyperprolactinaemia among infertile patients and its effect on sperm functions. *Andrologia* **28**, 197–202.

Peillon, F. & Racadot, J. (1969) Modifications histopathologiques de l'hypophyse dans six cas d'haemachromatose. *Annales Endocrinologiques (Paris)* **30**, 800–807.

Pont, A., Graybill, J.R., Craven, P.C. *et al.* (1984) High dose ketoconazole therapy and adrenal and testicular function. *Archives of Internal Medicine* **144**, 2150–2153.

Prader, A., Labhart, A. & Willi, H. (1956) Ein syndrom von Adipositas, Kleinwuchs, Kryptorchidism und Oligophrenie nach Myatonierartigem Zustard im Neugeborenalter. *Schweizer Medinische Wochenschrift* **86**, 1260–1261.

Redfar, N., Barter, F.C., Easley, R., Kolins, J., Javadpour, N. & Sherins, R.J. (1977) Evidence for endogenous LH suppression in a man with bilateral testicular tumours and congenital adrenal hyperplasia. *Journal of Clinical Endocrinology and Metabolism* **45**, 1194–1204.

Reifenstein, E.C. (1947) Hereditary familial hypogonadism. *Proceedings of the American Federation for Clinical Research* **3**, 86.

Rojdmark, S., Berg, A. & Kallner, G. (1988) Hypothalamic–pituitary–testicular axis in patients with hyperthyroidism. *Hormone Research* **29**, 185–190.

Rosewater, S., Gwinup, G. & Hamwi, G.J. (1965) Familial gynaecomastia. *Annals of Internal Medicine* **63**, 377–385.

Sexton, W.J. & Jarow, J.P. (1997) Effect of diabetes mellitus upon male reproductive function. *Urology* **49**, 508–513.

Siemons, L.J. & Mahler, C.H. (1987) Hypogonadotrophic hypogonadism in haemochromatosis: recovery of reproductive function after iron depletion. *Journal of Clinical Endocrinology and Metabolism* **65**, 585–587.

Snyder, P.J. (1985) Gonadotroph cell tumours of the pituitary. *Endocrine Review* **6**, 552–563.

Snyder, P.J. (1987) Gonadotroph cell pituitary adenomas. In: *Endocrinology and Metabolism Clinics*, Vol 16, No. 3 (ed. P.J. Snyder), pp. 755–764.

Snyder, P.J. (1993) Clinically non-functioning pituitary adenomas. *Endocrinology and Metabolism Clinics of North America* **22**, 163–175.

Sokol, R., McClure, R.D., Petersen, M. & Swerdloff, R.S. (1981) Gonadotropin therapy failure secondary to human chorionic gonadotropin-induced antibodies. *Journal of Clinical Endocrinology and Metabolism* **52**, 929–932.

Spratt, D.I., Finkelstein, J.S., O'Dea, L.S. *et al.* (1986) Long-term administration gonadotropin-releasing hormone in men with idiopathic hypogonadotropic hypogonadism. *Annals of Internal Medicine* **105**, 848–855.

Stewart-Bentley, M. & Wallack, M. (1975) Isolated FSH deficiency in a male. *Clinical Research* **23**, 96A.

Stocks, A.E. & Powell, L.W. (1972) Pituitary function in idiopathic haemochromatosis and cirrhosis of the liver. *Lancet* **ii**, 298–300.

Thomas, D., Touzel, R., Charlesworth, M., Wass, J.A.H. & Besser, G.M. (1987) Hyperprolactinaemia and microadenomas in primary hypothyroidism. *Clinical Endocrinology* **27**, 289–295.

Tincello, D.G., . Saunders, P.T. & Hargreave, T.B. (1997) Preliminary investigations on androgen receptor gene mutations in infertile men. *Molecular Human Reproduction* **3**, 941–943.

Tolis, G., Lewis, W., Verdy, M. *et al.* (1974) Anterior pituitary function in Prader–Labhart–Willi syndrome. *Journal of Clinical Endocrinology* **39**, 1061–1066.

Tsuchiya, H., Onishi, T., Imanaka, S. *et al.* (1985) Prolactin secretion in acromegalic patients before and after selective adenomectomy. *Journal of Clinical Endocrinology and Metabolism* **61**, 104–109.

Tweed, M.J. & Roland, J.M. (1998) Haemochromatosis as an endocrine cause of subfertility. *British Medical Journal* **316**, 915–916.

Urban, M.D., Lee, P.A. & Midgeon, C.J. (1978) Adult height and fertility in men with congenital adrenal hyperplasia. *New England Journal of Medicine* **299**, 1392–1396.

Wilson, J.D., Harrod, M.J., Goldstein, J.L. & MacDonald, P.C. (1974) Familial incomplete male pseudohermaphroditism, Type 1. *New England Journal of Medicine* **290**, 1097–1103.

Wischusen, J., Baker, H.W. & Hudson, B. (1981) Reversible male infertility due to congenital adrenal hyperplasia. *Clinical Endocrinology* **14**, 571–577.

10: Disorders of Ejaculation

Disorders of ejaculation are commonly found amongst the infertile male population and it is important that the clinician understands management of patients with these disorders.

The normal sexual response in the male

The sexual response in the human was initially described by Masters and Johnson in their classic works on this subject (Masters & Johnson 1966, 1970); indeed, it was these authors who provided the first real understanding of sexual dysfunction and allowed for the development of its rational treatment.

The sexual response in the human male can be divided into four main phases (Salkin 1994) and these phases are outlined below.

1 *Excitement*: this period involves the onset of erotic feelings and the beginning of erection. During this period, the scrotum thickens and the testes become elevated.

2 *Plateau*: this is seen near to orgasm and at this time the penis is firm and is extended to its maximum length. The secretion of mucoid substances from the urethral glands now occurs.

3 *Orgasm*: this consists of the occurrence of ejaculation itself. At ejaculation three to seven spurts of semen occur at intervals of around 0.8 s.

4 *Resolution*: in response to the sympathetic discharge that initiates ejaculation, the parasympathetic drive that induces erection is overcome and the penis after ejaculation rapidly detumesces. There now occurs a period of refractoriness to any further sexual stimulation.

In this section, the disorders of ejaculation will be discussed, but first one must examine the anatomy and physiology of ejaculation.

The anatomy of the posterior urethra

The posterior urethra is made up of two parts: the preprostatic and the prostatic urethra.

The preprostatic urethra is about 1–1.5 cm in length and has a stellate lumen. It extends from the bladder down to the superior edge of the prostate gland. Its wall is made up of smooth muscle arranged as circular fibres to form the internal sphincter, which merge inferiorly with the smooth muscle in the prostatic capsule. The internal sphincter is almost entirely innervated by sympathetic nonadrenergic fibres and thus differs from the nerve supply of the rest of the urethra and the bladder. Similar sympathetic nerves also supply the seminal vesicles, the smooth muscle in the prostatic capsule and the vas deferens, all of which contract at the time of ejaculation. Contraction of the internal sphincter around the preprostatic urethra at ejaculation prevents the retrograde flow of semen through the proximal urethra and into the bladder.

The prostatic urethra is about 3–4 cm in length and passes through the anterior half of the gland. It is continuous with the preprostatic urethra and emerges from the prostate gland at its apex. Down the length of the posterior wall of the prostatic urethra is an elevation known as the urethral crest. On either side of this crest is the prostatic sinus, in the floor of which lies the multiple orifices of the prostatic ducts. About half-way down the urethral crest is a small elevation known either as the verumontanum or the colliculus seminalis. On the centre of this elevation is the prostatic utricle and on either side of the prostatic utricle, and slightly cranial to it, lie the slit-like openings of the ejaculatory ducts. The prostatic utricle is some 6 mm in diameter and is seen as a small pit on the verumontanum. It is the remnant of the müllerian duct system in the male and one may find small patches of endometrial epithelium among the transitional epithelium that lines this small area.

At the distal end of the prostatic urethra is an outer layer of circular smooth muscle that forms the external sphincter.

The mechanism of ejaculation

Ejaculation is a much more complex phenomenon than erection and must now be considered in some detail.

Ejaculation can be divided into three major phases. These comprise: (i) the passage of the seminal fluid into the posterior urethra, a process known as emission; (ii) closure of the bladder neck; and (iii) the ejaculation of the contents of the urethra down the penile urethra and out through the external penile meatus.

The neurological control of ejaculation is complex. Afferent stimuli from the genitalia are initiated via the pudendal nerve (S2, 3 and 4) and enter the cord through both the thoracolumbar sympathetic fibres (T12–L3) and sacral parasympathetic outflow (S2–S4). The impulses are transmitted to the central nervous system and emission is initiated via the thoracolumbar outflow (T12–L3). It is via the hypogastric nerves that contraction of the caudal end of the epididymis, the vas deferens, the walls of the seminal vesicles and the capsule of the prostate gland take place (Fig. 10.1). At the same time, the internal sphincter contracts to prevent the retrograde flow of semen into the bladder. Because of the rhythmic contractions of the bulbocavernosus and ischiocavernosus muscles, also innervated by the pudendal nerve, the seminal fluid is milked down the penile urethra and out through the external penile meatus.

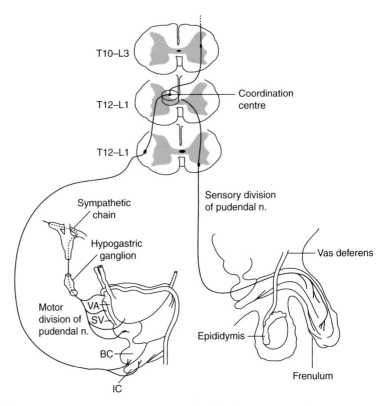

Fig. 10.1 A diagrammatic representation of the neurological control of both erection and ejaculation. Note the presence of the coordinating centre in the lower thoracic cord.

During emission, the secretions that make up semen are propelled into the urethra in a distinct order. The first of these secretions to arrive in the posterior urethra are the secretions of the testes and epididymides and these are followed by the secretions of the prostate. Last to arrive in the posterior urethra are the secretions of the seminal vesicles. The secretion of the mucoproteins by the urethral and bulbourethral glands frequently occurs prior to emission, thus providing lubrication for coitus. Thus, mixing of all the components that make up semen does not occur until the ejaculate reaches the exterior of the genital tract, a fact that must be remembered for those performing a semen analysis (Table 10.1).

As the secretions that make up the ejaculate are passed down the urethra in a distinct 'order', it is possible to separate out each major area of secretion into three separate fractions and the examination of these individual fractions can be useful diagnostically.

Disorders of ejaculation

There are three major disorders of ejaculation: premature ejaculation, retrograde ejaculation and ejaculatory failure. Retrograde ejaculation and

Table 10.1 Order of appearance of the secretions of the genital tract at ejaculation. These secretions can be separated out at ejaculation with surprising ease and this may be of value diagnostically

Secretions of the bulbourethral and urethral gland	5%
Testicular and epididymal secretions	5%
Secretions of the prostate	30%
Secretions of the seminal vesicles	60%

ejaculatory failure are also sometimes erroneously referred to as anorgasmia, but such nomenclature is unsatisfactory as, in many patients with either of these disorders, orgasm can be completely normal. Among patients with neurological disease, retrograde ejaculation may progress to ejaculatory failure. In such patients, retrograde ejaculation can be considered to be a less severe manifestation of total ejaculatory failure.

Premature ejaculation

This condition is one of the commonest disorders of sexual function. In premature ejaculation, the process of ejaculation is uncontrolled and occurs very quickly after the onset of the erection. Ejaculation may occur immediately on penetration or even before the penis has entered the vagina. However, erections are often difficult to obtain in these patients and indeed it is usually the problem with erections (Ozturk *et al.* 1997; Haensel *et al.* 1996) and the anxiety that goes with this problem (Strassberg *et al.* 1990) that initiates this disorder in the first place. The longer the problem with erection persists, the worse becomes the anxiety and the more marked becomes the premature ejaculation.

It is therefore important first to diagnose the cause of the ill-sustained erection, and this can of course be caused by all the many factors that cause complete erectile failure as well as less common conditions that interfere with erection, such as hypogonadism (Cohen 1997).

Treatment of premature ejaculation

In the treatment of premature ejaculation, it is first important to overcome the problems with erection, as otherwise all treatment of the premature ejaculation will fail. It is also essential to make a diagnosis of the causation of the initial erectile disorder and if possible treat that condition.

Several techniques have been used to overcome the problem of premature ejaculation.

The 'squeeze' technique

The first of these was devised by Masters and Johnson (Masters & Johnson 1970) and is known as the 'squeeze' technique (St Lawrence & Madakasira

1992). The patient or his partner squeezes the penis on erection and this often has an inhibitory effect upon ejaculation.

The 'stop–start' technique

Another method takes place without the patient's partner being present and is known as the 'stop–start' technique. The patient induces an erection by masturbation after which the erection is allowed to subside before being stimulated again in the same manner. Ejaculation is only allowed to take place after this stop–start erection has occurred four times. With the use of this technique on a regular basis, ejaculation can return to normal within 4–6 weeks.

Antidepressants

Another method of treatment of this problem is the use of antidepressants (Balon 1996). These drugs also have the advantage that they also reduce anxiety. Agents such as fluoxetine hydrochloride (Prozac, Eli Lilly), which inhibit serotonin uptake, are very effective at retarding ejaculation and are effective in the treatment of premature ejaculation (Kindler *et al.* 1997). Another drug that has been successfully used in the treatment of premature ejaculation is paroxetine (Aropax, SmithKline Beecham Pharmaceuticals) (Waldinger *et al.* 1997). Clomipramine hydrochloride (Anafranil, Novartis Pharmaceuticals) and sertraline hydrochloride (Zoloft, Roerig) are also reported as being successful in retarding ejaculation in men with this problem. A small dose of these agents can be taken a few hours before intercourse and can give very good results.

Retarded ejaculation

In this condition, erection is normal but the patient is unable to ejaculate intravaginally. Some men with this condition are even unable to ejaculate in the presence of their partner. This is basically a psychological problem and does not have a physical basis.

Retrograde ejaculation

Retrograde ejaculation is a not uncommon cause of infertility. It was at one time known as 'retrospermia' but is now always referred to as retrograde ejaculation.

In this condition, the semen at ejaculation passes back into the bladder rather than travelling down the urethra and out into the vagina. Patients with this problem will thus present with infertility and a persistently reduced ejaculatory volume. The ejaculate, however, is rarely totally absent as it must be remembered that some of the ejaculatory volume is made up of the secretions of the bulbourethral and the urethral glands whose secretions are directed into the penile and anterior part of the urethra. All patients with reduced ejaculatory volume should be suspected of suffering from retrograde ejaculation.

Causes of retrograde ejaculation

Idiopathic

In many patients with retrograde ejaculation, the cause cannot be determined. In many of the patients with this type of retrograde ejaculation, the lesion may involve an inadequate closure of the bladder neck at ejaculation. Such patients, however, show no abnormality on videocystometry (Jequier, unpublished). However, as bladder closure at ejaculation is different from that in operation to prevent urinary loss, one would probably not expect to see any such abnormality of bladder neck function, at least in relation to urinary continence.

Bladder neck incompetence

Retrograde ejaculation can follow any form of damage to the bladder neck, such as that occurring after transurethral resection, urethrotomy. Accidental damage to the bladder neck, which so often occurs in association with severe pelvic fractures, can also induce retrograde ejaculation. Congenital defects of the bladder neck such as bladder extrophy and hemitrigone may also give rise to retrograde ejaculation.

Damage or removal of the sympathetic chain

Because of the site of the sympathetic chain, any operation that takes place anteriorly or in close proximity to the lumbar spine may give rise to disorders of ejaculation (Fig. 10.2). In patients who have undergone lumbar sympathectomy, or even repair of an aortic aneurism, retrograde ejaculation is very common. Similar problems may also occur in men who have had excision of the para-aortic glands (Kedia *et al.* 1975) during procedures designed to extirpate conditions such as testicular cancer. During a retroperitoneal lymphadenectomy, it is, however, possible to avoid damage to the sympathetic chain provided that the tumour mass in that area is not too great (Arai *et al.* 1998). Such procedures may also induce the more serious condition of ejaculatory failure. Disorders of ejaculation including retrograde ejaculation may also occur after operations such as laparoscopic discectomy and after any operation that involves an anterior approach to the lumbar spine.

Retrograde ejaculation may also be the result of surgery in men with abdominal aneurysms and in men undergoing aortoiliac surgery (Machleder & Weinstein 1975) or rectal surgery. However in rectal surgery, such as an abdominoperineal resection, ejaculation can be preserved if care

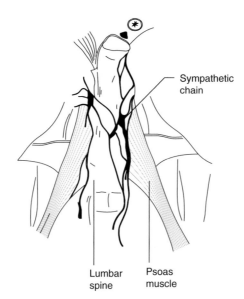

Sympathetic
chain

Lumbar
spine

Psoas
muscle

Fig. 10.2 A drawing of the
sympathetic chain and its close
relationship to the lumbar vertebrae.

is taken to preserve the presacral nerve (Maas *et al.* 1998), but this may not
be possible if the operation is being carried out as a cure for extensive malignant disease.

Pelvic surgery

Operations in the pelvis may also damage the hypogastric nerve plexus and
result in ejaculatory disorders (Fig. 10.3). Care must be taken in this area
not to cause damage or severance of the hypogastric nerves during this type
of surgery.

Diabetes mellitus

Retrograde ejaculation is a common complication of diabetes mellitus and
may occur in as many as 5% of young men with this condition (Greene &
Kelalis 1967). Retrograde ejaculation in diabetics is likely to have a neurological basis but the exact mechanism of its induction in diabetes has never
been elucidated.

Neurological disease

Retrograde ejaculation is a common accompaniment of many different
forms of neurological disease and indeed may be the presenting symptom
of these disorders. Thus, all men presenting at an infertility clinic should be
examined neurologically by the clinician. Common neurological disease
that can cause retrograde ejaculation include multiple sclerosis, motor
neurone disease and a variety of spinal cord disorders (Fowler 1998).

Traumatic diastasis of the pelvic symphysis may also cause a stretching

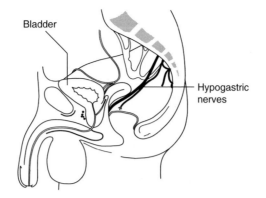

Bladder

Hypogastric
nerves

Fig. 10.3 The position of the hypogastric nerves as they cross the pelvic floor. They are susceptible to damage during many forms of pelvic surgery in the male.

of the lumbar plexus and a lumbar plexus neuropraxia that can also result in retrograde ejaculation. However, these changes are usually only temporary and will frequently resolve with the passage of time.

Spinal injury

Spinal cord injury almost always results in some form of disturbance of ejaculation but in men with incomplete lesions, the damage to ejaculation may be limited to the presence of retrograde ejaculation rather than the total ejaculatory failure that so commonly occurs in men with complete spinal transection. The whole problem of infertility in spinal cord injury will be discussed more fully in Chapter 12.

Urethral obstruction

Much more rarely, obstructive lesions may also result in retrograde ejaculation. Urethral stricture may also occasionally be a cause of retrograde ejaculation. The pressure within the posterior urethra caused by the emission can prevent closure of the bladder neck during ejaculation. Large ectopic ureteroceles are also known to cause retrograde ejaculation (Ng & Rickards 1994), as are the presence (and not just the surgery) of posterior urethral valves.

Other less common causes of retrograde ejaculation

There are also other rare causes of retrograde ejaculation and these include retroperitoneal fibrosis (Chally *et al.* 1998) and other causes of damage to the sympathetic chain. Operations such as lower lumbar interbody vertebral fusion runs the risk of inducing such damage (Christensen & Bunger 1997), as will many operations involving the pelvic organs. Retrograde ejaculation may also accompany hyperprolactinaemia (Ishikawa *et al.* 1993).

Abnormalities that mimic retrograde ejaculation

A wide variety of abnormalities may mimic retrograde ejaculation. Of these the most important include ejaculatory duct obstruction, where exclusion of the testicular and the seminal vesicular components of the ejaculate reduce its volume very considerably. Anomalous insertions of the ejaculatory ducts can also be mistaken for retrograde ejaculation. Such anomalies include the insertion of the ejaculatory ducts into the ureters (Redman & Suleiman 1976) and the fistulous connection between the ejaculatory ducts and the rectum that may occur following surgery in this area (Abramovichi *et al.* 1972).

Diagnosis of retrograde ejaculation

All patients with this condition must undergo careful history taking and a thorough clinical examination. Any second pathology must be excluded and such second pathologies are not uncommon in this group of patients. An example of a situation where two such pathologies may coexist is in the diabetic where vascular lesions may cause primary testicular disease while the neurological lesion may give rise to an ejaculatory disorder. In the absence of any second pathology, testicular size will be normal and the serum FSH will also be within the range of normal.

The diagnosis of retrograde ejaculation is made from the examination of postcoital urine (Crich & Jequier 1978).

The patient is asked to have intercourse or to induce ejaculation by masturbation. He is then instructed to empty his bladder and to take all of this urine to the laboratory for examination. The patient should be given a 24-h urine container for this purpose or some form of container that will hold at least 500 mL of urine. As contact with urine kills sperm very quickly, it does not matter if the urine sample is brought to the laboratory the following day if this is more convenient for the patient.

Examination of the postcoital urine specimen

The first part of the examination is to ensure that the urine in its container is very well mixed. As urine kills sperm very rapidly, the sperm will soon fall to the bottom of the container and will thus be excluded from the urine itself. As a sperm count will be performed on this urine, it is important to ensure thorough mixing.

Two 10-mL aliquots of urine are now removed and each is placed in a large test tube. The volume of the remaining urine is now measured using a large measuring cylinder and is then discarded. The total volume of the urine sample can then be easily estimated.

The two aliquots of urine are now centrifuged, the supernatant discarded and the pellet, which will contain sperm, is now resuspended in normal saline or phosphate buffer. A sperm count is now performed in duplicate on both of the resuspended sperm samples in the usual counting chamber. From these estimations, the total number of sperm in the ejaculate (i.e. in the urine specimen) can be calculated.

Number of sperm in 1 mL of saline = number of sperm in 10 mL of urine

Number of sperm in the urine specimen = (Volume of urine/10) × Sperm count

The total number of sperm in an ejaculate is then reported to the clinician as the mean of these four estimations made from these two aliquots of urine.

There will, of course, always be some sperm left in the urethra following normal antegrade ejaculation. These will appear in any urine sample examined after normal ejaculation. However, one should not find more than some 2–5 million sperm in a postcoital urine specimen from a man who does not have retrograde ejaculation.

A diagnostic problem may also arise however, in a man with retrograde ejaculation who is also azoospermic. In these circumstances, one makes the diagnosis of retrograde ejaculation by measuring one of the more stable seminal markers such as fructose or acid phosphatase in the postcoital urine specimen.

Another situation that may also cause diagnostic confusion is where the retrograde ejaculation is either intermittent or incomplete. To make this diagnosis, several samples of postcoital urine may need to be examined.

However, in most cases of infertility caused by retrograde ejaculation the diagnosis is usually easy to make and the examination of postcoital urine, carried out in the manner described above, should be a service offered by all laboratories carrying out semen analysis.

Methods of retrieving live sperm from men with retrograde ejaculation

Urine has a profoundly deleterious effect on sperm and frequently renders them immotile within a few moments of the initial contact (Crich & Jequier 1978). This appears to be because of the relatively low osmolality of urine in comparison with that of the seminal plasma. The variable pH may also exert an effect that may not be entirely countered by the huge buffering power of the protein in semen). However, the pH of the urine is unlikely to have very much effect upon the motility of the sperm in the ejaculate. Thus the contact between the semen and the urine in men with retrograde ejaculation is nevertheless very deleterious to the sperm and should be minimized.

There are, however, a number of ways in which this problem can be overcome.

The full bladder technique

This method has the advantage of simplicity but is frequently unsuccessful in men with severe damage or dysfunction of their bladder neck (Crich & Jequier 1978). The patient is simply asked to ejaculate while the bladder is very full. The high intravesical pressure exerted by the urine not only may itself prevent retrograde ejaculation but may also enhance the closing pressure of the bladder neck.

Using this technique, it is often possible to induce antegrade ejaculation in these patients, and pregnancies have been achieved during normal sexual intercourse using this technique alone. Although this method does not succeed in producing antegrade ejaculates in all men with retrograde ejaculation, its simplicity indicates that it should initially be tried out in most men with infertility due to this problem.

Passage of the clotted ejaculate into medium prior to liquefaction

Even if an antegrade ejaculate cannot be obtained using the full bladder technique, it is sometimes possible to use this method to prevent the ejaculate from entering the bladder.

For success, ejaculation must take place close to the laboratory. The patient is given a wide-necked semen pot containing medium such as human tubal fluid medium (HTFM) warmed to between 30 and 35°C. The function of the medium is to dilute the urine, correct the pH and provide the correct osmolality for the spermatozoa.

The patient is asked to ejaculate following masturbation, again when the bladder is uncomfortably full. Immediately after ejaculation, the patient is asked to pass the very first portion of urine into the semen pot containing the warmed medium. This fraction of urine will hopefully contain the unliquefied coagulum of semen. The ejaculate in the medium is then taken directly to the laboratory where the clot is washed with further medium to remove any urine that may surround it. The ejaculate is allowed to liquefy in its own time. Using this technique, it is often possible to collect good samples of semen that can be used for simple insemination.

Postejaculatory catheterization

In some men, especially those with severe damage to their bladder neck and who may also have problems with urinary incontinence, there is no simple means of overcoming their retrograde ejaculation. In such patients, one may have to resort to postejaculatory catheterization.

The patient is first asked to restrict fluids for around 6h and a dose of sodium bicarbonate may also be given in order to raise the pH of the urine.

A small silastic catheter (no. 5 French) is used for this procedure. No lubricant should be used as this is often harmful to the spermatozoa but the catheter can be moistened to aid insertion by using the medium itself. Some clinicians carry out a pre-ejaculatory bladder wash-out using 180 mL of 5% dextrose Ringer solution after which a small portion is left in the bladder. Some clinicians also instill the patient's serum into the bladder so as to increase the buffering power of the semen and also to enhance the osmolality of the urine.

The patient is then asked to ejaculate, after which the semen may be voided with the urine in the normal way, or postejaculatory catheterization with or without bladder wash-outs may be performed. If large numbers of sperm are obtained, they can be cryopreserved as this may reduce the need for this type of sperm retrieval.

However, it must be remembered that such procedures are invasive and are also unpleasant for the patient. They run the risk of inducing urinary tract infections and epididymo-orchitis. Even momentary contact with urine can damage sperm and these procedures may have to be repeated more than once to achieve a pregnancy. Despite all these problems, pregnancies can be produced using this technique and even postcoital intravaginal voiding of semen has reportedly once resulted in conception.

Vasal aspiration

This is a technique that is now used to collect sperm from patients with both retrograde ejaculation and ejaculatory failure (Hovatta *et al.* 1996) and is especially useful in the management of ejaculatory failure in the men with spinal injury. This technique can, however, also be used in men with retrograde ejaculation but sperm so harvested are too few in number to be used for insemination and therefore must be used in some form of assisted conception such as IVF.

Vasal aspiration may be carried out under either general or local anaesthesia. In the spinal cord-injured man, spinal anaesthesia is a very satisfactory form of analgesia.

Using a very small incision similar to that used for vasectomy, the vas is exposed and hemisected. A fine cannula is inserted into the proximal lumen and the vas is flushed with a culture medium such as HTFM until one can feel some distension of the cauda of the epididymis. The vas is then slowly and gently aspirated and with some pressure on the cauda it is possible to collect many millions of sperm. The vas is then closed using a fine suture and the skin closed over it.

Spermatozoa collected in this way can be cryopreserved and are probably best used within an IVF programme, as often too few sperm can be collected this way at least for repeated use as an inseminate.

Surgery in the management of retrograde ejaculation

Surgery may indeed be indicated in a few of these patients in whom the retrograde ejaculation is due to severe damage to the bladder neck by either past surgery or trauma. Such surgery may include tightening of the bladder

191

neck as in the Young–Dees operation or the Leadbetter technique in which a neourethra is formed. More recently, the use of a perivesical collagen injection has been described as a successful means of achieving antegrade ejaculation (Reynolds *et al.* 1998).

In some patients whose retrograde ejaculation may also be associated with severe urinary incontinence, diversion of the urine and removal of the bladder with total closure of the preprostatic urethra will, of course, also solve the problem of retrograde ejaculation.

Drugs in the treatment of retrograde ejaculation

Drug therapy would seem to be ideal for men with retrograde ejaculation as it is simple and noninvasive, but overall the results from the use of sympathomimetic agents are poor. These results may of course depend on the cause of the retrograde ejaculation. One would of course not expect good results from their use in a man with severe bladder neck damage while their application might give more favourable results in a patient with retrograde ejaculation due to a neurological disorder. Some success was at one time achieved using the antihistaminic and anticholinergic agent brompheniramine among diabetics with retrograde ejaculation (Andaloro & Dube 1975), but this agent did induce some quite nasty anticholinergic side effects such as a dry mouth and blurred vision. Drugs are today deemed to be of little value in the management of retrograde ejaculation.

The number of motile sperm obtained using any of these techniques may be too few to achieve a natural pregnancy and thus some form of assisted conception even using intracytoplasmic sperm injection may have to be considered in some patients with retrograde ejaculation. Indeed. the application of assisted conception to the problem of retrograde ejaculation has improved the pregnancy rate very considerably whatever means of collecting semen has been used (Okada *et al.* 1998).

Ejaculatory failure

In this condition, there is no emission and thus there can be no ejaculation. Retrograde ejaculation, especially when it is due to neurological disease, can, with time, progress to ejaculatory failure.

In this condition, there is no passage of any of the secretions that make up seminal fluid into the posterior urethra, i.e emission as well as ejaculation has failed. The sperm remain in the cauda epididymis, thus producing more major problems with fertility.

Causes of ejaculatory failure

Although ejaculatory failure can be idiopathic and can be caused by all of the neurological diseases, it in fact has only two common causes: diabetes mellitus and spinal injury.

Diabetes mellitus

Ejaculatory failure occurs in the diabetic patient and it may be preceded by retrograde ejaculation. The exact nature of the neurological disturbance that causes ejaculatory failure in the diabetic is unknown, but disorders of ejaculation are in general common, even in young men with this disorder.

Spinal injury

Spinal injury is one of the most common causes of ejaculatory failure that is seen in clinical practice. First, the higher centres are needed before ejaculation can take place and thus in any complete spinal cord lesion such an input will be absent. Second, the complexity of ejaculation and the fact that it requires two sites of input to the cord, i.e. the thoracolumbar and the sacral area, is doubtless why ejaculatory failure is almost the rule in men with complete spinal lesions.

Diagnosis of ejaculatory failure

The diagnosis is usually fairly obvious from the history as patients with this disorder often do not have a true orgasm and produce no semen at any time.

A careful history and clinical examination must be carried out to exclude any second pathology in these men. Among patients with spinal injury, especially among those men who self-catheterize, urinary infection is common and may give rise to an epididymitis. Thus, such men may not simply have ejaculatory failure but may also have an epididymal obstruction (Jequier 1997). The presence of epididymal distension or epididymal irregularities on palpation would indicate the presence of such an obstructive lesion.

It is, however, important to exclude retrograde ejaculation in some of these patients and so, whenever the diagnosis of ejaculatory failure may be in doubt, it is important to collect a postejaculatory sample of urine for examination.

Treatment of infertility caused by ejaculatory failure

There are several ways in which infertility caused by ejaculatory failure has been overcome.

Vibroejaculation

Some patients, particularly those with spinal injury, will produce an ejaculate in response to a vibratory stimulus directed against the glans penis. There are many vibrators on the market, which are sold as sex aids, but in general the amplitude of the vibration in these stimulators is insufficient to produce a response in a spinally injured man. It is thus better to purchase a vibrator specifically designed for such patients as in these instruments both the amplitude and the frequency of the vibration can be adjusted. The best of these specially manufactured vibrators is the Ferticare personal vibrator (Multicept Aps, Vallerodvaenge #2, 2860 Rungsted, Denmark) (Fig. 10.4). These vibrators give the best results when the peak-to-peak amplitude is about 2 mm and they are operated at around 80–100 Hz.

The vibrator is best placed on the underside of the glans close to the frenulum. By moving it slowly across the undersurface of this area of the penis, a 'trigger' area can often be found. Stimulation of this area results in increased penile tumescence and usually some increase in lower limb spasticity and clonus. The vibrator should be applied to the penis for about 3 min and if no ejaculate is obtained during that time further application can be tried after a rest interval of about 2 min. Most patients who are going to respond do so in the first one to two attempts at vibroejaculation.

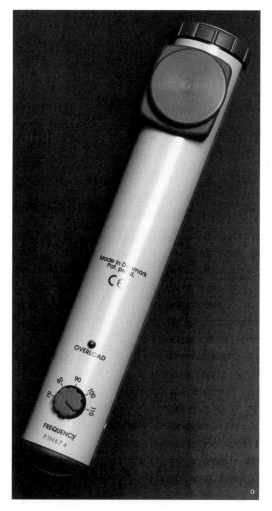

Fig. 10.4 The Ferticare (Multicept Aps, Denmark) vibrator, which may be used in an attempt to overcome ejaculatory failure. Both the amplitude and the frequency of the vibrations can be adjusted.

Patients with high spinal cord lesions respond better to vibratory stimulation than those with lower cord lesions. Oates has reported that of patients with cervical cord lesions, 75% will respond with satisfactory ejaculation while only 62% of those with thoracic cord injuries are able to produce an ejaculate after this type of stimulation. No ejaculate is obtained from those men with lesions below T12 (Oates *et al.* 1990). Overall, a success rate of around 70% should be obtained (Berratta *et al.* 1989).

It must, however, be remembered that even the vibrator can cause a prolonged rise in blood pressure at ejaculation in men with high spinal lesions. It is thus suggested that in men with high spinal cord lesions and preoperative dose of sublingual nifedepine of 20 mg is given to the patient about 1 h prior to the attempt at ejaculation. All men with spinal cord lesions above T6 should have their blood pressure measured, at least during the initial use of a vibrator.

However, not infrequently in these patients, even if an emission is induced and semen arrives in the posterior urethra, it may then be ejaculated in a retrograde manner, making collection of the semen difficult.

Electroejaculation

For many years, electroejaculation has been the standard way in which to retrieve sperm from men with ejaculatory failure. However, the quality of the semen so obtained has been poor (Ohl *et al.* 1989; Denil *et al.* 1996) and the pregnancy rate, by present day standards, is low.

Prior to an attempt at electroejaculation, it is important to treat all urinary tract infections, and some clinics routinely give antibiotics to the patient 5 days before this therapy. On the day before treatment, an enema is given to empty the lower bowel.

Patients can also be given 1.5 g of sodium bicarbonate 2 h prior to treatment to reduce the acidity of the urine should retrograde ejaculation or contamination of the ejaculate with urine occur.

The patients with ejaculatory failure because of high spinal cord lesions are at risk from autonomic dysreflexia and excessive rises in blood pressure during this procedure, and men with a history of this disorder are also best given sublingual nifedipine at a dose of 20 mg prior to the procedure. Whether or not these men have a general anaesthetic for this procedure depends upon the site of the lesion and the degree of sensory loss. It must be remembered, however, that sensory loss must be profound before this procedure can be carried out, and all patients with normal sensory function must have general anaesthesia for this procedure.

After the induction of anaesthesia, the patient is placed in the left lateral position and the probe placed in the rectum. Electroejaculators made by the G & S Instrument Company (National Rehabilitation Hospital, Washington, DC, USA) are the most commonly used. On the rectal probes, which are in different sizes, three electrodes are placed on the anterior surface and these are placed to face the posterior wall of the bladder and the prostate. The current is applied for some 5 s in increasingly wave-like patterns until ejaculation is complete. During the period of stimulation, an assistant places a container over the penis to collect the ejaculate, which often has to be milked forward from the posterior urethra out through the urethral meatus. Care must be taken not to induce rectal damage, which is a risk with these procedures, as rectal burns may occur.

Vasal aspiration and IVF

This form of treatment, although more complex than vibro- or electro-ejaculation, is now giving by far the best results in terms of pregnancy rates, at least among anejaculatory men (Hovatta *et al.* 1996) and in particular in men with spinal cord injury (Jequier 1997). However, this approach can be used for any man with ejaculatory failure, apparently with great success. One finding that is of interest among the men with spinal injury is that sperm function and the fertilization rate in IVF appears to be normal in these patients, indicating that the poor semen quality is likely to be a result of its method of collection rather than be a cause of the patient's infertility.

Sperm is collected by scrotal exploration and vasal aspiration and this is best carried out using either a general or a spinal anaesthetic, although a spinal cord block may also be employed. In men with high spinal cord lesions, a number of reflexes may be initiated, particularly reflex erection and the onset of clonus. These can be very embarrassing for the patient and for these reasons the author prefers the use of regional anaesthesia. A single-shot spinal anaesthetic also has the advantage that it greatly diminishes the risk of autonomic hyperreflexia.

A small incision is made over the vas as in a vasectomy. The isolated loop of vas is then isolated and hemitransected. A no. 22 intravenous cannula attached to a 2-mL syringe is inserted into the proximal vas and under pressure some medium such as HTFM is injected towards the cauda of the epididymis. The contents of the cauda are then aspirated into the syringe and this is aided by some pressure and milking of the cauda epididymis through the scrotal wall. When sufficient sperm have been collected, the vas is closed using a single 6/0 polydioxanone (PDS; Ethicon Ltd) suture. If no sperm can be aspirated, it is therefore possible that an epididymal obstruction may be present and this is common among men with spinal cord injury. Epididymal aspiration of sperm must then be carried out.

Following sperm collection, the vas is returned to the scrotum and the wound closed in the usual manner.

Using this technique it is possible to collect as many as 10–50 million sperm of good motility. All excess sperm can be cryopreserved, and it is our experience that this is the only procedure that will ever need be carried out on the anejaculatory patient. This technique can also be used on men with severe retrograde ejaculation in whom it is difficult to obtain an antegrade ejaculate or in whom postejaculatory bladder catheterization has caused complications.

These sperm can then be used within an IVF programme. If sperm motility is poor or if an obstruction is present and the sperm have been collected from the epididymis, then the technique of intracytoplasmic sperm injection can be used instead of classic IVF. This technique is associated with a clinical pregnancy rate of around 60% per cycle of treatment (Jequier 1997).

Thus, it is clear that much can be done for patients with disorders of ejaculation in relation to their fertility. However, it is important that the clinician understands the nature of the pathology that is causing the problem so that the correct management is applied to each of these different clinical problems.

Painful ejaculation

This is another disorder that is occasionally seen even in an infertility clinic. This is a diagnostically difficult problem as in the majority of men with this disorder no cause can be found. It may sometimes follow vasectomy but whether or not a significant number of patients have their pain resolved by vasectomy reversal is difficult to ascertain. There is no doubt, however, that this pain can be exceedingly distressing to the patients who suffer from this disorder.

The main source of the pain seems to involve the involuntary spasm of the pelvic muscles and these spasms may in fact be induced by certain psychosexual conflicts (Kaplan 1993). This type of pain has also been associated with the administration of the tricyclic antidepressants (Aizenberg *et al.* 1991), but how they could cause pain of such severity is unknown.

One interesting aspect of this problem is that in men with obstruction of the ejaculatory ducts pain is not usually a symptom, but painful ejaculation has been related to the presence of seminal vesicular calculi (Corriere 1997).

The cause and the treatment of this condition remains largely unelucidated.

Disorders of ejaculation are a surprisingly common cause of infertility in the male. Careful history taking is essential to provide an accurate diagnosis as many of the aetiologies of these disorders may be relatively easy to treat.

References

Abramovichi, H., Brandes, J.M., Paldi, E., Peretz, A., Peretz, B.A. & Gheresh, Y. (1972) Male sterility due to a fistula between the rectum and the common ejaculatory ducts: case report. *American Journal of Obstetrics and Gynecology* **114**, 840–841.

Aizenberg, D., Zemishlany, Z., Hermesh, H., Karp, L. & Weizman, A. (1991) Painful ejaculation associated with antidepressants in four patients. *Journal of Clinical Psychiatry* **52**, 461–463.

Andaloro, V.A. & Dube, A. (1975) Treatment of retrograde ejaculation with brompheniramine. *Urology* **5**, 520–522.

Arai, Y., Ishitoya, S., Okubo, K. *et al.* (1998) Nerve-sparing retroperitoneal lymph node dissecton for metastatic testicular cancer. *International Journal of Urology* **4**, 487–492.

Balon, R. (1996) Antidepressants in the treatment of premature ejaculation. *Journal of Sex and Marital Therapy* **22**, 85–96.

Berratta, G., Chelo, E. & Zanolla, A. (1989) Reproductive aspects in spinal cord injured males. *Paraplegia* **27**, 113–118.

Chally, P., Gopalakrishnan, G., Nath, V. & Kekre, N.S. (1998) Failure of emission in retroperitoneal fibrosis. *British Journal of Urology* **81**, 503.

Christensen, F.B. & Bunger, C.E. (1997) Retrograde ejaculation after retroperitoneal lower lumbar interbody fusion. *International Orthopaedics* **21**, 176–180.

Cohen, P.G. (1997) The association of premature ejaculation and hypogonadotrophic hypogonadism. *Journal of Sex and Marital Therapy* **23**, 208–211.

Corriere, J.N. (1997) Painful ejaculation due to seminal vesicle calculi. *Journal of Urology* **157**, 626.

Crich, J.P. & Jequier, A.M. (1978) Infertility in ejaculation. The action of urine on sperm motility and a simple method for achieving antegrade ejaculation. *Fertility and Sterility* **30**, 572–576.

Denil, J., Kupker, W., Al-Hasani, S. *et al.* (1996) Successful combination of transrectal electroejaculation and intracytoplasmic sperm injection in the treatment of anejaculation. *Human Reproduction* **11**, 1247–1249.

Fowler, C.J. (1998) The neurology of male sexual dysfunction and its investigation by clinical neurophysiological methods. *British Journal of Urology* **81**, 785–795.

Greene, L.F. & Kelalis, P.P. (1967) Retrograde ejaculation of semen due to diabetic neuropathy. *Journal of Urology* **98**, 693.

Haensel, S.M., Rowland, D.L. & Kallan, K.T. (1996) Clomipramine and sexual function in men with premature ejaculation and controls. *Journal of Urology* **156**, 1310–1315.

Hovatta, O., Reima, I., Foudila, T., Butzow, T., Johansson, K. & von Smitten, K. (1996) Vas deferens aspiration and intracytoplasmic injection of frozen–thawed spermatozoa in a case of anejaculation in a diabetic man. *Human Reproduction* **11**, 334–335.

Ishikawa, H., Kaneko, S., Ohashi, M., Nakagawa, K. & Hata, M. (1993) Retrograde ejaculation accompanying hyperprolactinaemia. *Archives of Andrology* **30**, 153–155.

Jequier, A.M. (1997) *Assisted conception in the treatment of male infertility caused by spinal injury*. Annual Meeting of the International Medical Society of Paraplegia, Perth, (Abstract).

Kaplan, H.S. (1993) Post-ejaculatory pain syndrome. *Journal of Sex and Marital Therapy* **19**, 91–103.

Kedia, K.R., Markland, C. & Fraley, E.E. (1975) Sexual function following high retroperitoneal lymphadenectomy. *Journal of Urology* **98**, 237–239.

Kindler, S., Dolberg, O.T., Cohen, H., Hirschmann, S. & Kotler, M. (1997) The treatment of comorbid premature ejaculation and panic disorder with fluoxetine. *Clinical Neuropharmacology* **20**, 466–471.

Maas, C.P., Moriya, Y., Steup, W.H., Kiebert, G.M., Kranenbarg, W.M. & van de Velde, C.J. (1998) Radical and nerve-sparing surgery for rectal cancer in the Netherlands: a prospective study. *British Journal of Surgery* **85**, 92–97.

Machleder, H.I. & Weinstein, M. (1975) Sexual function following surgical therapy for aorto-iliac disease. *Vascular Surgery* **9**, 283–287.

Masters, W.H. & Johnson, V.E. (1966) *The Human Sexual Response*. Little, Brown, Boston.

Masters, W.H. & Johnson, V.E. (1970) *Human Sexual Inadequacy*. Little, Brown, Boston

Ng, K.J. & Rickards, D. (1994) Ectopic ureterocele – a cause of retrograde ejaculation. *British Journal of Urology* **74**, 251–252.

Oates, R.D., Staskin, D.R. & Krane, R.J. (1990) Penile vibratory stimulation in the spinal cord injured male to induce ejaculation. *Journal of Urology* **143**, 344A (Abstract).

Ohl, D.A., Bennett, C.J., McCabe, M., Menge, A.C. & McGuire, E.J. (1989) Predictors of success in electro-ejaculation of spinal cord injured men. *Journal of Urology* **142**, 1483–1486.

Okada, H., Fujioka, H., Tastsumi, N. *et al.* (1998) Treatment of patients with retrograde ejaculation in the era of modern assisted reproduction technology. *Journal of Urology* **159**, 848–850.

Ozturk, M., Cetinkaya, M., Saglam, H., Adsan, O., Okin, O. & Memis, A. (1997) Erectile dysfunction in premature ejaculation. *Archivio Italiano di Urologia, Andrologia* **69**, 133–136.

Redman, J.F. & Suleiman, J.S. (1976) Bilateral vasal-ureteral communications. *Journal of Urology* **116**, 808–809.

Reynolds, J.C., McCall, A., Kim, E.D. & Lipschultz, L.I. (1998) Bladder neck collagen injection restores antegrade ejaculation after bladder neck surgery. *Journal of Urology* **159**, 1303.

Salkin, P. (1994) The role of the psychiatrist in the diagnosis and treatment of male sexual dysfunction. In: *Management of Impotence and Infertility* (eds E.D. Whitehead & H.M. Nagler), pp. 191–199. J.P. Lippincott Co., Philadelphia.

St Lawrence, J.S. & Madakasira, S. (1992) Evaluation and treatment of premature ejaculation: a critical review. *International Journal of Psychiatry in Medicine* **22**, 77–97.

Strassberg, D.S., Mahoney, J.M., Schaugaard, M. & Hale, V.E. (1990) The role of anxiety in premature ejaculation: a psychophysiological model. *Archives of Sexual Behaviour* **19**, 251–257.

Waldinger, M.D., Hengeveld, M.W. & Zwinderman, A.H. (1997) Ejaculation-retarding properties of parotexine in patients with primary premature ejaculation. *British Journal of Urology* **79**, 592–595.

11: Disorders of Erectile Function

Disorders of erectile function are among the most common andrological problems of all. Impotence becomes increasingly common among men as they age and may be present in varying severity in around 5% of men of 40 years of age or more (Feldman *et al.* 1994). Its frequency may rise to 25–30% at the age of 65 years (Furlow 1985) and at 75 years it is probably may be present in more than 50% of men. However, as erectile dysfunction correlates closely with increasing age, it thus should not present very frequently in an infertility clinic. However, the increase in the average age of patients requiring help with conception and the large numbers of men in second marriages who wish to start a second family makes the appearance of men with disorders of erection in an infertility clinic a not uncommon occurrence today.

It is thus important that those involved in the management of infertility have a good knowledge of all the causes of erectile failure and are very familiar with all the means that are available for its treatment.

Erectile dysfunction is defined as the inability of the male to attain and to maintain erection of the penis sufficient to permit satisfactory intercourse (NIH Consensus Conference 1993). It may have either organic or psychological aetiology. Contrary to a widely held notion that most impotence is caused by a psychological factor, in fact the incidence of organic causes of erectile dysfunction is double that of the psychological causes (Benet & Melman 1995). Other sexual dysfunctions may also precede or accompany erectile failure, and these include loss of libido, ejaculatory disturbances, particularly premature ejaculation, and even reduced orgasmic sensation. If the erectile failure precludes intercourse and intravaginal ejaculation, the patient may then present with infertility (Fabbri *et al.* 1997).

The cause of a patient's erectile failure can often be ascertained from a careful clinical history and clinical examination. As the treatment may depend for its success on an accurate clinical diagnosis, the clinical assessment of the patient with erectile failure is very important.

In order to understand the nature of erectile dysfunction, it is firstly important to have a good working knowledge of the anatomy of the penis and the erectile tissue that is contained within it.

The anatomy of the penis

The penis is made up of two parts: the root of the penis, which lies in the perineum, and the main body of the penis, which is free and pendulous and which is totally covered in skin.

The root of the penis

The root of the penis is made up of three masses of erectile tissue known as the two crura (right and left crus) and the central bulb of the penis, which lie on the urogenital triangle. Each crus penis is firmly adherent to both the sides of the pubic arch and the perineal membrane itself.

The crura

Each crus penis forms the posterior region of the corpora cavernosa while the bulb forms the posterior region of the more central corpus spongiosum. The erectile tissue in these structures thus forms a continuum into the shaft of the penis.

Each crus penis begins at the level of the inverted edge of the ischiopubic ramus and is covered by the ischiocavernosus muscle. As this elongated mass passes forward to enter the penile shaft as the corpus cavernosus it converges towards the crus of the opposite side. The two crura then pass downwards to become the corpora cavernosa within the shaft of the penis (Fig. 11.1).

The bulb of the penis

The bulb of the penis lies between the two crura and passes forwards towards the shaft of the penis and also narrows to become the corpus spongiosum. The bulb of the penis is covered by the bulbospongiosus muscle.

The prostatic urethra first pierces the perineal membrane to become the membranous urethra and at this point dilates to become the bulb of the urethra. The urethra then passes forwards and downwards to enter the bulb of the penis on its deep surface to enter the erectile tissue from where it will reach the corpus spongiosum. The urethra then passes down the penile shaft surrounded by the corpus spongiosum until it reaches another area of erectile tissue known as the glans penis (Fig. 11.1).

The shaft or the corpus of the penis

The shaft of the penis is variable in length but averages some 10–12 cm in length. It consists of three elongated masses of erectile tissue. The two corpora cavernosa, which lie in the upper half of the penile shaft, are joined by a tough fibrous septum. The single, more centrally placed corpus spongiosum lies in the depression on the undersurface of the two corpora cavernosa that is formed by their junction along the median septum. The corpus spongiosum contains the urethra in its centre.

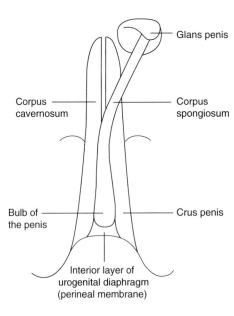

Glans penis

Corpus
cavernosum

Corpus
spongiosum

Bulb of
the penis

Crus penis

Interior layer of
urogenital diaphragm
(perineal membrane)

Fig. 11.1 A diagrammatic
representation of the erectile bodies
in the human penis. Note the
relationship between the two
corpora cavernosa and the corpus
spongiosum.

The glans penis

Towards the end of the penis, at a point known as the neck of the penis, the
corpus spongiosum expands into a structure called the glans penis. This
area of erectile tissue expands on to the dorsal surface of the penis and
overhangs the terminal urethra. The distal ends of the corpora cavernosa fit
neatly under this expanded glans. The navicular fossa of the urethra lies
within the glans and it is from here that the urethra terminates as the external meatus.

The nature of erectile tissue

Each of the three masses of erectile tissue within the penis are surrounded
by dense fibrous tissue, which is largely nondistensible and which, like its
counterpart that covers the testes, is known as the tunica albuginea. All the
corporeal bodies are surrounded by dense fascial tissue known as Buck's
fascia, from which extend fibrous septa between the corpora cavernosa and
the corpus spongiosum.

The erectile tissue itself is made up of cavernous spaces that are lined by
a flattened epithelium and are traversed by trabeculae. These trabeculae
are made up of collagen and smooth muscle. During erection there is a
massive increase in the blood flow through this erectile tissue that is associated with a relaxation of the smooth muscle in the trabeculae. As a consequence, the penis becomes engorged with blood. The arterial pressure
within the erectile tissue increases and puts the nondistensible fibrous covering of the erectile tissue under some tension. This tension impairs the
venous drainage of the erectile tissue, thus causing a considerable increase

in the arterial pressure within the erectile tissues. The expansion and distension of the erectile tissue within the penis thus 'straightens out' the penis resulting in the development of an erection.

The coverings of the penis

The skin of the penis is thin and dark in colour. It is loosely attached to the underlying tunica albuginea by thin fibrous tissue. At the neck of the penis, just posterior to the glans, it forms a major fold that overlaps the skin of the glans and which is called either the prepuce or the foreskin. This fold emerges from an area known as the corona, which is sited at the posterior edge of the glans penis.

The prepuce and the glans thus enclose a potential cleft called the preputial sac. On the undersurface of the distal penile shaft, beneath the prepuce, is a thin band of skin known as the frenulum. Around the corona on the undersurface of the prepuce are many sebaceous glands that secrete a substance called smegma.

Beneath the skin is a thin layer of loose connective tissue known as the superficial penile fascia. The penis is supported by two ligaments, both of which contain a high proportion of elastic fibres. The more superficial of these ligaments extends from the lower edge of the linea alba, splits into two halves and surrounds the penile shaft to end in the scrotal septum. Deep to this ligament is the more important triangular suspensory ligament, which extends from the front of the pubic symphysis and passes downwards and forwards to fuse with the penile fascia.

The blood vessels of the penis

The penis and the erectile tissue are supplied by two deep penile arteries. These arise as the terminal branches of the internal pudendal artery on either side. After giving off the perineal artery in Alcock's canal, these vessels pass forwards and upwards to penetrate the tunica albuginea of the corpora cavernosa along its dorsal surface.

On entering the erectile tissue, some of these cavernosal arteries become convoluted, when they are known as helicine arteries. The deep penile arteries on each side lie lateral to the veins and the dorsal nerves of the penis. The deep penile artery also provides a large branch to the bulb of the penis and these supply the glans and the skin of the penis.

There are very large numbers of arteriovenous shunts both within the erectile tissue as well as outside the tunica albuginea.

The venous drainage of the penis and its erectile tissue consists of many small vessels that emerge from the glans and the dorsal area of the corpora cavernosa as well as from the corpus spongiosum. These veins then join to form the deep dorsal veins, after which they drain mainly into the internal pudendal vein. Some venous blood may also drain into the prostatic plexus.

The nerve supply of the penis

The nerves of the penis arise from sacral segments S2, S3 and S4 and contain a large parasympathetic component. These nerves enter the penis via the pudendal nerve on either side. There is also a major contribution from the pelvic plexus. Persistent stimulation of the penile skin is also an important part of the maintenance of erection.

The neuroendocrinology of erection

The brain is a major sexual organ (Fabbri *et al.* 1997). Although androgens stimulate libido, the major force in inducing erection is the response to external erotic stimuli that are enhanced by tactile stimulation of the genitalia. These impulses are processed by the medial preoptic area of the hypothalamus. Many neurotransmitters are involved in this process and these include gonadotrophin-releasing hormone, corticotrophin-releasing hormone, melanocyte-stimulating hormone, prolactin, β-endorphin, neuropeptide Y and, in particular, oxytocin (Dorman & Malmsbury 1989).

Oxytocin is very important in the generation of sexual activity by enhancing sexual drive. Oxytocin-sensitive neurones are located in many areas of the hypothalamus as well as in the olfactory nucleus and the central amygdala together with the dorsal motor nucleus of the vagus. The sites of oxytocin action in the induction of an erection, at least in the rat, appear to be in the paraventricular nucleus of the hypothalamus and in the spinal cord itself (Arletti *et al.* 1992). There is some evidence in the human that there is an increase in oxytocin secretion by the pituitary during the orgasmic phase of sexual intercourse (Murphy *et al.* 1987).

The importance of oxytocin in erection is increased when it is realized that it reacts with vasopressin to generate neurophysin within the nerve fibres of the spinal cord that supply the muscles of the penis.

Another very important neuroendocrine mechanism in the generation of penile erection is the effect of nitric oxide. Nitric oxide (NO) is a powerful dilator of smooth muscle. It is formed from its precursor L-arginine by the action of the enzyme nitric oxide synthetase. Nitric oxide also activates guanyl cyclase to form intracellular guanosine monophosphate, which is a potent second messenger for smooth muscle relaxation. Thus, agents that inhibit the breakdown of guanosine monophosphate (such as the phosphodiesterase inhibitors) enhance erection considerably.

The mechanism of induction of erection

The mechanism of erection is complex, involving a close interaction between the neurological, the endocrine and, in particular, the vascular system (Andersson & Wagner 1995).

The initiation of erection is the result of sexual stimulation arising in the central nervous system and may be reinforced by tactile stimuli to the penis, especially in its most sensitive area, i.e. around the frenulum. The central nervous system is very important in the generation of an erection and its separation from the lower part of the spinal cord, as occurs in spinal injury, usually renders a patient impotent. However, lesions of the spinal cord below L2, often allow the patient to have cerebrally initiated penile erections.

The neurological drive in erection is complex and not clearly understood. It involves both the sympathetic as well as the parasympathetic nerve fibres. The sympathetic supply to the penis arises from the lower thoracic (T10) and upper lumbar (L2) and extends to the penis by means of the hypogastric nerves. These sympathetic fibres may mediate both erectile and antierectile effects.

The pudendal nerve (S2, 3 and 4) forms the main parasympathetic supply to the penis. It leaves the pelvis through the greater sciatic foramen and enters the pudendal (Alcock's) canal through the lesser sciatic foramen. It gives off the inferior rectal nerve and then divides into the perineal nerve and the dorsal nerve of the penis, which forms the main afferent pathway in the generation of a reflex erection. The pudendal nerve also forms a major sensory pathway from the penis, and section of this nerve may inhibit the generation of an erection.

In its flaccid state, the smooth muscle of the corpora, and of the penile arteries, is in a state of contraction. As the result of the central nervous system and also aided by tactile stimulation and the major action of nitric oxide, the penile arteries dilate and there is relaxation of the smooth muscle within the erectile tissue. This causes a great increase in the blood flow into the lacunae of the erectile tissue. There may be as much as an eightfold increase in the blood flow through the corpora (Shirai *et al.* 1976). Erection may also be enhanced by the contraction of the ischiocavernosus and bulbocavernosus muscles on the perineum, which helps to 'straighten out' the erectile tissue and thus support the erectile mechanism in general.

This great increase in arterial pressure causes the erectile tissue to expand and elongates the erectile bodies. This results in an increase in tension within the tunica albuginea and compression of the venous return, thus impeding the outflow of blood from the erectile tissue. In this way, the venous return is obstructed and the erection is maintained. As there are three major erectile bodies in the penis, namely the two upper corpora cavernosa and the lower corpus spongiosum, the penis in erection assumes a somewhat triangular shape. The glans penis also enlarges both in length and diameter during erection.

At ejaculation, the sympathetic drive, which both initiates and coordinates ejaculation, overcomes the parasympathetic drive that produces erection and thus at ejaculation detumescence occurs. Erection is thus very much a vascular event (Christ 1995) and is entirely dependent for its effectiveness upon a good blood supply to the erectile tissue and adequate veno-occlusion.

Disorders of erection can thus be the result of inadequate central drive, disruption of the neurological mechanisms that control erection, inadequate arterial blood supply to the erectile tissue of the penis, incompetent closure of the venous drainage of the penis during erection and disorders of the erectile tissue itself. Thus, it is clear that many different types of pathology will disrupt erection and these can now be considered in more detail.

The aetiology of erectile dysfunction

There are many different causes of impotence and it is important that the clinician is aware of these many different causes of erectile dysfunction.

Cavernosal smooth muscle dysfunction

This is the most common cause of impotence and was at one time known as idiopathic impotence. In this situation, the cavernosal smooth muscle is thought to be the primary cause of the problem. However, it is also likely that this form of impotence may relate to disturbances in the neuroendocrine control of erection, particularly of nitric oxide production. It is now known that many patients with this type of erectile disorder will respond well to the drug sildenafil (Viagra, Pfizer Ltd), which acts by enhancing nitric oxide production and increasing the production of guanosine monophosphate (Goldstein *et al.* 1998).

The erectile tissue may also become unable to relax due to the formation of fibrosis tissue within the erectile bodies. Such an occurrence may be seen in men undergoing long-term intracavernosal injection therapy. There may be inadequate release of the neurotransmitters as well as the precursor of nitric oxide. There may also be an abnormal communication between the erectile bodies as the result of surgery (Fabbri *et al.* 1997).

Arteriosclerosis

Any reduction in the arterial supply within the deep penile arteries can result in erectile dysfunction; indeed, it has been demonstrated that a 30% reduction in blood flow through these vessels will result in total erectile failure (Michael 1982)). Thus, impotence is a common associated problem in men with arteriosclerosis and is thus commonly found among men who are or who have been heavy cigarette smokers.

Damage to the penile arteries as the result of perineal surgery may also cause impotence. Recently, there have been discussions concerning the role of the bicycle saddle and the pressure it places on the perineum as a possible cause of erectile disturbance.

Psychogenic impotence

There are many psychological causes of erectile failure and this problem is frequently seen in men with various forms of anxiety. The sympathetic outflow is enhanced by fear and a state of anxiousness and will thus override the parasympathetic stimulus needed for erection. Such a mechanism may also be relevant to the problem of premature ejaculation.

Psychogenic impotence is usually associated with the presence of normal nocturnal or morning erections and is most commonly, but not exclusively, found in younger men

Psychogenic impotence may also be self-perpetuating: failure of erection because of anxiety generates more anxiety and an ever-increasing reduction in erectile function. Very careful history taking is important in these patients so that the cause of their problem can be elucidated. Professional psychological evaluation is also of great value in this group of patients.

Endocrine causes of erectile failure

The male sex hormone testosterone plays an uncertain role in the generation of impotence. Some men continue to produce erections while on antiandrogen therapy and are potent even after bilateral orchidectomy (Greenstein *et al.* 1995).

However, for the most part, falling testosterone production is associated with a reduction in both libido and erectile function. Poor testosterone secretion and a rise in the levels of sex hormone-binding globulin is associated with ageing and will produce a reduction in the free testosterone, which is the active component in the circulation (Hardy & Seckl 1994). Such changes may at least in part be responsible for the increased incidence of impotence with age.

Thus, measurement of the total testosterone, as occurs in the routine assay, may give little idea of the levels of active testosterone. For this reason, measurement of the levels of free testosterone and that of the sex hormone binding globulin will give the clinician a better idea of the androgen status of the patient than will routine estimation of the total testosterone.

Hyperprolactinaemia is also a well-known cause of erectile failure (Foster *et al.* 1990). Thus, in any condition where the serum prolactin is raised, such as acromegaly or any form of drug-induced rise in serum prolactin, impotence may also be a problem. Conditions such as renal failure may also give rise to hyperprolactinaemia.

It should also be remembered that abnormal forms of prolactin may exist in the blood that can give rise to very elevated levels of prolactin in the routine assay (Guay *et al.* 1996). These large and abnormal molecules of prolactin are poorly active biologically and thus have little effect on testosterone levels or upon sexual function. Thus, patients with this condition who present with impotence may produce diagnostic confusion and will not respond to treatment with any dopamine agonists. A similar problem may be seen in women with elevated prolactin levels and normal regular menstruation. The diagnosis of macroprolactinaemia is made by separation of the large molecules from those of normal size by passage of the patient's serum down a Sephadex column. This procedure can be carried out in most routine laboratories.

Neurological impotence

Many disorders of the nervous system can give rise to erectile dysfunction, but in most patients the presence of a neurological disorder is obvious to the clinician. Neurological conditions that cause loss of erectile function include all the peripheral neuropathies. Damage to the spinal cord as well as lesions of the cauda equina that are most frequently the result of intervertebral disc prolapse or more rarely may be caused by tumours may also be responsible for erectile failure.

Spinal lesions result in impotence by either causing damage to the reflex arc itself or by dissociating the central nervous system from these reflex arcs. Very occasionally, however, disorders such as multiple sclerosis can present with what appears, to a fertility clinic clinician, as erectile failure without any other neurological symptoms.

Prostatic surgery

The incidence of impotence after prostatic surgery is about 10% and it increases with age (Samdal *et al.* 1993). This is a serious complication of transurethral surgery in a younger man, and all patients must be warned of this possibility preoperatively. It is likely that the diathermy is mainly responsible for these changes as the neurological supply to the penis lies close to the verumontanum.

Drug-induced erectile failure

One of the most common group of drugs that may induce erectile failure are the beta-blockers (Buffum 1986). They are likely to have this effect by reducing the perfusion pressure into the penis, which, prior to treatment, may already have been compromised by the presence of arteriosclerotic changes in the major vessels or indeed in the deep penile arteries themselves. Such a phenomenon can, of course, be seen with any drug that causes a reduction in the blood pressure.

However, it is possible that the beta-blockers have a direct effect on smooth muscle. This theory is supported by the fact that treatment of high blood pressure with alpha-adrenergic receptor blockers does not produce erectile failure as frequently as do the beta-blockers, despite concomitantly reducing the blood pressure (TOMHS Research Group 1996). Indeed, treatment of mild hypertension with alpha-blockers such as doxazosin may in fact enhance sexual function.

Chronic illness

A variety of chronic illnesses can be associated with erectile dysfunction. Of these disorders, the best known are diabetes mellitus, hypertension, heart disorders and uraemia. Impotence can also be seen in men with depression (Feldman *et al.* 1994). In diabetes mellitus, autonomic dysfunction is likely to be the most common cause for erectile failure, but as hypertension and arteriosclerosis as well as renal disorders are common in these patients, more than one factor may be at work.

In men with hypertension, the problem is likely to be caused by generalized arterial deficiency (Carrier *et al.* 1994) but the drugs that are used to treat the hypertension, such as the beta-blockers, may also aggravate the problem.

The impotence that is seen in men with renal failure is sometimes but not always associated with a low testosterone and an elevated serum prolactin.

Impotence is also occasionally seen in men with peptic ulcer. Enhanced allergic responses may also be related to the presence of erectile failure (Wagner & Saenz de Tejada 1998).

Venogenic impotence

This type of impotence is caused by leakage of blood out of the penis as the result of an inadequate obstruction of the venous outflow by the tunica albuginea of the erectile bodies. The cause for this incompetence is largely unknown and indeed its very existence is questioned by many. It has been suggested, however, that venogenic impotence may be the result of changes in the fibroelastic component of the lacunar trabeculae, which prevents compression of the subtunical venules during erection rather than any anomaly of the tunica itself. The presence of the plaques caused by Peyronie's disease may also be associated with venogenic impotence (Kirby 1994).

Illicit drugs

These agents may also cause erectile failure and impotence is not infrequently found among narcotic addicts as well as among heavy users of cannabis. How these agents inhibit erection is not clearly understood but certainly the opiates are known to increase the secretion of prolactin, which will secondarily suppress testosterone production, while cannabis seems to have a direct effect upon the secretion of LH. Thus, the action of these drugs in causing impotence may indeed be endocrine.

Other drugs

Other agents that can cause erectile failure include the antihistamines, the antihyperlipidaemias and products such as ranitidine (Fabbri *et al.* 1997). Neurotoxic agents, in particular the heavy metals, are also known to cause erectile failure as are some of the chemotherapeutic agents.

The clinical evaluation of men with erectile failure

It is very important to evaluate these men carefully to come to a correct diagnosis and thus to apply the correct and appropriate treatment. Impotence is a very distressing symptom to most men, especially to young men, and a rapid and accurate diagnosis is essential in the management of these patients.

The clinical history

The nature of the onset of erectile failure is very important diagnostically. The gradual onset of impotence associated with loss of early morning erections is very suggestive of an organic cause of erectile failure, and if such impotence is of sudden onset and is associated with the maintenance of nocturnal and early morning erections one should be suspicious of a psychogenic cause.

Except in men with neurological disease or spinal injury, erectile failure is not often associated with any disturbance in ejaculation and libido may be normal. The presence of loss of libido in association with erectile failure can sometimes indicate an endocrine cause.

A history of vascular disease, of smoking, of alcohol intake and of hypertension is also important together with the presence of diabetes and hypercholesterolaemia. Any neurological problems of significance are usually self-evident. It must be remembered that occasionally impotence can be the presenting symptom of the demyelinating disorders such as multiple sclerosis.

A drug history is also important as there are many pharmaceutical products that induce hyperprolactinaemia as well as those that act directly upon the autonomic nervous system. Even agents such as the diuretics can raise the serum prolactin levels.

Impotence can also be induced surgically, and examples of this type of surgery include many forms of prostatectomy. However, erectile failure does not solely relate to the commonly performed operation of transurethral resection of the prostate. Radical prostatectomy is particularly prone to result in this complication, but nerve-sparing operations can reduce this postoperative problem to a minimum (Montorsi *et al.* 1997). Operations on the rectum and surgical procedures at the back of the bladder also run the risk of the occurrence of erectile failure postoperatively.

The physical examination

In men with erectile failure, a full clinical examination is very important. An apparent reduction in the quantity of facial and pubic hair may indicate a state of hypo-androgenization associated with a reduction in the serum testosterone.

An examination of the cardiovascular system together with measurement of the blood pressure is very important. It is of value to feel the peripheral pulses as a reduction in their amplitude may indicate the presence of arteriosclerotic change.

Evaluation of the nervous system should also be carried out including the peripheral reflexes. Perineal sensation must be tested so as to evaluate the normality of the S2–S4 dermatomes and the bulbocavernosus reflex must be elicited. Anal tone should also be tested.

The penis should also be carefully examined for the possible presence of Peyronie's disease and any such plaques should be recorded. The testes should be palpated and their size compared with the ovoids of a Prader orchiometer: a reduction in testicular size may indicate damage to the production of androgen.

Investigations

The blood tests that are indicated by the presence of impotence should include blood sugar and hormones such as testosterone and free testosterone, sex hormone-binding globulin, LH and FSH and prolactin. It is also of value to measure cholesterol and blood lipids.

The presence of nocturnal penile tumescence can be demonstrated using the Rigiscan device, which consists of a snap gauge band that breaks when nocturnal tumescence occurs (Ek *et al.* 1983). This device can be used at home and avoids the need for hospital admission overnight.

Colour Doppler imaging can also be of value in the investigation of erectile failure. Maximal smooth muscle relaxation is induced using a 20–40 µg dose of prostaglandin E_1, which is injected intracavernosally, and an increase in blood flow through the penile arteries should be identified. A reduced response could indicate the presence of an arterial insufficiency.

This technique can also be used to identify the presence of venogenic impotence. Exact sites of the venous leakage can be identified using a technique known as pharmacocavernosography, where an erection is induced using a saline infusion. A solution of normal saline is infused into the corpus cavernosum. If the flow of saline that is needed to create the erection is greater than 120 mL/min, and the flow needed to maintain it exceeds 20 mL/min, this indicates the presence of a venous leak. The site of these leaks can then be identified radiologically by adding contrast medium to the infusion.

The treatment of erectile dysfunction

The treatment of erectile dysfunction can be many faceted and may involve more than one regime.

Psychosexual counselling

This is an important form of treatment for all patients with psychogenic impotence. The cause of the problem must be identified and worked through with the counsellor. It is sometimes of value to have the partner attend these sessions but these decisions must be individualized to the patient concerned.

It must not be forgotten that organic impotence can give rise to a great deal of anxiety for the patient and thus psychogenic problems can soon superimpose themselves upon an organic problem. For this reason, the psychosexual approach is being increasingly used alongside pharmacological treatment.

Sildenafil (Viagra®)

Sildenafil, otherwise known by its tradename Viagra (Pfizer Ltd), is the newest form of treatment of many forms of impotence and is proving to be a very useful pharmacological agent.

As has been discussed above, normal penile erection necessitates the relaxation of the smooth muscle of the erectile tissue. In response to stimuli from the central nervous system and also from tactile stimuli to the penis itself, the cavernosal nerves and the endothelial cells release nitric oxide, which stimulates the formation of cyclic guanosine monophosphate (cGMP), and this action is catalysed by the enzyme guanylate cyclase. Sildenafil inhibits the action of cGMP-specific phosphodiesterase, which is the predominant enzyme that metabolizes cGMP in the erectile tissue (Goldstein *et al.* 1998). This results in a build-up of cGMP, which will enhance erections (Fig. 11.2).

Thus, sildenafil simply restores the natural erectile response to sexual stimulation. Unlike the other agents used in the treatment of impotence, it does not induce erections in the absence of the appropriate central nervous system and peripheral tactile stimuli that occur in the normal and potent individual.

Sildenafil is administered orally in doses of 25, 50 and 100 mg. It produces satisfactory erections in 72%, 80% and 85% of the patients treated, respectively (Goldstein *et al.* 1998). A single oral dose produces an effect that lasts for around 15 h. Thus, one dose will be effective for the patient throughout the night.

In the large Boston study cited above (Goldstein *et al.* 1998), only 5% of the patients in this study discontinued treatment because of a lack of

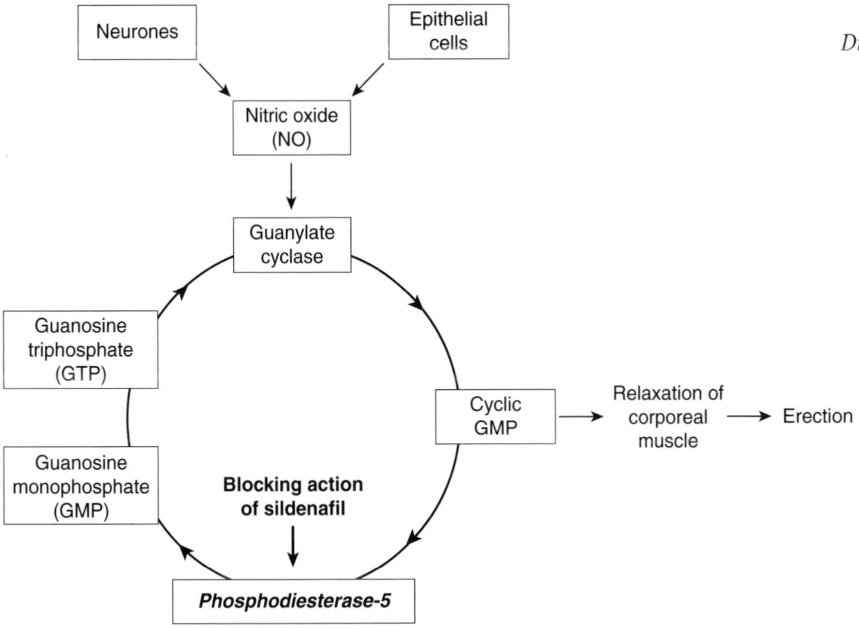

Fig. 11.2 A schematic representation of the mechanism of action of sildenafil.

effect and only another 2% discontinued treatment because of adverse effects.

Side effects after administration include nausea and vomiting, and in particular the development of headache. Flushing of the face as well as rhinitis were also reported.

Sildenafil, however, must never be used by a patient taking nitrites, or glyceryl trinitrate for angina, as these two agents in combination can cause a catastrophic fall in blood pressure and this hypotension can, at times, be lethal. Unaccustomed sexual activity can also cause problems. The cardiological fitness of the patients must also be assessed by the clinician before prescribing any drug that will restore potency.

Overall, sildenafil is well tolerated by most patients who find it a convenient and effective agent. It is proving to be very useful among men with quadriplegia whose limited hand movements make the use of the intracavernosal injections somewhat difficult. Theoretically, sildenafil may also be able to reduce the incidence of autonomic hyperreflexia, which can be associated with sexual activity in men with spinal injury.

It is of interest that this agent may also have a place in the treatment of sexual dysfunction in women.

Sildenafil is likely to replace most of the other agents used in the management of impotence and return the care of the patient with erectile failure to the family physician.

Mechanical devices

The cheapest device used for the treatment of erectile failure is the vacuum constriction device. The penis is inserted into the cylinder and the air is pumped out of the device with a small hand pump. Blood is thus sucked into the erectile tissue by the vacuum so formed. A constriction band is now slipped off over the end of the cylinder onto the base of the penis and thus the erection is maintained, after which the cylinder is removed (Fig. 11.3). The constriction band is removed at the completion of sexual activity.

This is a simple and effective means of inducing an erection and has few side effects when used correctly. It is largely used by older patients in long-standing relationships. It is, however, frequently unacceptable to the younger man (Guay 1995).

The vacuum device can also be used in conjunction with a prosthesis

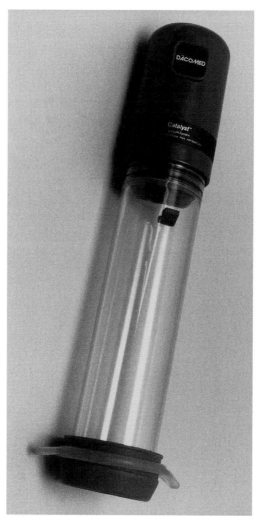

Fig. 11.3 An external vacuum device for the induction of an erection. A vacuum is induced within the cylinder and the plastic ring seen at the base of the device is slipped over the penis to maintain the erection.

where it can increase rigidity even when that prosthesis is an inflatable device (Soderdahl *et al.* 1997).

Intracavernosal injection therapy

The technique of intracavernosal injection began in 1982 when it was discovered that papaverine injected into the erectile tissue of the penis could induce an erection among impotent men (Virag 1982). It was then demonstrated that the alpha-blocker phenoxybenzamine could act in a similar manner (Brindley 1984). Today all these agents have been replaced by prostaglandin E_1 (Lea *et al.* 1996).

The use of intracavernosal injection therapy is now very likely to decline because of the success of the new oral agent sildenafil. However, for the small number of men who do not respond to this new agent, there will still be a place in the treatment of impotence with intracavernosal therapy.

The use of the intracavernosal injection technique in the management of erectile failure involves a short but nevertheless important training programme for the patient. Each man adopting this method for the treatment of his erectile failure must learn how to carry out the injection procedure itself, must understand the measurement of the dose and must be aware of the complications of this therapy. Adequate training can usually be achieved in around three clinic visits.

First visit

On the first visit, the dose of prostaglandin E_1 (Alprostadil, UpJohn Pharmaceuticals) is estimated and the first intracavernosal injection is given to the patient by the clinician. Men with neurogenic impotence are usually very much more sensitive to prostaglandin than those with other forms of erectile failure. The starting dose in most men should be low and probably should not exceed 20 μg although doses as low as 5 μg can be all that is needed in some men with neurological disorders. A common starting dose is thus 10 μg.

The prostaglandin is drawn up into the diabetic syringe, the skin at the side of the penis is cleaned and the needle is passed at right angles to the shaft of the penis into the corpus cavernosum. The prostaglandin solution is then injected into the corpus (Fig. 11.4). The patient is then asked to constrict the base of the penis with his forefinger and thumb in an attempt to prevent escape of the prostaglandin into the circulation. Pressure on the site of the injection is also useful to prevent any bleeding, which, however, is usually minor.

After some 3–5 min the erection will commence, and after some 10–15 min the rigidity of the penis is examined. If the erection is deemed to be satisfactory, a similar dose can be used at the next visit. If, however, the rigidity is not satisfactory, the clinician must never repeat the injection during the presence of any erection as this may cause serious bleeding to

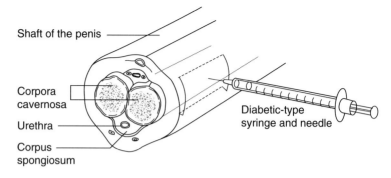

Shaft of the penis

Corpora
cavernosa

Urethra

Corpus
spongiosum

Diabetic-type
syringe and needle

Fig. 11.4 The site of the injection into the corpus cavernosum that is used for intracavernosal therapy in the induction of a penile erection.

occur through the second needle puncture site. On leaving the clinic, the patient is instructed to inform the clinician if the erection persists for more than 4 h as this constitutes the problem of prolonged erection known as priapism, for which treatment must be instituted.

Second visit

The results of the first injection are reviewed and the dose of prostaglandin E_1 are maintained or if necessary increased. If the period of the erection has been prolonged, the dose of vasoactive agent can be reduced and the quality of the erection is assessed.

At this visit, the patient is given instructions concerning the injection technique and the volume of fluid to be injected. The patient is also provided with some insulin syringes, some alcohol swabs and two or three ampoules of normal saline so that they can practise the injection technique at home during the next week. However, at the first or second visit, no active agent is given to the patient for use at home.

It is also important that the patient is given appropriate containers for used syringes in case these syringes should fall into the wrong hands. These containers must be brought to the clinic for disposal at the next visit.

Third visit

At this visit, the patient is asked to carry out self-injection using saline. The technique is examined. If the technique is unsatisfactory, the patient is given some more ampoules of saline for further practice at home. If his technique is satisfactory, the patient can now be given the active agent for use at home. The patient is, however, told not to inject himself more often than once each day.

In any clinic using intracavernosal therapy in the management of impotence, arrangements must be made to deal with the occurrence of priapism, and thus there should be a roster of clinicians on call to treat this problem should it arise. The patients should be given a telephone number where the on-call clinician can be contacted should prolonged erection occur.

It appears that intracavernosal prostaglandin E_1 produces satisfactory erections in around 70% of men (Lea *et al.* 1996). Penile pain is one of the more common complications occurring in or around 10% of all patients undergoing this treatment. It is also a cause of withdrawal from the treatment programme.

Complications of intracavernosal therapy for erectile failure

One of the long-term effects of intracavernosal injection therapy is penile scarring and the formation of fibrous tissue within the smooth muscle of the erectile tissue. These changes result in a decreasing effectiveness of the injection therapy (Chen *et al.* 1996). These changes, however, appear to be much less common after prostaglandin therapy than was the case when papaverine was more frequently used in the treatment of erectile failure. Other more minor complications include haematoma formation and ecchymoses at the site of the injection, which usually resolve after a few days. Cavernositis or infection of the corpora cavernosa as the result of these injections seems to be extremely rare.

Priapism as the result of intracavernosal therapy

Priapism, or prolonged erection, occurs in around 5% of patients undergoing this treatment and is its most important complication. Priapism is defined as an erection that persists for 4 h or more, and should always be treated. The first step in the management of this complication is to use a sedative such as valium and a warm shower, to which a number of patients will respond. If no response occurs (and this will be the case in many patients), a butterfly needle is inserted into one of the corpora cavernosa and 30–40 mL of blood are withdrawn. This can be replaced with a small dose of metaraminol tartrate at a dose of 10 mg, but great care must be taken to monitor the patient's blood pressure after using such medication. However, this particular drug must not be used in patients taking monoamine oxidase inhibitors. It is also important not to remove the butterfly needle until detumescence has occurred or severe bleeding from the site of the needle might occur. Almost all patients will respond to this treatment.

However, in men whose erections have persisted for more than 12 h, decompression of the erectile tissue may be needed and the formation of a cavernosal-spongiosus shunt may have to be induced surgically.

All patients undergoing treatment by intracavernosal injection should be warned of all these possible complications.

Topical and oral agents

It is now possible to use prostaglandin in a liposomal form as a topical treatment that is applied intraurethrally. This is known as a medicated urethral system for erection (MUSE) and was devised for the treatment of erectile failure (Lewis 1998).

This type of treatment, while not as effective as the intracavernosal injection, does indeed have a place in the management of all forms of impotence. It has proved to be especially useful in men with high spinal cord injury whose hand mobility is limited and where the injection technique may be difficult to master.

The effectiveness of this type of therapy can also be improved by adding a second agent to the prostaglandin E_1 and an example of this double therapy is the addition of the alpha-blocker prazosin (Peterson *et al.* 1998).

Oral prostaglandins have also been used in the management of erectile failure but are not very effective (Sato *et al.* 1997) and are certainly no longer the first line of treatment of these patients. Interestingly, despite the known effect of prostaglandins on the gut, few side effects are experienced by the patients taking such medication.

Penile prostheses

For men who do not respond to oral or intracavernosal treatment regimes, there are a series of prostheses that can be inserted into the erectile tissue of the corpora cavernosa. These prostheses can be semirigid or inflatable devices. The semirigid devices have the disadvantage that they are difficult to conceal but they are much less expensive and much easier to insert than the more complex inflatable devices.

The major disadvantage of all the prostheses is that their insertion effectively destroys the erectile tissue and thus the patient can never return to any form of pharmacological therapy for his erectile failure should he be dissatisfied with the prosthesis. Patients undergoing the insertion of a penile prosthesis must understand that natural erection will never again be possible. They must also know that tumescence of the corpus spongiosum or of the glans will not occur.

Because of the permanency of prosthetic therapy for impotence, careful counselling is needed prior to the insertion of any of these devices. The type of device that will be used must be demonstrated to the patient prior to its insertion as in this way the patient gets a good idea of its consistancy and the rigidity that it will produce. Discussions with another man who has already has a prosthesis in position may also be helpful to a patient contemplating the insertion of one of these devices.

The type of patient that does best with a penile prosthesis is a man with emotional stability and a good libido. They should be poor responders to pharmacotherapy or are men with a dislike for intracavernosal therapy and the penile injections that such treatment entails. The individuals who find this type of therapy acceptable and with whom it is successful are usually men over the age of 50 years. If ejaculation is normal prior to the insertion of the prosthesis, the patient can be reassured that ejaculation will continue to be normal.

Semirigid devices

These maleable but semirigid devices are made by several different companies. These companies include the Mentor Corporation in California and the Dacomed Corporation in Minnesota. These devices are made of polyethylene and can be bent into a position to simulate erection or flaccidity (Fig. 11.5). They also have the great advantage that they can be cut to the exact size of the corpora cavernosa of each individual patient.

The insertion of these devices requires skill and considerable experience, as a good fit of these devices within the corpora cavernosa is essential for their success as penile prostheses.

Inflatable devices

These devices are much more sophisticated than the semirigid devices and as a consequence are much more expensive. The are made up of two inflatable penile prostheses that are attached to a sump and to a small pump. Pressure on the pump fills and distends the penile prostheses with saline, thus causing distension and rigidity of the penis (Fig. 11.6). However, like

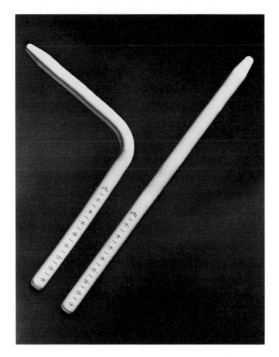

Fig. 11.5 An example of a semimalleable penile prothesis. These prostheses are inserted surgically into each of the corpora cavernosa. (Published by kind permission of Bennett Medical, Perth, Western Australia.)

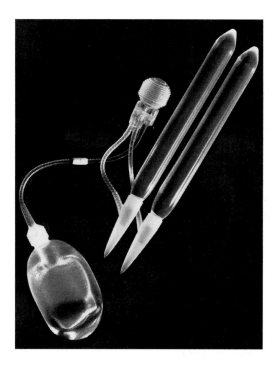

Fig. 11.6 An inflatable penile prosthesis that is commonly used in the treatment of erectile failure. The bulb that contains the fluid used in the distension of the two prostheses is placed in one scrotum. Pressure on the bulb both fills or deflates the penile protion of this device. (Published by kind permission of Bennett Medical, Perth, Western Australia.)

the malleable prostheses, the distension only involves the corpora cavernosa while the corpus spongiosum and the glans remain flaccid.

Despite these disadvantages, these devices make excellent prostheses, the only major problem with them being their price—which at the time of writing amounts to some A$4000–5000 (US$3000).

The insertion of these devices

Insertion of both these devices is usually carried out under general anaesthesia and must only be performed by urological surgeons with training in this technique.

Scrupulous attention to asepsis is essential so as to avoid any problem with postoperative infection. Great care must be taken in selecting the size of the prosthesis: a prosthesis that is too large can penetrate the tunica albuginea of the corpora cavernosa and will have to be removed. The stay in hospital after these procedures is short, and most patients can be discharged after 24 h, even after the insertion of the more complex inflatable prosthesis.

Complications of the insertion of penile prostheses

There are several important complications that relate to the insertion of penile prostheses.

The most serious complication of the insertion of a penile prosthesis is the problem of infection. This can occur both in the immediate postoperative period but also may be seen several months or even years after the insertion of the prosthesis, despite the use of prophylactic antibiotics. Infection of varying severity will occur in around 2% of these patients (Kabalin & Kessler 1988).

Severe infection will result in the extrusion of the device. Infection is more common following a reimplantation of the device or in men with recurrent urinary tract infections. Infection is thus more common when these devices are inserted into men with spinal cord injury and in men with diabetes mellitus (Bishop *et al.* 1992), in whom urinary infection is extremely common.

Tunical perforations

Perforation of the tunica albuginea of the corpora cavernosa can also occur. It may be the result of an intrinsically thin tunica, but it is more commonly caused by poor fitting of the penile prosthesis.

Once the tunica has been perforated, migration of the prosthesis can occur and perforation of the penile skin can then take place. These perforations need to be patched and Gore-Tex is commonly used for this purpose.

Perforation of the urethra

Perforation of the urethra is an uncommon complication and may present with a blood-stained penile discharge and haematuria. Should this complication occur, urinary diversion using suprapubic drainage is often necessary. The prosthetic device should be removed and not reinserted for several months, during which time the perforation in both the urethra and the tunica can be allowed to heal.

Glandular perforation

It is also possible that these devices may not only perforate the tunica of the corpora cavernosa but they can also perforate the glans. It is sometimes possible to repair these tears without removing the prosthesis.

Malfunction of the device

The inflatable penile prostheses are quite complex and thus malfunction can occur after their insertion. These malfunctions can include fluid leaks and pump failure. However, the failure of these devices is surprisingly infrequent.

Silicone prostheses can also shed small flakes of silicone into the surrounding tissues and these have even been found in the draining lymphatics (Barrett *et al.* 1991). However, this phenomenon does not seem to produce any problems of significance to the patient and the long-term benefits of these devices outweigh the possible hazards of silicone in the tissues.

Arterial surgery

Much impotence is caused by the presence of a reduced arterial input by the deep penile arteries. Patients who are especially at risk from this type of erectile failure include those with diabetes, hyperlipidaemia, heart disease and hypertension and also men who are heavy cigarette smokers (Virag *et al.* 1981). Trauma to the perineal area may also result in erectile problems, and recently there has been some informal discussion on the role of the saddle of the bicycle as such an agent.

Microvascular surgery aims to increase this blood flow and such surgery involves the by-pass of the arteriosclerotic obstruction of the cavernous arterial inflow. These procedures were first introduced some 20 years ago (Michal *et al.* 1977) and are still of at least some value to many impotent patients. This type of surgery has the opportunity to provide the patient with normal and nonpharmacologically assisted erections. The success of this type of surgery is high but these techniques require very careful patient selection.

The arterial input to the deep penile arteries can be evaluated in several ways.

The arterial input can be evaluated using the Doppler ultrasound. Focused and pulsed Doppler ultrasonography used in conjunction with the injection of a vasoactive agent such as prostaglandin E_1 into one of the corpora (Lue *et al.* 1985). This type of ultrasound can determine the changes that occur in the diameter of the cavernosal artery. Where there is arteriosclerotic damage, the diameter of the artery will only show minimal change. Alternatively, selective internal pudendal arteriography can also indicate the presence of arteriosclerotic change and can also site those changes with great accuracy.

A series of different operations can then be carried out on these patients (Hatzichristou & Goldstein 1994). Lesions that are proximal to the cavernosal artery and involve the internal pudendal artery are best treated by a microvascular anastomosis between the dorsal penile artery and the inferior epigastic artery.

Another alternative is to anastomose the inferior epigastric artery to one of the deep veins of the penis. This procedure will enhance perfusion of the erectile tissue via the venous outflow and thus provide a second 'arterial' supply to the corpora. This procedure is useful among patients with arterial lesions within the corpora themselves.

Another option is to use a segment of the deep dorsal vein to replace an occluded segment of the artery, and it is also possible simply to anastomose the deep penile artery to the deep vein and 'reverse' the input to the cavernosal tissue. The operation of choice will depend upon the site and the extent of the arteriosclerotic change in the penile arterial system.

Venous ligation

This type of surgery is useful in the management of impotence caused by venous leakage from the erectile tissue into the deep veins of the penis. The maintenance of an erection is dependent upon the generation of an intracorporeal pressure of around 100 mmHg. This pressure is generated by a good arterial input and thus venogenic impotence can occasionally occur as a consequence of arterial insufficiency and also as the result of poor relaxation of the erectile tissue.

The generation of venogenic impotence is thus complex. The assessment of these patients is difficult and requires great skill and experience on the part of the surgeon involved with their care.

Venogenic impotence is best diagnosed by using a technique known as pharmacocavernosography (Lewis 1994). In this technique two 19 gauge needles are placed into the corpora cavernosa on each side. One needle is attached to a manometer for the measurement of the intracavernosal pressure. Through the other needle is infused a solution of heparinized saline that has been prewarmed to body temperature. This fluid is infused at rate increments of 50 mL/min until an erection is achieved, after which the flow rate is decreased to a level that will maintain that erection. Through this needle is then added a vasoactive substance and the infusion is further reduced to a level that will, however, maintain the erection.

If the infusion rate needed to maintain the erection is greater than 50 mL/min then veno-occlusive dysfunction is likely to be present. The sites of any venous leakage can then be identified radiologically by injecting contrast medium through the infusion needle.

In the early management of veno-occlusive impotence, the practice involved the ligation of the deep dorsal vein of the penis alone. Today, however, this type of surgery involves complete penile dissection and the ligation of all the vessels that have been shown to be incompetent on pharmacocavernosography. This approach gives reasonably good results with improvement in around half the patients so treated (Lewis 1994).

Impotence is thus a complex disorder that is, because of the presence of an ageing population, becoming a common medical problem. It is not infrequently seen in an infertility clinic. The infertility clinician must therefore be aware of its presence and the common causes of erectile failure and their management.

References

Andersson, K.-E. & Wagner, G. (1995) Physiology of penile erection. *Physiological Reviews* **75**, 191–236.

Arletti, R., Benelli, A. & Bertolini, A. (1992) Oxytocin involvement in male and female sexual behavior. *Annals of the New York Academy of Sciences* **653**, 180–193.

Barrett, D.M., O'Sullivan, D.C., Malizia, A.A., Reiman, H.M. & Abell-Aleff, P.C. (1991) Particle shedding and migration from silicone genitourinary devices. *Journal of Urology* **146**, 319–322.

Benet, A.E. & Melman, A. (1995) The epidemiology of erectile dysfunction. *Urologic Clinics of North America* **22**, 699–709.

Bishop, J.R., Moul, J.W., Sihelnik, S.A., Peppas, D.S., Gormley, T.S. & McLeod, D.G. (1992) Use of glycosylated hemogolobin to identify diabetics at high risk for penile prosthetic infections. *Journal of Urology* **147**, 386–388.

Brindley, G.S. (1984) Pilot experiments on the actions of drugs injected into the human corpus cavernosum penis. *British Journal of Pharmacology* **87**, 495–500.

Buffum, J. (1986) Pharmacosexuology update: prescription drugs and sexual function. *Journal of Psychoactive Drugs* **18**, 97–106.

Carrier, S., Zvara, P. & Lue, T.F. (1994) Erectile dysfunction. *Endocrinology and Metabolism Clinics of North America* **23**, 773–782.

Chen, R.N., Lakin, M.M., Montague, D.K. & Ausmundson, S. (1996) Penile scarring with intracavernous injection therapy using prostaglandin E1: a risk factor analysis. *Journal of Urology* **155**, 138–140.

Christ, G.J. (1995) The penis as a vascular organ. *Urologic Clinics of North America* **22**, 727–745.

Dorman, W.A. & Malmsbury, C.W. (1989) Neuropeptides and sexual behaviour. *Neuroscience and Behavioural Review* **13**, 1–15.

Ek, A., Bradley, W.E. & Krane, R.J. (1983) Nocturnal penile ridgidity measured by the snap-gauge band. *Journal of Urology* **129**, 964–966.

Fabbri, A., Aversa, A. & Isodori, A. (1997) Erectile dysfunction: an overview. *Human Reproduction Update* **3**, 455–466.

Feldman, H.A., Goldstein, I., Hatsichristou, D.G., Crane, R.J. & McKinley, J.B. (1994) Impotence and its medical and psychological correlates: results of the Massachusetts male aging study. *Journal of Urology* **151**, 54–59.

Foster, R.S., Mulcahy, J.J., Callaghan, J.T., Crabtree, R. & Brashera, D. (1990) Role of serum prolactin determination in the evaluation of the impotent patient. *Urology* **36**, 499–501.

Furlow, W.L. (1985) Prevalence of impotence in the United States. *Medical Aspects of Human Sexuality* **19**, 13–17.

Goldstein, I., Lue, T.F., Padma-Nathan, H., Steers, W.D. & Wicker, P.A. (1998) Oral sildenafil in the treatment of erectile dysfunction. Sildenafil Study Group. *Journal of the American Medical Association* **338**, 1397–1404.

Greenstein, A., Plymate, S.R. & Katz, P.G. (1995) Visually stimulated erection in castrated men. *Journal of Urology* **153**, 650–652.

Guay, A.T. (1995) Erectile dysfunction—are you prepared to discuss it? *Postgraduate Medicine* **97**, 127–143.

Guay, A.T., Sabharwal, P., Varma, S. & Malarkey, W.B. (1996) Delayed diagnosis of psychological erectile dysfunction because of the presence of macroprolactinaemia. *Journal of Clinical Endocrinology and Metabolism* **81**, 2512–2514.

Hardy, K.J. & Seckl, J.R. (1994) Endocrine assessment of impotence—pitfalls of measuring serum testosterone without sex hormone-binding globulin. *Postgraduate Medical Journal* **70**, 836–837.

Hatzichristou, D.C. & Goldstein, I. (1994) Microvascular arterial bypass surgery for arteriogenic impotence. In: *Management of Impotence and Infertility* (eds E.D. Whitehead & H.M. Nagler), pp. 55–72. J.B. Lippincott, Co., Philadelphia.

Kabalin, J.N. & Kessler, R. (1988) Infectious complications of penile prosthetic implants. *Journal of Urology* **139**, 953–955.

Kirby, R.S. (1994) Impotence: diagnosis and management of male erectile dysfunction. *British Medical Journal* **308**, 957–961.

Lea, A.P., Bryson, H.M. & Balfour, J.A. (1996) Intracavernous alprostadil. A review of its pharmacodynamic and pharmacokinetic properties and potential in erectile dysfunction. *Drugs and Aging* **8**, 56–74.

Lewis, R.W. (1994) Venous ligation for venogenic impotence. In: *Management of Impotence and Infertility* (eds E.W. Whitehead & H.M. Naylor), pp. 73–92. J.B. Lippincott, Philadelphia.

Lewis, R.W. (1998) Transurethral alprostadyl with MUSE (medicated urethral system for erection) vs intracavernous alprostadil—a comparative study in 103 patients with erectile dysfunction. *International Journal of Impotence Research* **10**, 61–62.

Lue, T.F., Hricak, H., Marich, K.W. & Tanagho, E.A. (1985) Vasculogenic impotence evaluated by high resolution ultrasonography and pulsed Doppler spectrum analysis. *Radiology* **155**, 777–781.

Michael, V. (1982) Arterial disease as a cause of impotence. *Clinical Endocrinology and Metabolism* **11**, 725–748.

Michal, V., Kramar, R., Pospichal, J. & Hejkal, L. (1977) Arterial epigastrico-cavernous anastomosis for the treatment of sexual impotence. *World Journal of Surgery* **1**, 515–517.

Montorsi, F., Guazzoni, G., .Strambi, L.F. *et al.* (1997) Recovery of spontaneous erectile function function after nerve-sparing radical prostatectomy with and without early intracavernous injections of alprostadil: results of a prospective, randomised trial. Journal of. *Urology* **158**, 1408–1410.

Murphy, M.R., Seckl, J.R., Burton, S., Checkley, S.A. & Lightman, S. (1987) Changes in oxytocin and vasopressin secretion during sexual activity in man. *Journal of Clinical Endocrinology and Metabolism* **65**, 738–741.

NIH Consensus Conference (1993) Impotence. *Journal of the American Medical Association* **270**, 83–90.

Peterson, C.A., Bennett, A.H., Hellstrom, W.J. *et al.* (1998) Erectile response to transurethral alprostadil, prazosin and alprostadyl–prazosin combinations. *Journal of Urology* **159**, 1523–1527.

Samdal, F., Vada, K. & Lundmo, P. (1993) Sexual function after transurethral prostatectomy. *Scandanavian Journal of Urology and Nephrology* **27**, 27–29.

Sato, Y., Horita, H., Adachi, H. *et al.* (1997) Effect of oral administration of prostaglandin E1 on erectile dysfunction. *British Journal of Urology* **80**, 772–775.

Shirai, M., Nakmura, M., Ishii, N., Misuakawa, N. & Sawai, Y. (1976) Determination oftrapenile blood, using ^{99m}Tc-labeled autogenous red blood cells. *Tohuku Journal of Experimental Medicine* **120**, 377–383.

Soderdahl, D.W., Petroski, R.A., Mode, M., Schwartz, B.F. & Thrasher, J.B. (1997) The use of an external vacuum device to augment a penile prosthesis. *Techniques in Urology* **3**, 100–102.

TOMHS Research Group (1996) Incidence and disappearance of erectile problems in men treated for Stage 1 hypertension: the treatment of mild hypertension study. *European Urology* **30** (Suppl. 2), 38. (Abstract).

Virag, R. (1982) Intracavernous injection of papaverine for erectile failure. *Lancet* **ii**, 938 (Letter).

Virag, R., Zwang, G., Dermange, H. & Legman, M. (1981) Vasculogenic impotence: a review of 92 cases with 54 operations. *Vascular Surgery* **15**, 9–17.

Wagner, G. & Saenz de Tejada, I. (1998) Update on male erectile dysfunction. *British Medical Journal* **316**, 678–682.

12: Spinal Cord Injury and Infertility

Spinal cord injury is an uncommon but very serious injury. Its incidence in Australia is around 18 per million of the population and, of these injuries, some 40% are complete. Motor vehicle accidents are the major cause of this disorder, but they may also be the result of diving accidents, falls and even gunshot wounds. It must be remembered that spinal cord dysfunction may also be the result of surgery used to remove certain malignant or even benign spinal cord tumours, and can also be the result of vascular accidents to the arterial supply to the spinal cord.

This distribution of causes of spinal cord injury seems to be similar all around the world (Go *et al.* 1995). Certain sports, in particular rugby football, also have a sinister reputation for causing such lesions (Rotel *et al.* 1998). Less commonly, spinal cord injury can also be caused by suicide attempts in which individuals throw themselves off some elevated structure such as a building or a bridge. Permanent spinal injury, certainly where the lesion is complete and the whole diameter of the cord is involved, is a devastating injury for any individual and is an occurrence that changes their whole way of life for ever.

The majority of patients with these lesions are male and are between 16 and 35 years of age. Good data are available on this aspect of spinal cord injury as each state in the USA, as well as in Australia, keeps careful statistics on this problem (Gerhart 1991). As most men with spinal cord injury are young, fertility may be of great importance to them.

Such accidents also have important implications for the sexual activities of these young men as most spinal injuries will interfere with potency as well as with ejaculation. Reflex erections can often be induced among men with spinal cord injury, especially among those with higher lesions. However, both erection and ejaculation may be spared in some men with incomplete spinal cord lesions. Spinal cord injury is thus an important cause of both sexual dysfunction and of infertility; indeed, some 70% of all men with spinal cord damage suffer from ejaculatory failure and the incidence of natural fertility among men with spinal injury is low.

The treatment of the infertility in men with spinal injury must be rapid and effective. These patients have undergone enough trauma to themselves and to their way of life to tolerate years of unsuccessful treatment in order to achieve paternity. Thus, the method used must result in a pregnancy in a short time and the most effective way of achieving this objective is the way in which their infertility must be managed.

There are many problems in spinal cord injury that will affect many systems in the body, but particularly severe is the effect that it has on the urological and reproductive tracts. Although some aspects of spinal injury have been covered in the sections on disorders of ejaculation and of impotence, spinal injury produces such devastating results, in particular for the male patient, that a special section of the book has been set aside to examine this problem in more detail.

The causation of the disorders in erection and ejaculation in men with spinal cord injury

Around 70% of men with spinal injury will at least achieve occasional erections but only a minority will be able to ejaculate. However, these figures will vary according to the site of the spinal cord lesion. Thus, sexual difficulties, and in particular infertility, will be a very common occurrence among men with spinal injury. Suprasacral lesions may allow reflex erections, but only in an incomplete lesion will they occur as a psychological response. Cauda equina lesions are associated with a total absence of all erections. Disturbances in emission and ejaculation are a frequent accompaniment to spinal cord injury at all levels, and thus infertility in these men is very common.

The neurological control of ejaculation is fairly complex and involves sympathetic nervous system in two areas of the cord, namely T10–L3 and S2–S4. It appears that there is a 'co-ordination centre' in segments T12–L1 where the spinal cord integrates the sensory input from the genitalia and co-ordinates emission and ejaculation. Stimuli to the genitalia are carried to the cord via the pudendal nerve (S2–S4) but pass into the cord as sympathetic afferent nerves at the level of T12–L3. Afferent fibres also enter the cord via the parasympathetic nerves at the level of S2–S4.

Emission, namely the deposition of semen into the posterior urethra, is initiated via the thoracolumbar outflow and the hypogastric nerves. This results in the contraction of the caudal end of the epididymis and the vas deferens. This is followed by the contraction of the capsule of the prostate and then by contractions of the walls of the seminal vesicles. At the same time, the internal sphincter contracts and tightly closes the bladder neck, thus preventing the passage of each of the components of the seminal fluid from entering the bladder.

As soon as emission is complete, the motor components of the pudendal nerve induce rhythmic contractions in the bulbocavernosus and ischiocavernosus muscles, which propel the seminal fluids out of the external penile meatus in the process known as ejaculation.

The process of emission and ejaculation is thus controlled by both the sympathetic and the parasympathetic nervous system. These systems are integrated via the 'coordination' centre in the lower thoracic and upper lumbar cord. Any spinal cord injury at this level will therefore result in disordered or absent ejaculation. It also appears that contact between this area of the cord and the higher centres of the brain is also important for the normality of ejaculation. Therefore, an injury that results in damage to any area of the spinal cord is likely to interfere with the production of an ejaculate, and indeed spinal cord injury is by far the most common cause of ejaculatory failure.

The neurology of erection is a much simpler reflex that involves the parasympathetic fibres of the segments S2–S4. Sensory stimuli from the penis and genitalia enter the sacral plexus via the pudendal nerves. Further parasympathetic activity, via the nervi erigentes, causes an intense vasodilatation of the dorsal artery of the penis together with a relaxation of the muscle of the erectile tissue in the corpora of the penis. The erectile tissue now becomes distended with blood and the venous drainage is restricted thus causing the penis to become erect. Input from the cerebral cortex is also often needed for erection and thus loss of potency is also a frequent problem in men with spinal injury.

Damage to the autonomic nervous system in the absence of spinal cord injury

The spinal cord ends at the level of the lower border of L1, after which it becomes the cauda equina. When a vertebral injury is low and involves only the lower lumbar vertebrae, a major fracture dislocation of the lumbar vertebrae can occur without causing any major damage to the somatic nervous system. However, any displacement of the vertebrae can cause damage to the sympathetic chains that lie anteriorly on either side of the bodies of the vertebrae. Such an injury can thus give rise to disorders, particularly of ejaculation. Thus in some patients with this type of lower lumbar vertebral injury, failure of ejaculation may result.

Lumbar plexus neuropraxia

This is a surprisingly common cause of infertility among men with pelvic injury that may or may not be associated with incomplete spinal injury. It results from a diathesis of the pelvic symphysis. This diathesis allows a major opening of the pelvic side walls and stretches both the lumbar plexus and the sympathetic chain. As a consequence the neurology of ejaculation is disturbed and this lesion can result in either retrograde ejaculation or ejaculatory failure.

Provided that there has been no associated major spinal injury, these lesions are frequently only temporary but may take several months to resolve. The patient will also complain of weakness of his quadriceps and upper limb muscles. Erection is usually normal but ejaculation may be absent or retrograde. As the upper limb muscles regain their function, ejaculation will often concomitantly return, but it may take 9–12 months before all ejaculatory function returns to normal.

Urological problems in spinal cord injury

The incidence of urological injury among patients with spinal cord injury is high, especially when multiple injury is present. Thus, urological problems may begin with the injury itself. Even in the absence of traumatic injury, the bladder undergoes profound functional changes, and indeed the good management of the urinary tact may make a considerable difference to the prognosis for fertility in these men (Rutkowski *et al.* 1995).

Bladder atony

Immediately after a serious spinal injury involving a complete lesion, the bladder becomes atonic and remains in this state for several weeks (Gardner *et al.* 1986). However, this atonic state does not usually last, but other changes that can then result in pathological micturition may take over.

However, areflexia and atony can sometimes persist, and the patient then can only empty his bladder by intermittent self-catheterization. This technique of bladder emptying offers great advantages over an indwelling catheter. Men with spinal injury have little sensation and thus self-catheterization is well tolerated. Provided a good aseptic technique is observed and urinary acidification is maintained, urinary tract infections are few and the absence of an indwelling catheter reduces the incidence of bladder stones, urethritis and bladder contracture.

The reflex bladder

Some 6–8 weeks after a major spinal cord injury, detrusor activity returns to the bladder, and it can be triggered to undergo contraction either by overfilling or as a reflex by tapping on the abdomen. Abdominal strain-ing during micturition can also aid bladder emptying. This state of affairs provides the patient with a bladder that is under considerable control and, provided that it is not allowed to overfill, incontinence is not a major problem.

Detrusor dyssynergia

Sadly, this is a very common complication of spinal injury. These patients develop high-pressure voiding and incomplete emptying. As a result, urinary tract infection is common and the hydronephrosis and obstructive renal failure that may result can be life threatening. As a consequence, it is important to carry out urodynamic studies on these patients with spinal injury to exclude these potentially serious complications. Should the voiding pressure indeed be high, it may be necessary to consider perform-ing a sphincterotomy so as to decrease voiding pressure and enhance the completion of bladder emptying; however, such a procedure results in a dribbling incontinence, necessitating the use of a urinary condom. Also, should such a patient be able to ejaculate, then this operation will give rise to retrograde ejaculation.

Among patients with incontinence following a sphincterotomy, an artificial sphincter has been suggested as a possible means of treatment, but the cost of these devices frequently makes their use prohibitive. Selective nerve stimulation is now being carried out in certain centres and also appears to be effective in controlling bladder activity.

Occasionally among patients with very severe detrusor dyssynergia, it may be necessary to insert a mesh tube known as a 'Memocath', which holds the bladder neck open. Such a device will also induce retrograde ejaculation and its presence may also result in an obstruction of the ejaculatory ducts.

Urinary tract infection

This is a common complication among men with spinal injury. As has been stated above, this can be the result of inadequate bladder emptying or it can be the result of poorly performed self-catheterization. Some urologists recommend long-term antibacterial therapy, although the efficacy of such treatment has been questioned.

Calculi

Some 8% of men with spinal cord injury develop renal calculi. Bladder calculi can also form and are frequently caused by the presence of an indwelling catheter. These are managed in the usual way but the advent of extracorporeal shock wave lithotripsy (ESWL) makes the management of such stones among patients with spinal cord injury very much simpler.

Prostatitis

This disorder may also commonly occur in men with spinal injury and probably relates to the frequency of urinary tract infection. It may not be symptomatic but may be the site of white cell production. These white cells are the source of reactive oxygen species that can severely compromise the function of the sperm in an ejaculate.

Epididymitis

Epididymitis is a common problem amongst men with spinal injury, particularly in those men who undergo frequent urinary tract infections. As there is loss of sensation below the level of the lesion, such a disorder may pass unnoticed by the patient and may not even be apparent to the clinician. Epididymitis in any patient can, at times, induce the production of antisperm antibodies (Hirsch *et al.* 1990) and such an event can further compromise the fertility of the patient. Such pathology may of course also result in the occurrence of obstructive azoospermia and the production of azoospermic semen at electroejaculation.

From the above description of the many disorders of the urinary tract that spinal injury may induce, it is clear that passage of the semen through the lower urinary tract may cause damage to otherwise fertile spermatozoa. The lower urinary tract may also be the site of production of reactive oxygen species that are known to induce considerable damage to sperm function. Therefore, although the induction of ejaculation may seem a simple way of treating the infertility associated with ejaculatory failure in men with spinal injury, a poor pregnancy rate may also result from these methods of treatment.

Autonomic hyperreflexia

This is a serious complication of spinal cord injury of which all those clinicians who manage any aspect of spinal injury should be fully aware. Almost all patients with lesions above T6 will show signs of this problem at some time. Many stimuli will induce this condition but retention of urine is one of its more common causes. Other aetiological factors that can induce this dangerous condition include catheterization, testicular injury or torsion, vibroejaculation, electroejaculation and many other urological procedures.

This disorder is the result of a massive sympathetic and parasympathetic outflow and consists of severe and sometimes life-threatening hypertension, bradycardia, headaches, sweating above the level of the lesion, anxiety, piloerection and facial flushing. The treatment of this condition first necessitates rapid cessation of the causative stimulus. The hypertension needs to be controlled and this may be achieved by the use of nitroprusside. This can be administered at an initial dose of 1 mg/kg body weight by means of an intravenous infusion of a 5% dextrose solution. Other antihypertensives that can be administered intravenously may also be used, and an example of such an agent is hydralazine.

The use of a sublingual dose of 20 mg of nifedepine some 20 min prior to any urological procedure may be a very useful way to prevent the onset of autonomic hyperreflexia.

It must always be remembered that autonomic hyperreflexia can sometimes cause death to a patient with spinal cord injury.

The management of the sexual dysfunction in men with spinal cord injury

The major disability that results in sexual problems in men with spinal injury is the frequent occurrence of erectile failure. Sexual activity may also be made more difficult by the immobility that spinal cord injury imparts upon the patient, especially if the lesion has caused a complete spinal cord transection. As the majority of patients with spinal cord injury are young males usually between the ages of 16 and 35, then the management of their sexual disability should carry a high priority.

The management of impotence among these patients is similar to that applied to men with erectile failure that is unrelated to a spinal injury.

Erection can also be induced using the vacuum devices that are available commercially (Earle *et al.* 1996) and these are successful among men with spinal cord injury. Prostheses can also be inserted into men with erectile problems in spinal injury (Golji 1979) and these include the hydrostatic devices (Light & Scott 1981) as well as the simpler semimalleable implants. However, the cost of the hydrostatic devices tends to be prohibitive for many patients. This is of special importance to men with spinal cord injury, who are frequently trying to live on a meagre disability pension.

The most usual treatment for impotence among men with spinal cord injury is the use of an intracavernosal injection of prostaglandin E_2 (Wyndaele *et al.* 1986). In men with high lesions, this form of treatment may result in difficulties especially in men with limited hand movement. Men with neurological causes of impotence are also known to be especially sensitive to intracavernosal therapy and care must be taken in order to avoid the development of priapism. It is important to begin treatment of these patients with a low dose of prostaglandin.

The new intraurethral pessaries and creams that can induce erection may well prove to be valuable among this group of men whose limited hand movements make the use of intracavernosal therapy somewhat difficult. Medication in tablet form known as sildenafil (Viagra, Pfizer Ltd) has also already been used among men with spinal injury with a great deal of success (Derry *et al.* 1997).

Sexual intercourse for these men may also be aided by the use of explicit videos. Intercourse within a wheelchair and with the female partner sitting above the patient will also be of value to the spinal-injured male patient. However, such aids are probably only of assistance when the extent of the permanent damage to the cord is known and when the patient has come to terms with his injury. For a newly injured young man, great care must be taken in the use of such visual aids, which may, at least initially, do more harm than good to the young man with permanent spinal cord damage.

It must always be remembered that in a newly injured young male patient, the impairment of his sexual activity caused by his injury will be foremost in his mind. How he can perform sexually in the future will be one of the first questions that he will ask of his carers. These questions must be answered by capable and skilled individuals who have had much experience in this field of therapy. They must never be shrugged off as unimportant and such queries must be dealt with using care, skill and compassion.

Management of the ejaculatory failure in men with spinal injury

There are several ways in which ejaculatory failure may be overcome in the men with spinal injury.

The vibrator

This technique will only be of value when the lesion is above the level of T10, thus ensuring that the spinal reflex involved in emission and ejaculation is intact. If any part of the cord below this level has been involved in the injury, then the vibrator is unlikely to produce a response. However, if the vibration parameters are optimized, results can be good (Ohl *et al.* 1996).

A number of different vibrators are available for this purpose. Many commercial vibrators that are sold by sex shops can be used for this purpose, but frequently the amplitude of their vibration is insufficient to induce ejaculation in men with spinal cord injury. There are, however, some vibrators that are specially made for men with ejaculatory failure and one of these is the FertiCare Personal Vibrator (Multicept Aps, Denmark), which is the one given to patients with spinal cord injury by the author. This vibrator has a 'dial up' system that increases the number of vibrations per second and their amplitude. The Ling 201 vibrator may also be used for this purpose

The technique of penile vibratory stimulation is simple but even this procedure runs the risk of inducing the problem of autonomic hyper-reflexia and this must always be borne in mind. However, on removal of the stimulus, the hypertension usually disappears very quickly. All patients with lesions above T6 should have their blood pressure monitored during the procedure. The use of alpha-blockers administered prior to the procedure is not recommended as they will induce a sympatholytic effect.

The patient's bladder is emptied prior to the procedure. The tip of the vibrator is then placed in the area of the frenulum on the undersurface of the penis. The vibrator may be moved from side to side until there is a sudden increase in tumescence and this may be associated with some lower limb clonus. The semen that emerges is collected into a semen container and it is useful if this container is wide-necked so that no semen is lost at ejaculation. If a periurethral contraction occurs but no semen emerges from the external penile meatus, it is likely that retrograde ejaculation has occurred. The bladder can then be catheterized, washed out with medium and sperm retrieved.

Results, in terms of the pregnancy rate, when using the semen so obtained for simple insemination are not good, but this method of achieving a pregnancy is worth attempting provided that the semen is of good quality.

The electroejaculator

This method of obtaining an ejaculate may be used when vibratory stimulation has failed. Electroejaculation has been used for many years; it was in 1931 that Learmonth first used this technique to induce ejaculation in man. The first pregnancy achieved after electroejaculation of a man with paraplegia was by Thomas and colleagues in 1975 (Thomas *et al.* 1975).

The electroejaculator consists of a current generator and a series of rectal probes of different sizes (G and S Instruments, Duncanville, Texas, USA). The maximum voltage generated by this machine is 50 V and the voltage, milliamperage and the application of the current over time can be adjusted. The probes are made of polyvinyl chloride (PVC) and their diameters may very from 2.5 to 4 cm. On their ventral surface are electrodes that can stimulate the prostate, the vas and the seminal vesicles. These probes should also contain thermometers that give a reading of the rectal temperature and thus do much to prevent any thermal damage to the anterior wall of the rectum. As this apparatus is also capable of inducing autonomic hyperreflexia, careful preparation and management of the patient is essential.

The day selected for treatment must coincide with ovulation in their partner, and it is usually best for insemination to take place some 24 h prior to ovulation or 12 h after ovulation has been triggered using hCG.

The preparation of the patient for electroejaculation is very important. The procedure is always carried out under general anaesthesia when the lesion is incomplete but it is possible to carry out the procedure without anaesthesia in men in whom there is a complete spinal cord lesion and in whom the perianal region is insensate.

In order to alkalinize the urine and minimize any damage to the sperm by contamination of the semen by urine, all patients are given 1.5 g of sodium bicarbonate by mouth on the evening before treatment. Irrigation of the urethra may also be carried out just prior to stimulation using some suitable medium such as HTFM, which is itself commonly used in the preparation of semen for both IVF and intrauterine insemination. As retrograde ejaculation is a common occurrence in electroejaculation, it is important to minimize any damage to the sperm that is brought about by contact of the semen with urine. Some clinicians also instil medium into the bladder in an attempt to maintain the viability of the sperm and reduce contact of the semen with the urine.

In an attempt to prevent the occurrence of autonomic hyperreflexia, the patient is given 20 mg of nifedepine sublingually some 15–20 min prior to the electroejaculation. As the occurrence of autonomic hyperreflexia is a very real risk with this procedure, the blood pressure must be monitored very carefully, most particularly in a conscious patient.

The patient is best placed in the lateral position as this gives the clinician access to both the rectum and the penis. A semen collection pot is placed over the tip of the penis and the rectal probe inserted into the rectum with

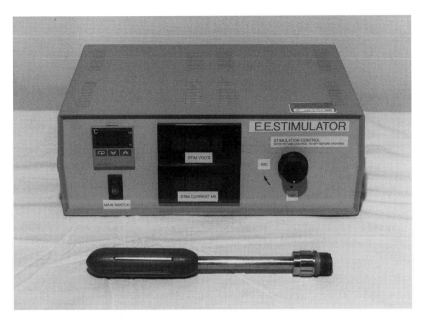

Fig. 12.1 A commonly used electroejaculator showing the voltage and wattage controls. A single rectal probe is shown, the longitudinal metal strips being the active electrodes.

the electrodes facing ventrally at the level of the prostate and the seminal vesicles. The initial stimulation begins at around 10 V and is allowed to last some 5 s. The voltage is then reduced to 5 V and stimulations are induced at a slowly increasing voltage for 5 s every 30 s. This procedure may also induce muscle spasms on stimulation.

Just prior to ejaculation, the penis often becomes fleetingly tumescent, and piloerection, sweating and goose pimples may be seen on the thighs. The ejaculate may of course pass directly into the bladder, and the fact that no ejaculate appears at the penile meatus does not mean that ejaculation has not taken place. If retrograde ejaculation is likely to have occurred, a catheter can be passed into the bladder and washed out with medium, rescuing many motile spermatozoa from destruction by urine.

After the electroejaculation procedure, a proctoscopy must be carried out in order to make sure that there has been no thermal damage to the mucosa on the anterior wall of the rectum. Rectal damage has occurred in a patient undergoing electroejaculation (Bennett *et al.* 1987).

The results of electroejaculation are very variable but better results are obtained from patients with lower spinal cord lesions than those with cervical lesions (Ohl *et al.* 1989). The presence of a sphincterotomy that has been performed in the past results in retrograde ejaculation and thus also jeopardizes the results. On average, however, a cumulative pregnancy rate of around 35% should be achieved in these men (Ohl 1993) using this method of semen production.

However, by standards of infertility treatment today, these results are not good and it is the author's view that assisted conception will give much better results in terms of pregnancy while producing less trauma to the patient.

Assisted conception in the treatment of infertility in men with spinal injury

Recently, the advantages of IVF, and in particular intracytoplasmic sperm injection, have become clear. With the high incidence of abnormalities in the seminal fluid obtained from men undergoing electroejaculation, the application of IVF to the problem of infertility in the male patient with spinal injury appeared to improve greatly the pregnancy rate in these patients (Randolph *et al.* 1990).

However, some of these patients have epididymal damage occurring as the result of past infection, and in these men, azoospermic semen will be obtained at electroejaculation. Such a problem will thus necessitate the collection of sperm from either the epididymis or from the testis.

In fact, it is usually possible to collect enough sperm from these men for several attempts of IVF or IVF/ICSI during the course of one small operation. In these men, their infertility usually relates only to their inability to ejaculate or to their acquired ductal obstruction. Thus, unless the testes have been involved in a situation of multiple injury or there has been previous pathology present prior to the patient's accident, the expected pregnancy rate should be good. It would thus seem that the application of ICSI to these men should improve the pregnancy rate greatly. Indeed it could even be suggested that the vasal or epididymal collection of sperm should be applied to most men with ejaculatory infertility.

The collection of sperm in these men is usually simple. The patients are anaesthetized either using a general anaesthetic or if the spinal lesion is high, then a spinal anaesthetic is ideal. In both situations, anaesthesia can be used to prevent autonomic hyperreflexia, to obliterate clonus (thus making the procedure easier for the surgeon) and will also prevent the occurrence of reflex erections, which the patients frequently find very embarrassing. If no obstruction is present, vasal washout of sperm is simple and provides many millions of sperm that can be cryopreserved. If an obstructive lesion is present, then sperm can be collected from the epididymis or from the testis itself.

The pregnancy rate on a small number of patients with spinal injury treated by IVF and ICSI has been excellent, producing a pregnancy rate of some 65% per cycle of treatment (Jequier 1997). One thus wonders whether this form of treatment should always be recommended to many of the patients with infertility related to spinal cord injury.

It is thus clear that in men with spinal injury, the application of assisted conception gives excellent results with the least trauma to the spinally injured male patient. It is certainly the method advocated by the author.

References

Bennett, C.J., Ayers, J.W.T., Randolph, J.F. *et al.* (1987) Electroejaculation in paraplegic males followed by pregnancies. *Fertility and Sterility* **48**, 1070–1072.

Derry, F., Glass, C., Fraser, M. *et al.* (1997) Sildenafil (Viagra); an oral treatment for men with erectile dysfunction caused by traumatic spinal injury—a 28-day double-blind, placebo controlled, parallel-group, dose–response study. *Neurology* **48**, A214. (Abstract).

Earle, C.M., Seah, M., Coulden, S.E., Stuckey, B., G. & Keogh, E.J. (1996) The use of the vacuum device in the management of erectile impotence. *International Journal of Impotence Research* **8**, 237–240.

Gardner, B.P., Parsons, K.F., Machin, D.G., Gallaway, A. & Krishnan, K.R. (1986) The urological management of spinal cord damaged patients: a clinical algorithm. *Paraplegia* **24**, 138–147.

Gerhart, K.A. (1991) Spinal cord injury outcomes in a population-based sample. *Journal of Trauma* **31**, 1529–1535.

Go, B.K., DeVivo, M.J. & Richards, J.S. (1995) The epidemiology of spinal cord injury. In: *Spinal Cord Injury* (eds S.L. Stover, J.A de Lisa & G.G. Whiteneck). Aspern Publishers Inc, Gaithersburg, MD, pp. 21–55.

Golji, H. (1979) Experience with penile prosthesis in spinal cord injury patients. *Journal of Urology* **121**, 288–289.

Hirsch, I.H., Callaghan, H.J., Sedor, J. & Staas, W.F. (1990) Systemic sperm autoimmunity in spinal-cord injured men. *Archives of Andrology* **25**, 69–73.

Jequier, A.M. (1997) *Assisted conception in the treatment of male infertility caused by spinal injury.* Annual Meeting of the International Medical Society of Paraplegia, Perth (Abstract).

Light, J.K. & Scott, F.B. (1981) Management of neurogenic impotence with inflatable penile prostheses. *Urology* **26**, 341–343.

Ohl, D.A. (1993) Electroejaculation. *Urologic Clinics of North America* **20**, 181–188.

Ohl, D.A., Bennett, C.A., McCabe, M., Menge, A.C. & McGuire, E.J. (1989) predictors of success in electro-ejaculation of spinal cord injured men. *Journal of Urology* **142**, 1483–1486.

Ohl, D.A., Menge, A.C. & Sonksen, J. (1996) Penile vibratory stimulation in spinal cord injured men: optimized vibration parameters and prognostic factors. *Archives of Physical Medicine and Rehabilitation* **77**, 903–906.

Randolph, J.F., Ohl, D.A., Bennett, C.J., Ayers, J.W.T. & Menge, A.C. (1990) Combined electroejaculation and *in vitro* fertilization in the evaluation and treatment of anejaculatory infertility. *Journal of In Vitro Fertilization and Embryo Transfer* **7**, 58–62.

Rotel, T.R., Lawson, J.S., Wilson, S.F., Engel, S., Rutkowski, S.B. & Ablett, C. (1998) Severe cervical cord injuries related to Rugby union and league football in New South Wales. 1984–96. *Medical Journal of Australia* **168**, 379–381.

Rutkowski, S.B., Middleton, J.W., Truman, G., Hagen, D.L. & Ryan, J.P. (1995) The influence of bladder management on fertility in spinally injured men. *Paraplegia* **33**, 263–266.

Thomas, R.J., McGleish, G. & McDonald, I.A. (1975) Electro-ejaculation of the papaplegic male followed by pregnancy. *Medical Journal of Australia* **2**, 798–799.

Wyndaele, J.J., De Meyur, J.M., De Sy, W.A. & Clossens, H. (1986) Intracavernous injection of vasoactive drugs for treating impotence in spinal cord injury patients. *Paraplegia* **24**, 271 (Abstract).

13: Vasectomy-related Infertility

Vasectomy-related infertility is now becoming a common and thus important cause of secondary childlessness. As the incidence of marriage break-up approaches 50% in the Western world, it should be no surprise that vasectomy (a form of permanent birth control) is often regretted. As men tend to marry women younger than themselves, a family is often desired by the second wife. For this reason, problems of infertility arise because of the presence of the now unwanted vasectomy. Indeed, unwanted vasectomy is fast becoming one of the most common causes of infertility seen in an infertility clinic (Jequier 1998).

There are, however, many religions that reject the use of any form of permanent contraception and the Muslim faith and the Roman Catholic Church are well known for their prohibition of this procedure. Despite this, vasectomy now forms an important means of contraception, even in countries such as Brazil (Foreit *et al.* 1989).

Sterilization, both male and female, is now a commonly used form of contraception; it has been estimated that in the USA around 30% of couples may use some form of sterilization procedure, be it vasectomy or tubal occlusion, as a means of birth control. In Western Australia, about 1 in 500 adult males has had a vasectomy (Jequier, unpublished). The rate for requests for reversal of vasectomy has been estimated to be around 7.5% for Australia as a whole (Baker 1991). In the author's private fertility clinic, 10% of all requests for fertility treatment involve vasectomy-related infertility. Thus, regretted vasectomy is fast becoming an important cause of infertility.

Reasons given for carrying out a vasectomy

The most common reason by far for requesting a vasectomy is that both partners consider that their family is complete (Howard 1978). As vasectomy is a simple operation and can be carried out under local anaesthesia, it is an attractive option as a means of permanent contraception. Another common reason for request of a vasectomy is the female partner's poor acceptance of many forms of female contraception together with her nonacceptance of female sterilization. A very small number of patients elect to undergo vasectomy when they do not wish to have any children at all. Occasionally, this operation is done simply for genetic reasons.

The operation of vasectomy

If one is going to treat the infertility associated with vasectomy, then it is important to understand the ways in which the original operation may be carried out.

This procedure may be carried out either under general anaesthesia or by using a local anaesthetic.

The first step is to identify the vas deferens at the back of the neck of the scrotum and then to manoeuvre it up to the undersurface of the skin on the anterior surface of the scrotal neck. Local anaesthetic, usually marcaine and adrenaline (epinephrine), is now injected into the skin and the subcutaneous tissue. When this anaesthetic has become effective, a small incision is made in the skin to expose the muscle and fascial sheath that covers the vas. This sheath is now incised taking care not to damage the vasal artery that lies along side the vas.

The vas is now exposed and a loop of vas is now gently pulled out through the incision where it is held in position using a pair of Babcock forceps. There are a number of different ways in which the vasectomy may be carried out.

Simple clamp and tie

This is by far the most commonly used method of performing a vasectomy. Clamps are applied to the vas on either side of the Babcock forceps and the intervening portion of the vas is excised. This small segment is then usually sent for histological examination to confirm occlusion of the vas. The cut ends are then tied using an absorbable suture such as 3/0 catgut or polyglactin (Vicryl, Ethicon Ltd), although many surgeons recommend the use of a nonabsorbable suture such as silk or nylon (Hendry 1994). The cut ends are then usually folded back onto each end of the vas and retied. The cut ends are then dropped back into the scrotum and the skin closed with a small subcuticular stitch (Fig. 13.1).

Some surgeons recommend that a fascial interposition is made prior to closure as this is said to reduce the recanalization rate after vasectomy (Esho & Cass 1978).

Diathermy to the proximal cut end of the vas

In this technique (Schmidt & Free 1978), a diathermy needle is inserted into the lumen of the proximal end of the vasa and the epithelium of this portion of the vas is then coagulated. The distal cut end of the vas is not tied. This is said to make subsequent reversal much easier.

Open-ended vasectomy

For this procedure, the proximal end of the vas is not tied but is simply left

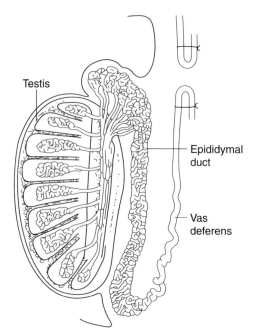

Testis

Epididymal
duct

Vas
deferens

Fig. 13.1 A diagrammatic
representation of the testis, the vas
deferens and the common site of a
vasectomy.

open. This allows the sperm to spill out around the cut end of the vas post-operatively. These sperm generate the formation of a sperm granuloma around the proximal end of the vas (Silber 1978). The distal cut end of the vas is tied in the usual way. This technique is said to enhance the success of reversal rates and may help to reduce epididymal damage after the vasectomy.

'No scalpel' vasectomy

In this technique, a very small skin incision is made using scissors. The cut ends of the vas are tied in the usual way and a small fascial interposition is carried out. The tiny incision in the skin does not need any form of suturing.

Vasal washouts

In this technique the distal portion of the vas, and in particular the ampullae of each vas, may be washed out with either saline or some spermicidal agent prior to ligation of each of the cut ends. This technique reduces the time taken to achieve sterility postvasectomy. However, it does nothing to prevent recanalization nor does it enhance or reduce the chances of fertility after reversal.

Complications of vasectomy

There are of course complications to the operation of vasectomy.

Haematoma formation

The most common postoperative problem is haematoma formation (Barnes *et al.* 1973), which may become obvious within an hour or two of the procedure. Early evacuation of the clot is important for rapid recovery. Delay in any action allows the blood to extravasate into the scrotal connective tissue and this considerably delays healing and causes a great deal of discomfort to the patient.

Infection

Infection of a vasectomy wound is rare, although this can occur as secondary infection within a haematoma. Diabetic patients may also be more susceptible to infection following vasectomy.

Postvasectomy pain

Postvasectomy pain is thankfully a relatively rare complication of this operation but when it occurs it can be very difficult to treat. Clinical examination reveals no obvious pathology as this condition is thought to be caused by damage and probable neuroma formation in the perivasal nerves, but in almost all cases the cause of the pain cannot be determined. This can, however, also be the symptom of a spermatic granuloma (*vide infra*). Occasionally, even among patients with no abnormal physical signs, epididymectomy seems to resolve this problem.

Granuloma formation

Despite careful ligation of the proximal end of the vas, spermatozoa can leak out of the proximal cut end of the vas. Within the connective tissue, the sperm induce an inflammatory reaction with the formation of a sperm granuloma. These granuloma can sometimes be the source of postoperative pain that can on occasions be severe (Schmidt 1979). The development of canaliculae in the space between the cut ends of the vas has also been described, and these tiny channels may even result in a small number of sperm reappearing in the ejaculate some time after a vasectomy (Fig. 13.2). These sperm, however, are never in sufficient numbers to result in a pregnancy. Sperm from these granulomata may also enter the lymphatic systems that drain this area. Sperm have even been seen in the para-aortic lymph nodes of a patient following a vasectomy (Ball *et al.* 1982).

Antisperm antibody formation

If any breach is made in the integrity of the male genital tract and spermatozoa are allowed to spill out, there is a risk of the formation of antibodies

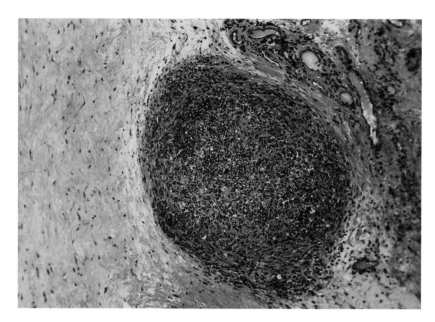

Fig. 13.2 A histological section of a sperm granuloma found during vasectomy reversal at the site of a vasectomy. Note the small canaliculi that have formed to one side of the granuloma. It is possible that these could be the means of transfer of small numbers of sperm into the distal vas.

that are directed against the spermatozoa. Indeed, the presence of sperm antibodies is common after vasectomy and may occur in as many as 60–80% of men within 1 year of this procedure (Hellema & Rumpke 1978).

These antibodies are of the immunoglobulin A (IgA) and IgG immunoglobulin subgroups. The IgA subgroup antisperm antibodies are commonly found in the secretions of the mucus-producing components of the male genital tract. Following vasectomy, 60% of men develop anti-sperm antibodies and these antibodies usually persist even after the vasectomy has been reversed; indeed, the antibody titre may increase after any attempt at reversal (Sutherland *et al.* 1984).

Damage to the epididymal duct and its function

Long-term vasectomy can result in damage to the epididymal duct. This damage may give rise to poor function of its luminal epithelium and may be the reason why asthenozoospermia is so common after vasectomy reversal; it is common to have a good sperm count but very poorly motile sperm after such a procedure. The second problem that can arise is an actual rupture of the epididymal wall, resulting in the extravasation of sperm into the surrounding connective tissue (Silber 1979). These ruptures are often referred to as postvasectomy 'blow-outs'.

Recanalization of the vas

Recanalization of the vas and a return of fertility is a well-recognized complication of vasectomy that may occur in around 0.5% of all such operations (Barnes *et al.* 1973). Such recanalization can occur several months after the vasectomy. The ends of the vas may come together and rejoin; as Rolnick showed many years ago, the vas is surprisingly efficient at achieving recanalization (Rolnick 1924).

The presence of a double vas

This is not an uncommon entity and, rather than recanalization, it may be the cause of persistent sperm in an ejaculate following a vasectomy. This anomaly usually only involves the proximal (scrotal) ends of the vasa deferentia. It is present in around 0.1% of men undergoing vasectomy (Barnes *et al.* 1973).

Other diseases that may be associated with vasectomy

It has long been said that vasectomy may increase the incidence of heart disease amongst men undergoing this procedure. The first suggestion of this relationship was reported in primates that appeared to have an increased incidence of aortic atheroma after vasectomy (Alexander & Anderson 1979). However, no such relationship between coronary artery occlusion in the human has been demonstrated (Wallace *et al.* 1981).

Vasectomy has also been related to an increase in the incidence of prostate cancer. How vasectomy might cause prostate cancer is unknown and indeed this relationship has been seriously questioned.

Reasons for request for reversal

The most common reason for a request for reversal of vasectomy is remarriage (Howard 1982; Jequier 1998). Other reasons include loss of a child or, more commonly, loss of a pregnancy soon after a vasectomy. For these reasons and because of the fact that the majority of childhood deaths occur at or soon after birth, vasectomy should not be carried out for at least 1 year after the completion of a pregnancy.

Occasionally a vasectomy is perceived by the patient to have induced impotence and request for reversal in these circumstances is not that uncommon. Quite how a vasectomy could cause a loss of erectile function is difficult to understand, and this problem is thus likely to have a major psychological component.

Some couples, of course, simply have a change of heart about having further children and, for this reason, careful counselling is necessary before the vasectomy is carried out.

Vasectomy reversal

It would appear that vasectomy reversal is requested by between 7% and 10% of all men who have undergone this procedure, but this figure may vary greatly in different parts of the world. This is much higher than the request for reversal sought by women, which is probably only around 1–2%.

The basic procedure used in the reversal of vasectomy is the operation of vasovasostomy.

Incisions used for a vasovasostomy

Bilateral incisions in the neck of the scrotum

These incisions are made over the site of the vasectomy on each side in the neck of the scrotum. This is a simple and very commonly used approach to vasectomy reversal. However, it has the disadvantage that it does not allow the inspection of any other part of the distal genital tract, but it has the advantage that it provides a minimum disturbance of the surrounding tissue and considerably reduces the danger of postoperative bleeding.

Midline scrotal incision

This may also be used and has the distinct advantage in that it allows inspection of the epididymis and the identification of epididymal 'blow-outs' that would render any vasovasostomy useless in terms of future fertility. However, this approach involves a much greater degree of tissue disruption and the incidence of postoperative bleeding is likely to be much greater. This incision also allows a wider field for exploration, especially if one is unsure on palpation of the exact site of the original vasectomy.

Subpubic incision

This incision has been used in the past but has now largely been abandoned (Kelami 1978). A transverse incision is made across the upper symphysis pubis and the testes are then exteriorized out through the incision. Although this has the advantage of allowing an inspection of the epididymis on either side, it is an approach that has largely been abandoned today.

The operation of vasovasostomy

For most surgeons, this operation is considerably facilitated by the use of some form of magnification for this procedure, but this does not necessarily mean that the procedure has to be carried out using the operating microscope. Many recommend the use of the operating microscope (Silber 1977) but good results are obtained without its use (Belker *et al.* 1991). Magnification of around ×4 is usually sufficient for this procedure and thus an operating loupe can be used.

Approach to the cut ends of each vas deferens

There may be a considerable gap between the cut end of each vas and there are even some surgeons (who are thankfully rare) who remove the whole of the scrotal vas in the course of a vasectomy, making the reversal very difficult indeed.

The ends of the vas can usually easily be palpated and may be blown out by the presence of a sperm granuloma at the proximal cut end. Each end may also be surround by fairly dense adhesions and it is usually possible to identify the proline thread that was used to carry out the original vasectomy. Using gentle sharp dissection, each end of the vas deferens is freed from its coverings and the surrounding adhesions. The fibrous tissue between the cut end of the vasa can now excised. Each cut end of the vas is now grasped using a Babcock forceps.

Each end of the vas is now pared back using small incisions across the end of each vas until the lumen is exposed. On exposing the lumen of the proximal cut end of the vas, the seminal fluid will ooze out into the wound. The site of the past vasectomy must be completely excised to leave clean undamaged vasal tissue for use in the vasovasostomy. At this point, it is important to control all bleeding very carefully.

A sterile microscope slide should now be placed on the cut end of the vas and the smear covered with a cover-slip, after which the slide must be examined for the presence of spermatozoa. If the fluid that oozes out of the proximal cut end of the vas is thick, this usually (but not reliably) indicates the presence of large numbers of spermatozoa within it. It is, however, important to check this fluid microscopically before proceeding with a vasovasostomy. If there are no sperm in the fluid that exits the cut end of the vas and there is no evidence of 'blow-outs' in the epididymis then a vasovasostomy *may* be worth doing, as occasionally sperm can reappear in the ejaculate after a reversal despite these negative findings.

However, if no sperm are present in this smear then it is very likely that some other lesion, in particular a postvasectomy epididymal 'blow-out', is present making the success of this vasectomy reversal very unlikely. Such a situation may necessitate the use of an epididymovasostomy instead of the planned vasovasostomy.

When the lumen of the distal end of the vas deferens is cut open, it is also useful to inject saline down the vas to exclude a secondary obstruction distal to the site of the vasectomy. Some authors at this point also inject saline down the distal end of the vas prior to vasovasostomy as this will indicate patency of the vas deferens distally. However, it is possible that this technique may increase the risk of infection.

A single-layered technique

The vasovasostomy can now be carried out. Either a microscope or a loupe may be used, and many surgeons stress the need for the use of the operating microscope (Silber 1978). However, the lumen of the vas is very obvious and results of vasectomy reversal have not been shown by some authors to be any better using any higher magnification (Belker *et al.* 1991), especially if a single-layer technique is used. The self-healing qualities of the vas have been known for many years (Rolnick 1924).

The removal of all scar tissue and fibrous tissue from around the cut ends of the vas prior to anastomosis is very important for success. Using healthy well-vascularized tissue for the anastomosis and ensuring good apposition of the cut ends of each vas deferens is likely to be all that is needed to achieve patency at the site of a past vasectomy.

The ends of the vas are now sutured together using either fine (6/0) proline or PDS. The anastomosis is best carried out in one layer. If the operating microscope is used, the anastomosis is usually performed using 10/0 proline; if using the loupe, larger 6/0 sutures are usually employed. Between three and four sutures are used in each layer and extend through the whole thickness of the vasal wall to enter the lumen. It is best to insert all the sutures before tying them or visualization of the lumen of the vas deferens will be lost. After closing the vasovasostomy, two or three anchoring sutures can be inserted to ensure stability of the anastomosis.

The use of any form of stent in a vasectomy reversal has now been abandoned as the results after the use of stents is poor. Whether these poor results are caused by an inflammatory change or leakage of sperm near the vasovasostomy is unclear.

The anastomosed vas is now dropped back into the wound and the incision closed. It is very important to ensure that complete haemostasis has been achieved before closure.

A double-layered technique

This technique is very likely to improve apposition of the cut ends of the vas, but there is little evidence that in fact it is needed to achieve good results at vasectomy reversal. However, it may be the better operation when there is a major discrepancy between the size of the vasal lumen proximally and distally. This operation is, however, best carried out using an operating microscope.

Two layers of sutures are used, one for the mucosa of the vasal lumen and the second for the vasal wall. An 8/0 or 9/0 proline suture is best used for this procedure.

Each cut end of the vas deferens is cleaned of its surrounding fibrous tissue and adhesions and is then held in a Silber clamp, which maintains the ends of the cut vas deferens in apposition. This instrument allows rotation of the cut ends of the vas and facilitates the insertion of the two layers of sutures.

An inner layer of three sutures is now placed to include the mucosa and the inner layer of the muscle wall of the vas. These sutures are tied as soon as they are inserted. The site of the anastomosis needs irrigation as seminal fluid may continue to seep out of the proximal cut end of the vas and interfere with visualization of the mucosal edges. A total of six sutures, this time using 6/0 proline are then inserted into the muscular coat of the vas, inserting three stiches on each side of the vasovasostomy. The rotational facility afforded by the Silber clamp is of great help in this procedure.

Testicular biopsies in relation to vasectomy reversal

Some authors suggest that a testicular biopsy should be taken whenever a vasectomy reversal is carried out. This procedure prolongs the operations and enhances the risk of haematoma formation postoperatively. However, a rough estimate of the expected sperm count can be made from counting the number of spermatids present in a number of seminiferous tubules (Silber & Rodrigues Rigau 1981). If the spermatid numbers do not correlate with the sperm count in the semen, it is possible that there is some degree of obstruction present that could indicate a repeat attempt at reversal. However, it must be remembered that there is some focal change in testicular histology even among otherwise normal men. Also, such a change may be more marked with advancing age. It is not the author's policy to carry out testicular biopsies on all men when carrying out a vasectomy reversal.

It must also be remembered that histological changes can occur as the result of the initial vasectomy. A common example is the presence of interstitial oedema that is frequently found in testicular biopsies taken from men undergoing vasectomy reversal (Fig. 13.3).

Closure of the scrotal wound

The anastomosis is dropped back into the wound, haemostasis is completed and the scrotum closed. The scrotal skin can be closed using silk sutures or, better still, using a fine rapidly dissolving polyglactin subcuticular suture.

Postoperative care

Most patients are kept in hospital overnight and are discharged home the following day. As ejaculation causes contraction of the wall of the vas deferens and this could disrupt the newly formed vasovasostomy, intercourse is best avoided for about 10 days postoperatively. Some 5–7 days off work, especially if work involves a great deal of physical activity, is also recommended.

A semen sample is requested 6 weeks postoperatively and thereafter at 2-monthly intervals to ensure that the vasovasostomy has been successful.

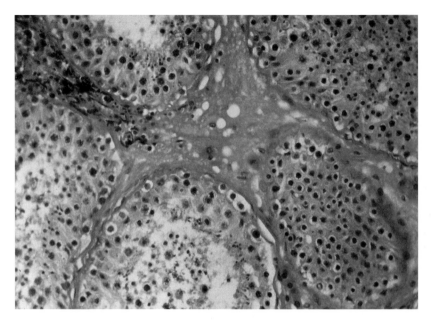

Fig. 13.3 A testicular biopsy showing marked interstitial oedema. This testicular biopsy was taken from a man undergoing vasectomy reversal.

It may take as long as 6 months for an ejaculate to return to normal after a vasectomy reversal.

Difficulties encountered during a vasovasostomy

There are many difficulties that may be encountered during the performance of a vasectomy reversal.

Excess vas excised at the past vasectomy

This can result in difficulty in apposing the two cut ends of the vas at vasectomy reversal. It has been suggested that by opening the inguinal canal and mobilization the distal end of the vas towards the scrotum can be of assistance in this situation. However, the vasal or epididymal aspiration of sperm and their use within an IVF/ICSI programme is more likely to result in fertility than would any operation of this sort.

Past excision of the vas into its convoluted section

This problem does not make the vasovasostomy impossible but just makes it technically more difficult. The wall of the convoluted portion of the vas is much thinner than that more distally, and thus it may not be so easy to make the anastomosis as secure as is the case when the anastomosis is more distal.

The presence of 'blow-outs' in the epididymis

These lesions indicate the presence of a rupture in the epididymal duct as the result of prolonged distension after vasectomy. Spillage of sperm out of the epididymal duct causes an inflammatory reaction around the area of the rupture and occasionally may result in the formation of a sperm granuloma. These lesions thus cause a second site of obstruction within the epididymal duct (Silber 1979). These changes are particularly common in men with a long-standing vasectomy, i.e. of over 5 years, and result in a poor prognosis for reversal.

The management of men with these changes can be twofold. One can either carry out a vasoepididymostomy or one can collect sperm by aspiration of the epididymal duct and use it within an IVF/ICSI programme.

The presence of an obstructive lesion distal to the vasectomy

This is not a very common phenomenon but can occasionally occur. If such an obstruction is clearly present when the distal end of the vas is flushed with saline, then there is clearly no point in carrying out a vasovasostomy until the site of this obstruction has been identified and the feasibility of its treatment has been assessed. In this situation, it will be necessary to carry out a vasogram and identify the site of this lesion. If the lesion is close to the site of the vasectomy it may be possible to carry out a second vasovasostomy on the same vas.

If, however, this lesion is at a distance from the original vasectomy, then it may be simpler and more effective from the fertility point of view to collect sperm from the proximal end of the vas deferens. Should it be necessary, these spermatozoa can be used at a later date within an IVF programme. Alternatively, one could deem that the vasectomy is inoperable unilaterally and rely on the vasovasostomy on the opposite side for a positive ejaculate. It must be remembered, however, that failure to relieve an obstruction within the reproductive tract can result in the persistence of a high titre of antisperm antibodies in both the serum and in the semen.

The need for a 'crossed vasovasostomy'

Very rarely one may find two different lesions on each side in men undergoing vasectomy reversal. This may include a 'blow-out' on one side and a distal obstructive lesion on the other. This of course is not a common occurrence but may be seen among these men undergoing either vasectomy reversal or surgery for other forms of ductal obstruction on rare occasions.

The easy way around this problem is to carry out a 'crossed vasovasostomy', where the distal end of one vas is anastomosed to the proximal end of the vas on the opposite side. One vas is passed through the scrotal septum and the anastomosis performed in one scrotum only.

Complications of vasovasostomy

There are several important complications of vasovasostomy and these are very similar to the complications of vasectomy. However, these complications arise more frequently after a vasectomy reversal than they do after a vasectomy, which is a more complex procedure.

Haematoma formation

The most important complication of this procedure is of course haematoma formation. In order to prevent this, it is important to be scrupulous in achieving haemostasis at all stages of the procedure.

Scrotal pain

As with vasectomy it is also possible for the patient to develop scrotal pain postoperatively, which may be very difficult to treat and may necessitate an epididymectomy.

Increasing titres of antisperm antibodies

During the procedure of vasovasostomy, the genital tract is opened and sperm may spill into the surrounding tissues. It is possible therefore that the titre of antisperm antibodies may rise following this procedure and this may impede the fertility of the patient (Thomas *et al.* 1981).

Asthenozoospermia

It is not uncommon after a vasectomy reversal for there to be a large number of sperm in an ejaculate, but their motility is too poor to ensure fertility. This phenomenon may be the result of damage to the epididymal wall by the distension induced during the period of the obstruction. Thus, it is not uncommon for men who have had vasectomy reversals to end up achieving pregnancies by IVF/ICSI even when the vasectomy reversal appears to have been successful, at least in terms of sperm numbers in the ejaculate. This situation may be further compromised by the presence of antisperm antibodies.

Overall results of vasectomy reversal

As a good general rule, the results of vasectomy reversal decline with increasing time since the original vasectomy, i.e. the longer the vasectomy interval, the worse the results of any reversal, and this applies to both the quality of the semen and the subsequent pregnancy rate. This phenomenon is likely to be a result of damage to the excurrent duct system, especially epididymal function, after the vasal ligation.

The overall success in terms of pregnancy rate is very variable and such results may relate to both the length of the vasectomy interval and the method of performing the vasectomy reversal. It would appear that the longer the time between the vasectomy and its reversal, the poorer are the results both in terms of patency and pregnancy rate. Results will of course also depend upon the operation used to carry out the initial vasectomy. Although success may occur in men undergoing vasectomy reversal after long vasectomy intervals (the longest vasectomy interval with a successful reversal is claimed to be 23 years), results decline with increasing time since the initial vasectomy. However, factors that may influence the success of reversal include the length of vas removed, the presence of a granuloma at the site of the vasectomy and also the method used to carry out the vasectomy.

The application of advanced reproductive technology (ART) to the problem of vasectomy-related infertility

The success of ART to the management of vasectomy-related infertility has been striking. The application of ICSI enables one to overcome the asthenozoospermia that so often accompanies vasectomy reversal and allows one to use sperm aspirated from the epididymis from men with failed reversal or where there are epididymal 'blow-outs' present. Indeed, so successful has this technique been in producing pregnancies that it has been suggested that this technique should be used instead of vasectomy reversal; this concept allows for a good pregnancy rate to be achieved but provides good contraception between such pregnancies. The many techniques that may be used for epididymal aspiration will be described in the chapter on assisted reproduction.

When a man wishes to have a vasectomy reversed, one important decision that should be made is whether it would be more cost effective to undergo a reversal or whether it would be more effective to proceed to epididymal aspiration of sperm and IVF and ICSI. This decision will of course depend on the relative chances of success for each of these methods in an individual patient together with their relative costs. The availability and the cost of each of these procedures will of course vary in different locations and in different countries (Pavlovich & Schlegel 1997), and thus one has difficulty in making any rules about the management of such patients.

There is no doubt that where a vasectomy has been carried out and has resulted in the production of sperm showing gross asthenozoospermia, IVF and ICSI are indicated. Likewise, where the semen contains high titres of antisperm antibodies, IVF and ICSI are also probably the most effective treatments.

The most important question of course is whether the reversal is worth doing at all, and whether it might be both simpler and cheaper to simply perform IVF, ICSI and epididymal aspiration of sperm without performing any initial vasectomy reversal. It is the author's practice to consider the application of assisted reproduction as an initial means of treatment in any patient whose vasectomy interval is more than 5 years and in all patients in whom Bayle's sign is positive and where there is clear clinical evidence of an epididymal 'blow-out'. However, these are simply guidelines that can be adjusted according to the cost factors that exist in different countries and localities around the world.

References

Alexander, N.J. & Anderson, D.J. (1979) Vasectomy: consequences of autoimmunity to sperm antigens. *Fertility and Sterility* **32**, 2253–2260.

Baker, H.W.G. (1991) Failed vasectomy reversal: an epidemic of preventable infertility. In: *Proceedings of the Annual Meeting of the Fertility Society of Australia*, Lorne, Victoria, Australia (Abstract No 18).

Ball, R.Y., Naylor, C.P.E. & Mitchinson, M.J. (1982) Spermatozoa in an abdominal lymph node after vasectomy in a man. *Journal of Reproduction and Fertility* **66**, 715–716.

Barnes, M.N., Blandy, J.P. & England, H.R. (1973) One thousand vasectomies. *British Medical Journal* **4**, 216–221.

Belker, A.M., Thomas, A.J., Fuches, E.F., Konnak, J.W. & Sharlip, I.D. (1991) Results of 1469 microsurgical vasectomy reversals by the vasovasostomy study group. *Journal of Urology* **145**, 505–511.

Esho, J.O. & Cass, A.S. (1978) Recanalisation rate following methods of vasectomy using interposition of fascial sheath of vas deferens. *Journal of Urology* **120**, 178–179.

Foreit, K.G., de Castro, M.P. & Franco, E.F. (1989) The impact of mass media advertising on a voluntary sterilization program in Brazil. *Studies in Family Planning* **20**, 107–116.

Hellema, J.W.J. & Rumpke, P. (1978) Sperm autoantibodies as a consequence of vasectomy. 1. Within one year post-operation. *Clinical and Experimental Immunology* **31**, 18–29.

Hendry, W.F. (1994) Vasectomy and vasectomy reversal. *British Journal of Urology* **73**, 337–344.

Howard, G. (1978) Motivation for vasectomy. *Lancet* **i**, 794–795.

Howard, G. (1982) Who asks for vasectomy reversal and why? *British Medical Journal* **285**, 490–492.

Jequier, A.M. (1998) Vasectomy-related infertility: a major and costly medical problem. *Human Reproduction* **13**, 1757–1759.

Kelami, A. (1978) 'Infra-pubic' approach in operative andrology. *Urology* **12**, 580–581.

Pavlovich, C.P. & Schlegel, P.N. (1997) Fertility options after vasectomy: a cost effective analysis. *Fertility and Sterility* **67**, 133–141.

Rolnick, H.C. (1924) Regeneration of the vas deferens. *Archives of Surgery* **9**, 188–203.

Schmidt, S.S. (1979) Spermatic granuloma: an often painful lesion. *Fertility and Sterility* **31**, 178–181.

Schmidt, S.S. & Free, M.J. (1978) The bipolar needle for vasectomy. 1. Experience with the first 1000 cases. *Fertility and Sterility* **29**, 676–680.

Silber, S.J. (1977) Microscopic vasectomy reversal. *Fertility and Sterility* **28**, 1191–1202.

Silber, S.J. (1978) Vasectomy and vasectomy reversal. *Fertility and Sterility* **28**, 57–60.

Silber, S.J. (1979) Epididymal extravasation following vasectomy as a cause of failure of vasectomy reversal. *Fertility and Sterility* **31**, 309–315.

Silber, S.J. & Rodrigues Rigau, L.J. (1981) Quantitative analysis of testicle biopsy: determination of partial obstruction and prediction of sperm count after surgery for obstruction. *Fertility and Sterility* **36**, 480–485.

Sutherland, P.D., Matson, P.L., Masters, J.R. & Pryor, J.P. (1984) Association between infertility following reversal of vasectomy and the presence of sperm agglutinating activity in semen. *International Journal of Andrology* **7**, 503–508.

Thomas, A.J., Pontes, J.E., Rose, N.R., Segal, S. & Pierce, J.M. (1981) Microsurgical vasovasosotomy: immunologic consequences and subsequent fertility. *Fertility and Sterility* **35**, 447–450.

Wallace, R.B., Lee, J., Gerber, W.L., Clarke, W.R. & Laver, R.M. (1981) Vasectomy and coronary disease in men less than 50 years old: absence of association. *Journal of Urology* **126**, 182–184.

14: The Microbiology of Semen and Infections of the Male Genital Tract

Genital tract infections can in themselves be a cause of infertility and they can also cause infertility by the damage they do to the testes, the excurrent ducts of the testes and to the accessory glands of the genital tract.

Such infections may manifest themselves in obvious ways clinically with pain, fever and the presence of blood in an ejaculate. Infection can also be asymptomatic and may present to the clinician as an excess of white blood cells in a semen sample, a condition known as pyospermia. In infective conditions involving the genital tract, these white cells are often present in semen in aggregates and this appearance is usually diagnostic of a genital tract infection. All semen samples that show an excess of white cells must be sent for microbiological culture.

It must also be remembered, however, that neutrophils can frequently be found in normal semen samples especially those from older men and from men with benign prostatic hypertrophy when the source of these cells is the prostate itself.

Care must be taken in the diagnosis of pyospermia. It is impossible to differentiate white blood cells from immature germ cells without staining the cells, and it is often difficult to tell the difference between these two types of cells without access to a peroxidase stain. All too frequently patients are administered expensive courses of antibiotics when there is in fact no evidence of infection, but where germinal cells are mistaken for white blood cells.

The positive identification of white blood cells in semen

Before the diagnosis of an infection can be confidently made, the white blood cells in semen must be accurately identified and this is performed by the demonstration of peroxidase in the cells believed to be leucocytes. The demonstration of peroxidase can be carried out in several ways.

Benzidine cyanosine stain

This stain colours the white blood cells brown and allows them to be positively identified from any germinal cells that may be present in a semen sample. This method is more fully described in Chapter 5, which deals with the analysis of semen. It is a simple staining technique and is a very accurate way of differentiating white blood cells from all the other types of cells

254

that may be present in semen. Its routine use in semen analysis is to be recommended.

Fluorescein-conjugated antiperoxidase antibody

The enzyme peroxidase is a protein and thus an antibody can easily be raised against it. The use of an antiperoxidase antibody is a very simple but much more expensive way of demonstrating the presence of peroxidase in the cells in semen.

The Papanicolaou stain

White blood cells can usually be differentiated from germinal and other types of cells in semen using this stain, but it is difficult and a great deal of experience is required to carry this out successfully. Although the Papanicolaou stain is excellent for defining the morphology of spermatozoa, mistakes are easily made when attempting to differentiate white blood cells from germinal cells (Fig. 14.1). It is thus much better to use the benzidine cyanosin stain routinely for the demonstration of white blood cells.

Reporting the presence of white blood cells in a semen sample

The density of neutrophils in semen can be reported in a number of different ways. First, they must be accurately identified in the ways described

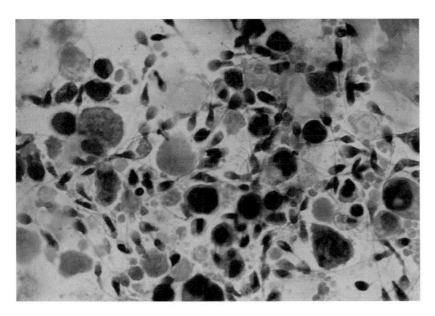

Fig. 14.1 A photomicrograph showing a severe pyospermia from a patient with a genital tract infection.

above. If the smear is now examined at a magnification of around ×400 then the number of white blood cells present in one such field will equal their concentration in semen in millions per millilitre of semen. Thus, white cells can be reported as the number per high power field or as millions per millilitre of semen. Either way is acceptable provided that the clinician is left in no doubt about the accuracy of the report or of the abnormal number that are present in the semen.

The concentration of white blood cells in an ejaculate can also be calculated from the sperm concentration. Thus, if there are 50 million sperm per millilitre and there is one white blood cell for every 10 sperm then the concentration of white cells will be 5 million per millilitre. Also, if the total number of white blood cells in an ejaculate needs to be known, then the concentration of white cells per millilitre is simply multiplied by the ejaculatory volume.

A concentration of more than 1 million white blood cells (or more than 1 white blood cell per high power field at a magnification of ×400) is generally considered to be abnormal and will thus constitute pyospermia.

Identification of the sites of an infection in the genital tract

There are four main sites of infection within the male genital tract. These are the testis/epididymal complex, the seminal vesicles, the prostate and the bulbourethral and urethral glands. There are a number of different techniques by which the source of the white blood cells and thus the site of the infection can be identified.

The split ejaculate

The site of production of the neutrophils and thus the probable site of a genital tract infection can be more accurately identified using a split ejaculate.

During emission and ejaculation, the components of the ejaculate enter the posterior urethra and pass down the penile urethra in a predetermined sequence. The first part of the ejaculate to be expelled are the secretions of the urethral and paraurethral glands and these lubricate the urethra to aid the expulsion of the main part of the ejaculate. The next portions of the ejaculate to exit the urethra are the testicular and epididymal secretions and these are followed by the secretions of the prostate. The last or third part of the ejaculate is made up of the secretions of the seminal vesicles. It is possible for a patient to collect the three major portions of the ejaculate as three separate aliquots of seminal fluid as it emerges from the external urethral meatus.

In order to collect an ejaculate in three parts, the patient is provided with three semen containers that are taped together (Fig. 14.2). The patient is asked to produce the semen in three parts, each spurt of semen being col-

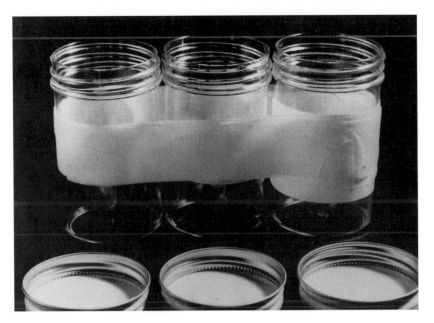

Fig. 14.2 Three semen pots that have been taped together to be used for the collection of three separate portions of the ejaculate.

lected in one of the three pots. It may take a small amount of practice for a patient to be able to produce a good separation of the three parts of an ejaculate but this in fact can be fairly easily achieved by most men.

Each fraction is now examined individually both microscopically and microbiologically, and in this way the site of any infection can be more precisely demonstrated and its causative organism identified.

The technique of split ejaculate production can be applied to many other aspects of andrology; it has even been used to track the site of entry of drugs into the male genital tract and of toxins into the seminal fluid.

Expressed prostatic secretions

A method of demonstrating a specific prostatic infection is by the use of expressed prostatic secretions. These are obtained by the collection of a discharge from the penile urethra and from the passage of urine after prostatic massage per rectum. The patient lies on his left side on the examination couch while the posterior wall of the prostate is massaged digitally per rectum. A container is held over the external urethral meatus to collect any discharge and after the massage the first few millilitres of urine are collected, as these will contain the bulk of the prostatic fluid produced by the massage. These samples are then sent to the laboratory for both cytological and microbiological examination. In this way, the site of the prostate as a source of infection and the nature of the organism that causes this infection can be identified.

Common organisms that can infect seminal fluid

It must firstly be remembered that a number of organisms that may be found in semen are never the cause of a genital tract infection, even in the presence of pyospermia. The most common example of this phenomenon is the presence of skin commensals that can so commonly contaminate a semen sample produced by masturbation. However, a very large number of organisms have been described in semen in relation to a genital tract infection and the causation of infertility.

The bacterial infections

There are many different bacterial infections that can invade the male genital tract.

Gram-negative bacilli

The most of common group of organisms that are found in semen are *Escherichia coli* and other related Gram-negative bacilli. *E. coli* is often found in the semen of patients with urinary tract infection and thus the organism may relate to contamination of the semen by the small amounts of urine that are always present in the urethra.

However, *E. coli* also colonizes the prostate in men with chronic urinary tract infection and in this way it may become an infective agent within the semen itself.

E. coli may also cause infertility by inducing sperm agglutination and also by stimulating the production of sperm surface-specific IgA. The finding of agglutinated sperm in the semen of a patient with pyospermia would thus very strongly indicate the presence of an *E. coli* infection.

E. coli can also damage the surface of spermatozoa by means of the action of complement on the cell membrane. This damage may result in severe impairment of sperm function.

Enterococci

Organisms such as *Streptococcus faecalis* may also occasionally be found in semen in association with pyospermia. These organisms are however, frequently found as commensals within the anterior urethra. It must not be assumed that, even in the presence of pyospermia, that they are the causative organism of any infection in the genital tract nor are they necessarily the cause of any pyospermia that may be present. Thus, culture of this organism in semen is not necessarily diagnostic of the presence of infection within the genital tract.

Staphylococci

Pathogenic staphylococci are a very rare cause of genital tract infection. However, the skin commensal *Staphylococcus epidermidis* is frequently present on the skin and may also be found in the terminal portion of the penile urethra.

Again, it must not be assumed that because an organism is cultured from semen, its presence is diagnostic of genital tract infection nor that this organism is the cause of that infection.

Neisseria gonorrhoeae

For the most part, gonoccocal infection in men produces severe symptoms and obvious physical signs. For these reasons, it is an easy diagnosis to make clinically. Dysuria and penile urethral discharge are the rule in this disorder. It will thus only rarely be picked up during the routine evaluation of infertility and pyospermia.

As in other body fluids, these organisms are seen as Gram-negative intracellular diplococci. Despite its infrequent finding among infertile men, its presence should always be sought in a urethral swab and in the semen of men with pyospermia.

Mycobacterium tuberculosis

Tuberculosis is an uncommon finding among infertile men in the Western world (Ferrie & Rundle 1983) but is not infrequently found among infertile men from the developing countries.

In the male, tuberculosis may cause infertility by inducing obstructive lesions in various sites in the genital tract including the epididymal duct. Tuberculous seminal vesiculitis and tuberculous involvement of the prostate can also occur. The changes in the semen from such infection may be azoospermia, reduced seminal volume, haematospermia and also pyospermia.

Tuberculous infection of the genital tract is frequently associated with concomitant infection of the urinary tract and thus this problem may also present with haematuria as well as pyuria. Culture of the semen for *Mycobacterium tuberculosis humanis* should always be carried out in any patient who has pyuria alongside pyospermia.

Mycoplasma *and* Ureaplasma urealyticum

Both *Mycoplasma hominis* and *Ureaplasma urealyticum* will colonize the male genital tract and thus can be cultured in semen samples. However, there is considerable doubt as to whether these organisms actually cause lesions in the genital tract that will result in infertility. There is some evidence in the literature that the treatment of patients with these organisms in their

259

semen with appropriate antibiotic therapy will improve sperm motility and may thus enhance fertility.

Chlamydia trachomatis

Chlamydia trachomatis may also be found in semen and is becoming an increasingly common cause of epididymo-orchitis in young men (Grant *et al.* 1987). Such infections frequently result in obstructive azoospermia. This organism is often as difficult to detect as it is very resistant to culture.

However recent use of the polymerase chain reaction (PCR) in the detection of this organism has aided diagnosis considerably. It must also be remembered that chlamydial infection can be present in the semen of an otherwise asymptomatic patient, although it will nevertheless cause significant changes to the semen analysis (Weidner *et al.* 1996). The presence of this organism in the genital tract may even induce the presence of anti-sperm antibodies (Eggert-Kruse *et al.* 1996).

Trichomonas vaginalis

This protozoon can be found colonizing the anterior urethra and may even be found within the prostate. It can thus be detected in a sample of semen. *Trichomonas* does not seem ever to be a cause of either pyospermia or infertility in the male although there is some evidence that its presence in semen may cause a minor reduction in sperm motility.

Candida albicans

Candida albicans may also be found in semen. It usually only colonizes the area around the foreskin and as a consequence can often be detected in smegma. When it is found in semen, it is usually simply a contaminant but it can rarely cause infertility in the male. However, in patients with an immune deficiency, *Candida* can cause an epididymitis (Docimo *et al.* 1993).

Viral infections

Viruses can also invade the male genital tract and can at times cause infertility.

HIV

Many viruses can be found in semen, the best known of which is the human immunodeficiency virus (HIV). Although HIV probably does not *per se* cause infertility, its presence in semen must always be suspected by all laboratory personnel involved in semen analysis. Appropriate protection from potential infection of laboratory staff by this virus must be used at all times.

Hepatitis B and C

The hepatitis viruses may also be present in semen and, like HIV, are very rarely themselves a cause of infertility. However, hepatitis B infection has been described as a cause of orchitis (Molitor & Warrens 1985).

Cytomegalovirus

This virus has also been identified as a cause of infection in the male genital tract but appears only to have a minor effect on fertility. This virus can, however, be found in the semen from sperm donors (Mansat *et al.* 1997) and this may cause problems in the subsequent pregnancies among the women receiving such semen as part of a donor insemination programme.

Variola

Variola, the smallpox virus, has now disappeared but has been a well-known cause of lesions of the epididymal duct and a cause of obstructive azoospermia in the past (Phadke 1973). The worldwide eradication of this infection has made this disorder of historical interest only.

Genital herpes

This virus can frequently be isolated from seminal fluid (De Ture *et al.* 1976) and although it is clear that the male genital tract can be a reservoir of this infection and it can also cause urethral and penile ulcers, there is little evidence that it has any deleterious effect on testicular or epididymal function.

Human papillomavirus (HPV)

The human papillomavirus may also be identified in semen but has never been shown to be a cause of infertility in the male.

Other rare virus infections

Uncommon viral infections of the testis include the Coxsackie group (Freij *et al.* 1970) and infectious mononucleosis (Ralston *et al.* 1960), and even dengue fever. These infections can produce an orchitis but the true diagnosis is often overlooked due to the difficulties in identification of these organisms.

Other much rarer infections of the male genital tract

A number of other rare infections may involve the male genital tract. These include brucellosis (Afsar *et al.* 1993), leprosy (Pareek & Tandon 1985), syphilis (Persaud & Rao 1977), actinomycosis (Scorer 1952) and bilharzia (Mitry *et al.* 1986). More rare still are infections by filariae, cytomegalovirus (McCarthy *et al.* 1991) and coccidiomycosis organisms (Connor *et al.* 1975), but these infections occur mostly among immunocompromised patients.

These are all very uncommonly seen in the Western world and all present as chronic granulomata of the testes and/or the epididymis.

Other noninfective causes of epididymo-orchitis

Inflammatory changes in the epididymis or the testis may also very occasionally be caused by infiltration by sarcoidosis (Winnaker *et al.* 1967). In a small number of patients with Behçet's disease, the epididymis may also be involved (Kirkali *et al.* 1991).

The methods of culture of organisms in semen

The culture of the organisms that may be found in semen can be difficult. Firstly semen has a high pH (7–8) which does not provide optimal culture conditions for most organisms. Semen also contains large amounts of lysozymes and zinc, both of which are powerfully bacteriostatic.

Semen that is sent for culture must be fresh as bacteria quickly die in semen containing these antibacterial substances. Thus, the rapid application of the semen to the various culture media will yield a higher rate of positive cultures that will occur from older samples.

The first step in the microbiological examination of a sample of semen is to make a smear and perform a Gram stain. The presence of a predominant type of organism may aid decisions concerning the methods of culture of the semen sample. Such stains may also detect the presence of contaminants such as *Candida albicans*.

In general, the methods used for the culture of seminal fluid are simple and four main media only are used (Table 14.1).

Blood agar

Blood agar inoculated with neat semen will be sufficient to identify most organisms that may be present in seminal fluid. These organisms include the Gram-negative bacilli such as *E. coli*, the enterococci and the staphylococci. If the blood agar is cultured in both air and in carbon dioxide enriched air, then *Neisseria gonorrhoeae* will also be identified.

Table 14.1 A summary of the media that are commonly used in the microbiological examination of semen together with some of the most common organisms that they will identify

Medium	Organisms cultured
Blood agar	Gram-negative bacilli, enterococci, staphylococci
New York City medium	*Neisseria gonorrhoeae*
CLED medium	Many of the gut organisms including the enterococci
Monolayer tissue culture	*Chlamydia*
PCR	*Chlamydia*, viruses

New York City medium

This medium, when inoculated in carbon dioxide-enriched air, is a good culture medium for the identification of *Neisseria gonorrhoeae*. If this infection is suspected from the presence of Gram-negative intracellular diplococci on the smear, this is the medium of choice for use in the culture of the semen sample.

Cystine–lactose–electrolyte-deficient medium (CLED)

This is a particularly good medium for the identification of *E. coli* and many other gut organisms. It is also an excellent medium for the culture of the lactose-fermenting bacteria such as the enterococci.

Monolayer tissue culture

Some organisms such as *Chlamydia* require tissue culture for the identification. The use of simple tissue monolayer cultures makes this a simple and accurate way to identify the chlamydial organisms. However, *Chlamydia* is now also more easily identified using a variety of immunoassay techniques, and even PCR technology is now in standard use for this purpose

Infections of the male genital tract

Infections of the male genital tract remain a common cause of infertility and it is important to have an understanding of their presentation and the nature of the damage that these infections can induce particularly on the excurrent duct system of the testes.

Acute bacterial orchitis and epididymo-orchitis

Orchitis is an infection of the testis that frequently involves the epididymis. The inflammation that occurs in the testis will result in oedema, and as the seminiferous tubules are enclosed within the poorly distensible tunica albuginea this oedema will result in ischaemia of the testis and loss of spermatogenic function even when the condition is unilateral (Osegbe 1991). Similarly, a primary inflammation of the epididymis will also often result in the involvement of the testis producing the condition of epididymo-orchitis

Acute bacterial epididymo-orchitis presents as a rapidly increasing painful swelling of the testis and epididymis. It is also often occurs bilaterally and results in marked swelling, particularly of the epididymis. A secondary hydrocele also soon forms, thus making the swelling even more obvious. There is also often a tenderness of the prostate on rectal examination.

Making the diagnosis

The most important differential diagnosis of epididymo-orchitis is testicular torsion. Doppler ultrasonography can be helpful diagnostically (Stage *et al.* 1981) but often the scrotum is so tender that this investigation is difficult to carry out. Similarly, technetium scanning can also help diagnostically, but it may take too long to set up this investigation and in a country hospital such an investigation may not be available. If there is any doubt about the diagnosis, then surgical exploration is indicated.

The causative organism can be identified from culture of a urine sample or a urethral swab but a more accurate diagnosis is made from an aspirate of the epididymis.

Treatment

The treatment of this condition must be immediate as delay will increase the chances of abcess formation. The treatment of a bacterial epididymo-orchitis is bed rest and systemic antibiotic therapy and very adequate analgesia, the latter being very important, as this is an extremely painful condition for the patient. Scrotal support is also helpful.

The antibiotic used will depend upon the nature of the infection. Gonococcal epididymo-orchitis is best treated with intramuscular ceftriaxone followed by a course of doxycycline (Berger 1994), while the therapy of choice for a chlamydial infection is vibramycin at a dose of 100 mg 12-hourly after an initial dose of 200 mg. Many of the gut organisms will also respond well to ceftriaxone. However, therapy of this condition must be prolonged and continued treatment as an outpatient is essential using oral antibiotics such a amoxicillin or ciprofloxacin.

Complications

Despite treatment the complications of a bacterial epididymo-orchitis may be serious. An epididymal or testicular abscess can sometimes form which will present as a fluctuant swelling that will require drainage. Damage to the epididymal duct is almost the rule in patients with a severe epididymo-orchitis and this can frequently give rise to obstructive azoospermia. The ischaemia that results from the testicular swelling will also damage sperm production and may even result in atrophic testes with damage to Leydig cell function as well as to sperm production.

Viral orchitis

Mumps orchitis is the most common viral infection of the male genital tract. It never occurs prior to puberty but after puberty may complicate an attack of mumps parotitis. The orchitis usually appears a few days after the onset of the parotitis and is bilateral in around 25% of these patients. The formation of a hydrocele is also a common phenomenon around the inflamed testes. Again, the ischaemia that is induced by the inflammation results in damage to sperm production in more than 50% of men with this condition. Thus, particularly if the orchitis is bilateral, infertility is a very common complication.

In the past, attempts were made to reduce intratesticular tension by surgically incising the tunica albuginea during the phase of acute orchitis. This did not, however, greatly help the late effects of mumps orchitis as the ischaemia was usually already well established prior to hospital admission and before such surgery could be carried out.

Again it must be remembered that testicular torsion can occur in relation even to mumps, and thus the diagnosis of mumps orchitis should never be assumed. If there is any doubt about the diagnosis, then surgical exploration is indicated.

There is little treatment to offer patients with mumps orchitis apart from symptomatic relief of the extreme discomfort of the problem. Incision of the tunica albuginea will relieve the pain caused by the tension within the testis but there is little evidence that this procedure will improve the prognosis for future fertility.

Chronic orchitis and epididymitis

There are a number of different causes of chronic orchitis and epididymitis.

Chronic bacterial epididymitis

Unfortunately, a severe attack of acute epididymitis can lead to the development of a relapsing chronic lesion and may continue to recur even after vasectomy. The epididymis shows chronic inflammatory changes that may eventually result in the formation of epididymal abscesses.

The treatment of this condition usually involves the prolonged use of antibiotics, but in men with abscess formation epididymectomy may have to be carried out. Epididymectomy is a difficult procedure, especially where there has been extensive inflammation. It is therefore important to identify and preserve the testicular artery, which lies behind the epididymis, during such surgery as damage to the artery at this site will itself result in testicular atrophy.

Sperm granulomata of the epididymis

These granulomatous lesions are not the result of infection but are one of the most common chronic lesions of the epididymis. They are usually the result of vasectomy where in time the epididymal duct becomes distended with sperm and the wall eventually ruptures in a condition often familiarly known as postvasectomy 'blow-outs' (Silber 1978). These lesions do not usually cause any symptoms but can occasionally cause pain.

Tuberculous epididymitis and orchitis

This disorder can occasionally have an acute onset but for the most part this is a chronic condition. It affects the epididymis but can also preferentially involve the distal portion of the vas deferens and in particular the epididymis. Very rarely, the prostate may also be involved. Caseating lesions of the testis can also occur and these lesions may necessitate orchidectomy.

The diagnosis is made by finding the presence of calcification in and around the vas and seminal vesicles. The epididymis feels hard and irregular and may also show evidence of calcification on X-ray or ultrasound.

This type of infection severely damages the structures that it involves and obstructive azoospermia is the major cause of infertility in these men. These lesions are never amenable to any form of remedial surgery.

Tuberculous infection of the genital tract is commonly associated with infection in the renal tract, and its presence must be sought in all infertile men with these lesions. Thus, an intravenous pyelogram is an important investigation in any patient with a tuberculous infection of the genital tract.

Syphilis

Gumma of the testis was at one time a common problem but is very rarely seen today. It will present as a mass which clinically is difficult to distinguish from a tumour (Persaud & Rao 1977). The best treatment of this lesion is orchidectomy.

Bilharzial epididymitis and orchitis

This chronic granulomatous lesion is caused by infection with *Schistosoma* and may be most commonly found in Africa and Arabia. Damage to the testis may occur because of vascular obstruction. The mass is firm and is difficult to distinguish from a tumour (Mitry *et al.* 1986). Frequently, both the epididymis and the testis are involved. The best treatment is epididymectomy but if the testis is involved then orchidectomy is best carried out.

Brucellosis

Infection of the male genital tract with this organism is very rare but, when it occurs, it produces a mass in the testis, which, like many other of the chronic infections, is indistinguishable from a tumour. This infection is thus usually only identified after orchidectomy and may be confirmed immunologically.

Actinomycosis

This fungal infection affects the testis and forms a lesion containing many sinuses leading towards the central infective mass (Scorer 1952). The treatment is orchidectomy under tetracycline cover.

Infective disorders of the vas deferens

The vas deferens can also be involved in a number of genital tract infections.

Neisseria *infection*

Severe gonoccocal infection can cause multiple strictures in the vas as well as lesions in the epididymis. Thus, in any attempt to carry out remedial surgery on an epididymal obstruction caused by this type of infection, a vasogram to exclude other obstructive lesions in either vas is very important.

Tuberculous lesions of the vas deferens

Tuberculous infection can also cause multiple strictures of the vas. Many of these lesions are associated with caseation and thus calcification is a common accompaniment of this type of infection. This calcification can easily be identified on either a pelvic X-ray or on transrectal ultrasound.

Vasitis nodosa

This is an inflammatory rather than an infective condition of the vas that occurs after a vasectomy. These lesions are the result of the extraluminal extension of the epithelium of the vas extending out into the surrounding connective tissues together with the presence of a sperm granuloma. They can even produce lesions on the skin of the scrotum (Balogh & Argenyi

1985) and such lesions may become secondarily infected. Vasitis nodosa is, however, a rare complication of vasectomy.

Infective disorders of the seminal vesicles

The seminal vesicles may also be the site of infection. Untreated infection, especially that due to *Neisseria gonorrhoeae*, can cause infection of the seminal vesicles. However, the ease with which this infection responds to treatment makes seminal vesiculitis caused by this organism a rarity today.

Another infective agent that tends to involve the seminal vesicles is tuberculosis. This latter agent will produce severe damage to the seminal vesicles, which on X-ray may show the presence of obvious calcification. Nonspecific infection of the seminal vesicles may also occur and can be related to obstruction of the duct of the seminal vesicles causing retention of their secretions.

Occasionally, obstruction can also be brought about by the presence of stones in the duct of the seminal vesicles (Hendry *et al.* 1990). Stones are in fact quite common in the seminal vesicles but rarely cause any symptoms unless they induce obstruction in the ducts of the seminal vesicles.

If an infection in the seminal vesicles is allowed to go untreated, then abscess formation may occur, but this is an uncommon phenomenon today.

In men with infection, both the volume and the constituents of the seminal vesicular secretions will be altered. As the seminal vesicular secretions make up around 60% of the total ejaculatory volume, the seminal volume may become considerably reduced. The fructose content will also be decreased and this will result in asthenozoospermia. If the ejaculatory ducts are also involved in the infective process and this is a common accompaniment of this problem, then the semen volume will be low and the seminal fluid sample will be azoospermic.

Prostatitis

Infection of the prostate can be acute or chronic and may occasionally present in an infertility clinic.

Acute prostatitis

This condition commonly presents with perineal pain and because of the swollen prostate gland some difficulty in micturition may also be present. In men with a severe infection, rigors may occur. Severe prostatitis is also commonly associated with an acute epididymitis and this combination will give the patient a great deal of pain and will make him very ill indeed.

Rectal examination will reveal the presence of a very tender and somewhat tense prostate. The causative organism can almost always be identified from the microbiological examination of a urine sample and this condition needs prompt and effective antibiotic therapy as septicaemia is a complication of this condition. Treatment consists of ciprofloxacin intra-venously and this can be changed to oral therapy after 48 h. On recovery, antibiotic therapy should be continued for at least a further 6 weeks.

Delay in treatment may result in a prostatic abscess and this is best treated by drainage transurethrally. Acute prostatitis is unlikely to be seen in men attending an infertility clinic but may occur among men with recurrent urinary problems such as patients with spinal cord injury. It is, however, important that the gynaecologists involved in the treatment of infertility in men who are at risk from prostatitis are aware of its symptomatology even though they would not of course be expected to treat this problem.

Chronic prostatitis

Patients with this problem may present with recurrent urinary tract infection. The patient may also complain of perineal pain or even some pain on ejaculation. In an infertility clinic, this condition may also present as pyospermia. However, on rectal examination, the prostate gland frequently feels normal and tenderness may be minimal. Transrectal ultrasonography is not helpful diagnostically and the best way to make the diagnosis of chronic prostatitis is by identifying the causative organism.

However, it is more difficult to isolate the causative organism in this condition than is the case in acute prostatic infection. The best means of carrying this out in men with chronic prostatitis is by the examination of the urine but this time this examination follows a prostatic massage. The patient cleans the penis and the external urethral meatus with sterile water and passes the few millilitres of urine into a sterile container. A small midstream sample is then collected in a second container. The clinician then carries out a rectal examination and performs a prostatic massage. The prostatic secretions that appear at the urethral meatus are collected in a third container. A further few millilitres of urine are then passed into a fourth container. All four containers are now sent for microbiological examination.

The prostatic massage can itself be therapeutic as it often resolves or improves the symptoms of this condition.

The treatment will depend upon the nature of the causative organism but the most commonly used antibiotics include ciprofloxacin or trimethoprim (Berger 1994). Therapy must be prolonged and is best continued for 4–6 weeks. It must be remembered that, even in men with chronic prostatitis, abscess formation can occasionally occur.

Tuberculous infection of the prostate

This is a rare condition that is very uncommonly seen in the Western world. The tuberculous infection forms a granuloma in the prostate that can clearly be identified on transrectal ultrasonography. The diagnosis can be confirmed by biopsy. The treatment of this condition is medical and this granuloma will resolve after effective antituberculous therapy.

Occasionally, however, the caseating mass may discharge posteriorly into the rectum resulting in a fistula (Teklu & Ibrahim 1990).

Brucellosis of the prostate

Like tuberculosis, this is a very rare condition that also forms a granuloma within the prostate (Aygen *et al.* 1998). On occasions it may even lead to abscess formation. Like tuberculosis, its presence induces calcification within the area of the granuloma. It is also best treated by antibiotic therapy.

Urethritis

Urethritis is the most common infective disorder of the male genital tract and there are several different causes of this disorder.

Chlamydia trachomatis *urethritis*

This can cause distressing symptoms that include both pain on micturition and urethral discharge. If it goes untreated, it can result in an epididymitis that can have serious consequences in relation to the patient's fertility. This disorder can also result in the infection of the patient's female sexual partner and induce salpingitis, with equally serious affects on .fertility.

Chlamydial urethritis is best diagnosed using an endourethral swab for culture of *Chlamydia* and a smear should be taken for a Gram stain. Treatment of this condition is antibiotic therapy and consists of doxycycline 500 mg twice daily for 7 days. The patient's sexual partner should also be treated in the same way.

Gonococcal urethritis

Infection by *Neisseria gonorrhoeae* results in severe urethritis in the male together with an obvious purulent urethral discharge. It is again diagnosed on culture of an endourethral swab and by the presence of Gram-negative intracellular diplococci in a Gram-stained smear. It commonly coexists with a chlamydial infection. It is best treated using ceftriaxone 250 mg intramuscularly and doxycycline orally twice daily for 7 days (Berger 1994). The doxycycline is added to overcome any concomitant chlamydial infection. As with chlamydial infection, the patient's sexual partner should also be treated concurrently as chlamydial infection can cause salpingitis, which also has an equally deleterious effect upon fertility.

This is a difficult problem to treat but may frequently be the result of undiagnosed or recurrent chlamydial infection. Erythromycin 500 mg four times per day for 3 weeks is recommended for the treatment of this problem.

Penile infective problems

There are a number of different infections of the penis that, although they do not cause infertility, should be considered in this section so that they can be recognized in an infertile male patient.

Herpes simplex type II

This viral infection causes acute pustular lesions on the penis that are commonly recurrent. These lesions finally ulcerate and become infective. Acyclovir ointment limits the duration of the symptoms. In more severe cases, oral acyclovir in doses of 200 mg five times per day may be more effective than topical therapy.

Candidiasis

This infection occurs commonly under the foreskin and is seen most frequently in diabetics. It is best treated by local fungicides but if recurrence is a problem then circumcision may be indicated.

Syphilis

This is now a rare cause of penile infection in the heterosexual patient. The chancre of primary syphilis appears as a papule, which then forms an ulcer with the characteristic undermined edges. A swab taken from this ulcer will demonstrate the presence of *Treponema pallidum*. Serological testing at this early stage is often negative.

Chancroid

This lesion is caused by the bacterium *Haemophilus ducreyi* and results in ulceration of the penis and prepuce. These ulcers often become secondarily infected and obvious enlargement of the local lymph nodes is seen. These ulcers can frequently be mistaken for the primary chancres of syphilis.

The organism can usually be identified from the exudate within the ulcer and their best treatment is by antibiotic therapy. The antibiotics of choice in the treatment of this condition include tetracycline 500 mg four times per day for 3 weeks or erythromycin 500 mg four times per day also for 3 weeks. It is also important to treat the patient's sexual partners.

Acute balanitis

This is a simple bacterial infection occurring in uncircumcised men with poorly retractile foreskin. In diabetics, however, this can result in a severe cellulitis. Treatment is simple cleansing and antibiotic therapy appropriate to the infective organism, but in severe infections that produce marked oedema then drainage of the preputial space may be required. Circumcision is indicated at a later date. However, if the infection is intractable then it may be necessary to carry this out even in the presence of an acute infection.

Lymphogranuloma venereum

This disorder is caused by the presence of *Chlamydia trachomatis* and is associated with ulceration of the penis and a gross lymphadenopathy of the draining lymph nodes. It is a rare disease in the Western world but is common in the tropics. It is best treated by tetracycline or erythromycin in doses of 500 mg four times per day for at least 3 weeks.

Lymphogranuloma inguinale

This is another disease seen usually only in the tropics. It results in the presence of shallow painful ulcers that are filled with mononuclear cells that contain the organism *Donovania granulomatis*. The diagnosis is easily made by examining a Gram-stained smear taken from these ulcers. They respond well to treatment with one of the tetracyclines.

References

Afsar, H., Baydar, I. & Sirmatel, F. (1993) Epididymo-orchitis due to brucellosis. *British Journal of Urology* **72**, 103–105.

Aygen, B., Sumerkan, B., Doganay, M. & Sehmen, E. (1998) Prostatitis and hepatitis due to Brucella mellitensis: a case report. *Journal of Infection* **36**, 111–112.

Balogh, K. & Argenyi, Z.B. (1985) Vasitis nodosa and spermatic granuloma of the skin; an histologic study of a rare complication of vasectomy. *Journal of Cutaneous Pathology* **12**, 528–533.

Berger, R.E. (1994) Infection of the male reproductive tract. *Current Therapy in Endocrinology and Metabolism* **5**, 305–309.

Connor, W.T., Drach, G.W. & Bucher, W.C. (1975) Genitourinary aspects of disseminated coccidiomycosis. *Urology* **113**, 82–88.

De Ture, F.A., Drylie, D.M., Kaufman, H.E. & Centifanto, Y.N. (1976) Herpesvirus type 2: isolation from seminal vesicles and testes. *Urology* **1**, 541–544.

Docimo, S.G., Rukstalis, D.B., Rukstalis, M.R., Kang, J., Cotton, D. & DeWolf, W.C. (1993) Candida epididymitis: a newly recognized opportunistic epididymal infection. *Urology* **41**, 280–282.

Eggert-Kruse, W., Buhlinger-Gopfarth, N., Rohr, G. *et al.* (1996) Antibodies to *Chlamydia trachomatis* in semen and relationship with parameters of male infertility. *Human Reproduction* **11**, 1408–1417.

Ferrie, B.G. & Rundle, J.S.H. (1983) Tuberculous epididymo-orchitis. A review of 20 cases. *British Journal of Urology* **55**, 437–439.

Freij, L., Norriby, R. & Olsson, B. (1970) A small outbreak of Coxsackie B5 infection with two cases of cardiac involvement and orchitis followed by testicular atrophy. *Acta Medica Scandinavica* **187**, 177–181.

Grant, J.B.F., Costello, C.B., Sequiera, P.J.L. & Blacklock, N.J. (1987) The role of *Chlamydia trachomatis* in epididymitis. *British Journal of Urology* **60**, 355–359.

Hendry, W.F., Levison, D.A., Parkinson, M.C., Parslow, J.M. & Royle, M.G. (1990) Testicular obstruction: clinico-pathological studies. *Annals of the Royal College of Surgeons of England* **72**, 396–407.

Kirkali, Z., Yigitbasi, O. & Sasmaz, R. (1991) Urological aspects of Behçet's disease. *British Journal of Urology* **67**, 638–639.

Mansat, A., Mengelle, C., Chalet, M. *et al.* (1997) Cytomegalovirus detection in cryopreserved semen samples collected for therapeutic donor insemination. *Human Reproduction* **12**, 1663–1666.

McCarthy, J.M., McLoughlin, M.G., Shackleton, C.R. *et al.* (1991) Cytomegalovirus epididymitis following renal transplantation. *Journal of Urology* **146**, 417–419.

Mitry, N.F., Satti, M.B., Tamini, D.M. & Metawaa, B. (1986) Testicular schistosomiasis. *British Journal of Urology* **58**, 721–727.

Molitor, P.J.A. & Warrens, A.N. (1985) Acute orchitis associated with hepatitis B infection. *British Medical Journal* **291**, 940. (unrefereed report)

Osegbe, D.N. (1991) Testicular function after unilateral epididymo-orchitis. *European Urology* **19**, 204–204.

Pareek, S.S. & Tandon, R.C. (1985) Epididymal lesion in leprosy. *British Medical Journal* **291**, 313.

Persaud, V. & Rao, A. (1977) Gumma of the testis. *British Journal of Urology* **49**, 142.

Phadke, A.M. (1973) Smallpox as an aetiologic factor in male infertility. *Fertility and Sterility* **24**, 802–804.

Ralston, L.S., Saiki, A.K. & Powers, W.T. (1960) Orchitis as a complication of infectious mononucleosis. *Journal of the American Medical Association* **173**, 1348–1349.

Scorer, C.G. (1952) Actinomycosis of the testis. *British Journal of Surgery* **40**, 244–247.

Silber, S.J. (1978) Epididymal extravasation following vasectomy as a cause of failure of vasectomy reversal. *Fertility and Sterility* **31**, 309–315.

Stage, K.H., Schoenvogel, R. & Lewis, S. (1981) Testicular scanning: clinical experience with 72 patients. *Journal of Urology* **125**, 334–337.

Teklu, B. & Ibrahim, A. (1990) Tuberculosis of prostate. *Saudi Medical Journal* **11**, 74–75.

Weidner, W., Floren, E., Zimmermann, O., Thiele, D. & Ludwig, M. (1996) Chlamydial antibodies in semen search for 'silent' chlamydial infections in asymptomatic andrological patients. *Infection* **24**, 309–313.

Winnaker, J.L., Becker, K.L., Katz, S. & Matthews, M.J. (1967) Recurrent epididymitis in sarcoidosis: report of a patient treated with corticosteroids. *Annals of Internal Medicine* **66**, 743–748.

15: Infertility and the Presence of Antisperm Antibodies

It has been known for many years that spermatozoa can induce the formation of antibodies not only between species but within one species and more particularly within an individual. Indeed nearly 100 years ago, both Metchnikoff and Metalnikoff demonstrated the antigenicity of sperm from both experimental animals and from humans.

However, it was not until 1954 that both Rumpke and Wilson (Rumpke 1954; Wilson 1954) each separately reported that the formation of antisperm antibodies could be a cause of infertility in the male. These two workers reported the presence of sperm-agglutinating and sperm-immobilizing antibodies in the sera of a small number of men with infertility.

It was also shown that these patients with antisperm antibodies in their serum demonstrated the occurrence of spontaneous agglutination of the spermatozoa in their semen. It is thought that the antibody holds different parts of the sperm together and so induces agglutination (Fig. 15.1). That sperm autoimmunity is a cause of infertility is now well established, as the presence of sperm autoimmunity can be demonstrated in some 5–10% of infertile couples (Clarke *et al.* 1985).

Antisperm antibodies can also be present in the serum of infertile women and thus may also be present in cervical mucus. Their presence in cervical mucus can induce a further means by which penetration of this mucus by the sperm can be impaired.

Immunity to sperm may thus be an important cause of infertility and is a subject that is vital to the proper evaluation of childlessness in an infertile couple. Although sperm autoimmunity as the sole cause of infertility in a couple is relatively uncommon, the detection of antisperm antibodies in serum but more particularly in semen is an essential part of a semen analysis.

The antigens on sperm and the induction of antisperm antibodies

The production of spermatozoa begins at puberty long after the maturation of the immune system has been completed. The testis, however, is an immunologically privileged site that is protected from access by both lymphocytes and macrophages. Thus, under normal circumstances, the male genital tract does not allow the generation of specific antibodies against spermatozoa. Likewise, the very entry of sperm into the female genital tract

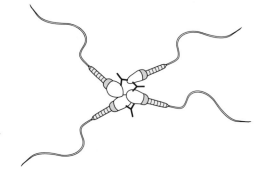

Fig. 15.1 A diagrammatic representation of the way in which sperm, in this case the sperm heads are held together by antisperm antibodies in the semen.

also only rarely induces the presence of antisperm antibodies even though the cervix and the uterus are fully immunocompetent.

Why sperm, for the most part, fail to elicit an immune response even in the female genital tract is a difficult question to answer. It has however, been reported that T-suppressor lymphocytes are present both in the upper epididymal region and also in semen and these cells may provide the semen, and indeed the sperm with an immunosuppressive mechanism that impedes the production of antisperm antibodies (El-Demiry & James 1988). This does not, however, explain the apparent lack of any immune response to sperm that occurs in the female even after many years of coitus with the same partner.

The source of antigen for any immune response to sperm lies on their surface. These antigens are largely glycoproteins and crossreactivity may occur between these antigens and the antibodies that they may induce. Thus, the presence of individual antigens on different areas of the sperm surface cannot be inferred from simple binding studies. Likewise, some antisperm antibodies can cross react with other tissues and even with some bacteria.

Antisperm antibodies are formed by two major immunoglobulins: namely the IgA and IgG subgroups. Secretory IgA is present in many secretions such as saliva and mucus and in the many genital tract secretions from the prostate, the seminal vesicles and bulbourethral and the urethral glands. It is also clear that even the epididymis may be capable of local IgA secretion as antibody production by the epididymis has been shown to be increased after vasectomy.

Secretory IgA is generated by plasma cells and is complexed with a protein known as the secretory component to form an IgA–secretory component complex. This complex is then transported locally into and across the epithelial cell to be then released into the secretions of that cell.

This mechanism is of course of value in the protection of the genital tract from infection. In situations where infection can occur, the organ involved increases its secretion of IgA. In, for example, men with prostatitis caused by an *Escherichia coli* infection, prostatic production of IgA is greatly increased and this IgA is also anti-*E. coli* specific. However, this IgA production can also be generated against the various antigens on the surface of spermatozoa. As IgA is generated locally, its titre in semen will be much higher than that in serum and indeed there is in practice little correlation between the levels of sperm-specific IgA in serum and semen. Thus, it must be remembered that even the total absence of antisperm antibodies of the IgA subgroup in serum does not exclude the presence of high titres in semen that are highly relevant clinically.

The second type of immunoglobulin that may be involved in the generation of antisperm antibodies is the IgG subgroup. IgG is derived from serum and appears in semen as a transudate from serum. As this group of antisperm antibodies arises from serum, the titres in serum will correlate much more closely with those in the semen.

The third type of immunoglobulin that may present as antisperm antibodies is the IgM subgroup. This subgroup is much less commonly seen than either IgA or IgG in this context, but nevertheless such antibodies may occur in relation to immunological infertility. As this type of antibody is also derived from serum, the titre of IgM seen in serum will correlate reasonably well with that in semen.

Thus, in order to establish the presence of antisperm antibodies of the IgG and the IgM subgroups it is sufficient to measure these titres in serum; but high levels of the IgA subgroup may well be present in semen without this being apparent in serum. It is therefore of much more value from the clinical standpoint to examine the antisperm antibody titre of all three immunoglobulin sperm-specific subgroups in semen rather than in serum.

Means by which antisperm antibodies may impair fertility

However, the manner in which this infertility is induced by these antibodies is less clear. There are a number of different ways in which antisperm antibodies can interfere with fertility.

Spontaneous agglutination of the sperm within the ejaculate

In some but not all patients the presence of antisperm antibodies may induce agglutination of the sperm within an ejaculate (Fig. 15.2). This agglutination may be tight and thus can prevent the passage of the sperm out of the ejaculate and into the cervical mucus. This contact between sperm can be tail-to-tail, or less frequently head-to-head, or even a mixture of the two. This type of agglutination makes the counting of the sperm very difficult and it may be impossible to assess the number of sperm in an ejaculate when this phenomenon is present. However, it must also be remembered that antisperm antibodies can be present in high titre in semen without there being any evidence of sperm agglutination.

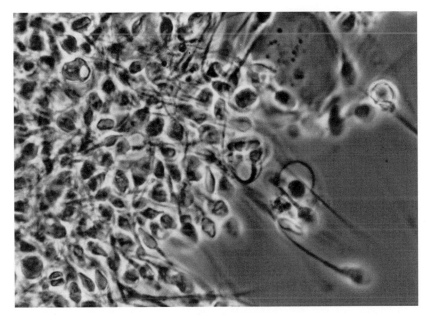

Fig. 15.2 A photomicrograph showing severely agglutinated sperm in the semen of a man known to have a high titre of antisperm antibodies in his semen.

When agglutination is present it is often recorded in a semen analysis in the following way:

+ = less than 1/3 of total spermatozoa involved in agglutination;

++ = 1/3–2/3 of total spermatozoa involved in agglutination;

+++ = 2/3 or more of total spermatozoa involved in agglutination.

Thus, a semen report on a semen analysis showing this problem may read: 'Agglutination ++, tail-to-tail'. The small numbers of sperm that may agglutinate to particulate matter and cellular debris is a normal finding and should be ignored.

Failure of penetration of the cervical mucus

There is now little doubt that the presence of antisperm antibodies in semen reduces the ability of the sperm to enter and to traverse the cervical mucus (Bronson *et al.* 1987). This appears to be caused by the activity of the Fc portion of the immunoglobulin that is coating the sperm and which impedes the passage of the sperm through the cervical mucus. The sperm may remain motile in the cervical mucus but may exhibit the 'shaking phenomenon' that is characteristic of the presence of antisperm antibodies on their surface (Kremer & Jager 1980). It is of interest that this effect can be removed by treating the sperm with a Fab preparation of IgG that enables the sperm to swim through cervical mucus without impediment. It is therefore suggested that human cervical mucus contains some form of receptor for the Fc portion of the immunoglobulin molecule.

Damage to the sperm surface by the induction of complement activity

It has been shown in the past that some antisperm antibodies have cytotoxic activity (Hamerlynck & Rumpke 1968) and thus their presence may, via the complement cascade, damage the surface membrane of the sperm and thus impair its function. However, it has been suggested that ejaculates containing antisperm antibodies may contain a higher proportion of acrosome-reacted sperm than those not containing antisperm antibody. The possible premature induction of the acrosome reaction by antisperm antibodies could thus also give rise to problems with binding of the sperm to the zona pellucida.

Interference with the binding of sperm to the zona pellucida

For penetration of the egg and the occurrence of fertilization, binding of the sperm to the zona pellucida must first take place. It is thus possible that coating of the sperm and particularly the head of the sperm by immunoglobulin could interfere with this phenomenon.

From experiments using sperm coated with and without antisperm antibody, it is clear that the presence of the immunoglobulin does indeed impair sperm binding to the zona pellucida (Mahoney *et al.* 1991). These immunoglobulins therefore interfere not only with natural conception, but also with fertilization within an IVF programme (Clarke *et al.* 1985). This problem may therefore be an important means by which antisperm antibodies induce infertility in the human.

Sperm–oocyte interaction in the presence of antisperm antibodies

An interesting experiment reported by Aitken and colleagues (Aitken *et al.* 1988) demonstrated that the addition of IgG from human sera containing sperm surface-specific antibody actually enhanced the penetration by sperm of the zona-free hamster egg. Thus it would appear that the presence of immunoglobulin on the surface of the sperm facilitated the adherence of the sperm to the oolema. However, this finding has certainly not been confirmed in humans, in whom the binding of sperm to the oolemma and its subsequent penetration are clearly reduced in the presence of antisperm antibodies (Liu *et al.* 1991).

Tests for the presence of antisperm antibodies

In the past it has been customary to use a number of different tests that indicate the nature and the activity of these antisperm antibodies. It was at one time deemed important to know whether the action of these antisperm antibodies was to immobilize sperm to act in a cytotoxic capacity or if they could induce sperm agglutination. However, today this differentiation of the antibodies is not considered necessary and thus only three methods of identifying and quantifying the presence of such antibodies are in common use at the present time. These three tests are outlined below.

The immunobead test (direct and indirect test)

Direct test

This is today by far the most common method of identifying the presence of antisperm antibodies and allows one to determine the subgroups of immunoglobulins involved in both semen and serum. For this test, the washed spermatozoa under test are incubated with freshly prepared latex beads (Biorad Laboratories Chemical Division, Richmond, CA, USA) that are coated with antibodies to one of the three immunoglobulin subgroups. When an immunoglobulin is present on the surface of the sperm, that sperm will bind to the bead by that part of the sperm that is coated with the specific immunoglogulin. These beads can be purchased commercially as a kit.

Spermatozoa are incubated in three separate tests using immunobeads that are coated with IgA, IgG or IgM. It is, however, also possible to purchase beads that are coated with all three immunoglobulin subgroups. In this way the presence or absence of antisperm antibodies of one or of all three of the subgroups of inmmunoglobulins can be identified, and to some extent quantified.

The number of motile sperm that are adherent to the beads indicate the presence of antisperm antibodies. Only motile or live sperm must be recorded as dead sperm may stick to these beads nonspecifically. From microscopy, it is also possible to determine whether the sperm are adhering to these beads by the head, by the midpiece or by the tail.

The results are expressed according to the percentage of motile sperm that are adherent to the beads. If more than 50% of the motile sperm are adherent to the beads, this is likely to have clinical significance in relation to a complaint of infertility. The World Health Organization (WHO 1992), however, has suggested that immunobead tests should be reported in the following manner:
< 20% = negative
20–49% = positive
> 50% = clinically significant.

Indirect test

It is possible to determine the presence of antisperm antibodies in serum or in any other body fluid using the indirect immunobead test. Spermatozoa that are known not to be coated with antisperm antibody are incubated with the fluid under test, e.g. a patient's serum. The sperm are then carefully washed and further incubated with the immunobeads after which the percentage of motile sperm that are bound to the beads is estimated as in the direct test.

The immunobead test is now the most commonly used test to detect the presence of antisperm antibodies. The direct test is used to determine the presence of these antibodies on the sperm themselves while the indirect test is employed to determine the presence of antisperm antibodies in any other body fluid, most particularly for their presence in serum. This test has the advantage that it is relatively cheap and is easy to perform.

The mixed antiglobulin reaction test (MAR)

This test was at one time very popular but its use has declined rapidly since the introduction of the immunobead test. This test also suffers from being a fairly complex reaction to carry out and is also expensive both in reagents and in the time taken to complete it.

The MAR test is based on the Coombs' reaction (Coombs *et al.* 1973), which is used in haematology to crossmatch blood, but which was applied to the detection of antisperm antibodies. This was further modified in 1978 (Jager *et al.* 1978) and was put into routine clinical practice in 1982 (Hendry *et al.* 1982a).

In this test, rhesus-positive red blood cells are first incubated with a suspension of anti-D followed by incubation with antibodies directed against the two immunoglobulins IgG or IgA that will adhere to their coating of anti-D. These treated red cells are then incubated with the sperm under test and if these sperm carry the antisperm antibody of either the IgA or the IgG immunoglobulin subgroup then they will adhere to these treated red cells (Fig. 15.3).

The test is reported as follows:

'0' = Negative – no motile mixed agglutinates, all sperm swimming freely, occasional nonmotile mixed agglutinates.

'1' = Positive – 10–90% of the motile sperm forming mixed agglutinates.

'2' = Strongly positive – 90–100% of the motile sperm are attached to red blood cells, very few freely motile sperm.

This test is probably clinically relevant when more that 50% of the motile sperm are adherent to the red blood cells.

This test has the advantage that the red blood cells can be prepared well in advance of the test and can be stored for 1 month. It also indicates the presence of the clinical relevant antisperm antibodies of the IgA and IgG classes and can also be carried out indirectly by incubating normal sperm with the serum or the semen of azoospermic men. It has the disadvantage that, in comparison with the immunobead test, it is long winded and tedious to carry out and the reagents that are needed such as anti-D and the anti-immunoglobulin preparations are expensive. Although this test continues to be used in some laboratories, it has now largely been abandoned.

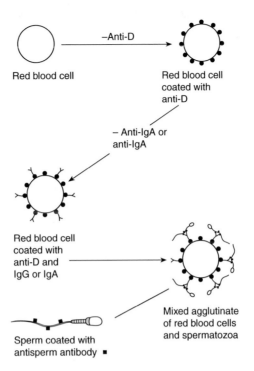

Fig. 15.3 A diagram of the MAR test.

The enzyme-linked immunosorbent assay (ELISA)

An ELISA for antisperm antibodies, as well as small numbers of radio-immunoassays, has been devised to identify the presence of antisperm antibodies both on the surface of semen and in the semen and in other body fluids such as serum. Indeed, a number of kits are now commercially available for these purposes. However, these kits tend to be relatively expensive and their ability to withstand shipment and storage may make them unreliable. This method of detecting antisperm antibodies has not been adopted by many laboratories.

Clinical conditions that induce the formation of antisperm antibodies

It has been known for many years that it is easy to induce the formation of antisperm antibodies by the immunization of laboratory animals with either sperm or with testicular homogenates. Such immunization experiments can not only result in the production of antisperm antibodies but may also give rise to an immune orchitis with total loss of sperm production. Indeed, the injection of sperm intramuscularly has even been carried out in the human with the consequent production of antisperm antibodies (Mancini *et al.* 1965).

It would appear therefore that the placement of spermatozoa outside the genital tract could itself induce the generation of antibodies against such sperm. Thus, injury to the testis or to the genital tract would appear to be an important manner in which sperm antibodies can be generated.

Likewise, damage to the testis and loss of the blood–testis barrier can also be an important cause of antisperm antibody formation. Such damage to the blood–testis barrier may even be induced by an obstructive lesion of the excurrent ducts of the testis such as vasectomy, so losing the testis its privileged immunological status.

Vasectomy and vasectomy reversal

Probably the most common cause of antisperm antibodies among the infertile male population is the operation of vasectomy. Vasectomy-related infertility is now a common cause of infertility and may make up as much as 10% of all the infertile male patients attending an infertility clinic (Jequier 1998). Antisperm antibodies may be found in 75% of such patients. Such antibodies may persist even after an apparently successful vasectomy reversal and thus their presence may jeopardize the pregnancy rate. The incidence of antisperm antibodies after vasectomy reversal may be as high as 50%.

Obstructive lesions of the excurrent ducts

Obstructive lesions may also result in the generation of antisperm antibodies, but their incidence in this type of pathological obstruction is not as high as that seen after vasectomy. This may relate to the fact that, in pathological obstruction, there is only infrequently a breach in the integrity of the lumen of the genital tract that of course always occurs at vasectomy. Interestingly, the incidence of antisperm antibodies in men with congenital absence of the vas is low (Patrizio *et al.* 1989), probably for the same reason. However, the presence of antisperm antibodies in serum can be induced by repeated epididymal sperm aspiration in men with congenital absence of the vas (Jequier, unpublished). It is also of interest that antisperm antibody formation is a particular feature of unilateral obstruction of the genital tract (Hendry *et al.* 1982b).

Testicular trauma, testicular torsion and testicular biopsy

Damage or injury to the testis can result in the induction of antisperm antibodies both in serum and in the semen. This is likely to be a result of ischaemic damage to the testis that will compromise the integrity of the blood–testis barrier. Measurement of antisperm antibodies should be carried out on all patients who give a history of testicular injury or torsion.

The role of testicular biopsy in the induction of antisperm antibodies is more controversial. Some authors report that testicular biopsy will indeed induce the formation of antisperm antibodies while others refute this. With the now clear evidence of testicular damage and haematoma formation that can occur after testicular biopsy (Schlegel & Su 1997), and the fact that even minor ischaemic change to the experimental testis may result in serious damage to spermatogenesis (Markey *et al.* 1994), it must now be conceded that testicular biopsy is indeed a cause of antisperm antibody formation.

Genital tract infection

Antisperm antibody formation can also be induced by infection in particular by infection with *Chlamydia* (Soffer *et al.* 1990). Prostatitis has long been known to be associated with the presence of antibodies and this may be a mechanism in the causation of infertility in the older patient. Antisperm antibodies can also be caused by viral infections, such as mumps, that may cause serious and permanent damage to the seminiferous tubules and the spermatogenic epithelium.

Other possibilities

As has been indicated above, semen and indeed sperm themselves are known to have immunosuppressive activities. It is thus possible that in disorders such as the autoimmune diseases this immunosuppressive activity could be reduced.

The incidence of antisperm antibodies among homosexual men is also increased. However, whether this is because of the deposition of sperm into the intestinal tract or is due to the relatively high incidence of genital tract infection in these individuals is not clear.

Antisperm antibodies in the cervical mucus

The antisperm antibodies that may be present in cervical mucus are usually of the IgG or the IgA subgroups.

Antibodies of the IgG subgroup in the female are most easily detected in serum but such an assay will not, however, have provided an adequate assessment of the presence of antisperm antibodies of the IgA subgroup, which may also be present at this site.

In order to detect the presence of antibodies in cervical mucus, the mucus must first be solubilized in phosphate-buffered saline and the proteolytic enzyme bromelain solution (Mortimer 1994). Interestingly, this enzyme does not appear to distort the measurement of the antisperm antibodies in such a solution even though such an enzyme must alter the configuration of the immunoglobulin molecule. This solution can now be used in any of the assays used to detect antisperm antibodies. It can also be used in the indirect immunobead assay.

The presence of antisperm antibodies in cervical mucus may be indicated by an abnormal postcoital test or by observing the 'shaking' phenomenon on examining the mucus. These antisperm antibodies may also be detected more formally by using either the sperm–cervical mucus penetration (SCMP) test or the sperm–cervical mucus contact (SCMC) test, both of which were described by Kremer (Kremer 1965).

The SCMP test

In this procedure, the midcycle mucus that is showing a good *spinnbarkeit* is aspirated into a narrow tube. One end of this narrow tube is dipped into the semen sample while the other is sealed using a nontoxic wax. The mounted tube is now laid horizontally in a Petri dish together with some moistened filter paper to provide humidity. This is incubated for 1 h at 37°C, after which the capillary tube is examined microscopically and the distance travelled into the mucus by the sperm is then measured in millimetres. In the absence of antibody or of any other factor that should impede their progress, the sperm should be able to travel at least 50 mm through the mucus in 1 h.

The SCMC test

In this test, the mucus is spread out on a slide and a sample of semen is placed over the mucus. The mixture is then covered with a cover-slip and the slide incubated for 1 h at 37°C in relatively moist conditions. The mucus under the cover-slip is then examined microscopically and the presence or absence of the 'shaking' phenomenon can be ascertained.

It must always be remembered that the presence of an abnormal postcoital test does not necessarily indicate the presence of antisperm antibodies. An abnormal postcoital test can also be caused by many factors including a poor midcycle oestrogen rise, poor mucus production, or even the presence of a cervical infection.

Treatment of infertility caused by the presence of antisperm antibodies

There are three major ways in which infertility caused by antisperm antibodies has been treated in the past.

Corticosteroid therapy

Two forms of corticosteroid therapy have been devised for the management of infertility caused by antisperm antibodies: one using low-dose steroids and the second using high-dose therapy.

In the low-dose regime, 10–20 mg of prednisolone daily was administered over a period of 3–6 months, but it did not appear to produce a satisfactory reduction in antibody levels.

In 1977, Shulman suggested the use of steroids in a much higher dose and recommended the use of methyl prednisolone at a daily dose of 96 mg for 7 days (Shulman 1977). Both the semen analysis and the ability of the sperm to penetrate cervical mucus was noted (Hendry *et al.* 1979). However, one patient on this therapy developed an avascular necrosis of the head of the femur (Hendry 1982) after which the high-dose regime was largely abandoned.

Intrauterine insemination

It was at one time thought that washing of sperm improved chances of conception. However, as most naturally occurring antigen–antibody reactions usually have an affinity constant (K_1) of around 10^7–10^9 L/mol, it would be very unlikely that simple washing would ever be sufficient to remove a significant amount of antibody adherent to the surface of the sperm.

However, in men with immunological infertility, not all of the sperm may be affected by the presence of antibody. Thus, as pregnancies can be achieved with smaller numbers of sperm than would otherwise be needed for natural conception, a pregnancy rate, using intrauterine insemination, of around 35–40% over six cycles has been achieved and this was probably higher than that which would have occurred naturally (Bronson 1994). Such a cumulative pregnancy rate, however, would only result in a pregnancy rate per cycle of treatment of less than 10%.

Assisted reproduction (IVF/ICSI)

The treatment of choice today, at least for severe forms of immune infertility, is certainly IVF and ICSI. Using these techniques, most clinics are now achieving pregnancy rates of around 30–40% per cycle of treatment. The use of assisted reproduction overcomes all the sperm transport problems that may be induced by the presence of antisperm antibodies and the possible effects of any antisperm antibodies that may be generated by the female are likewise overcome. If ICSI is used within the cycle of IVF, all the problems of sperm–zona binding, as well as those associated with the acrosome reaction and penetration of the zona and the oolemma, are overcome.

The major problem with IVF/ICSI is that it is expensive and problems relating to a possible increase in sex chromosome and autosomal anomalies together with other congenital abnormalities have, as yet, not been excluded. However, it is now a very useful means of overcoming immune infertility and will doubtless continue to be used for this purpose.

References

Aitken, R.J., Parslow, J.M., Hargreave, T.B. & Hendry, W.F. (1988) Influence of antisperm antibodies on human sperm function. *British Journal of Urology* **62**, 367–373.

Bronson, R.A. (1994) Immunologic infertility: significance and treatment options. In: *Management of Impotence and Infertility* (eds E.D. Whitehead & H.M. Nagler), pp. 390–408. J.B. Lippincott, Philadelphia.

Bronson, R.A., Cooper, G.W. & Rosenfeld, D.L. (1987) Autoimmunity to spermatozoa: effect on sperm penetration of cervical mucus as reflected by post coital testing. *Fertility and Sterility* **41**, 609–614.

Clarke, G.W., Elliott, P.J. & Smaila, C. (1985) Detection of sperm antibodies in semen using the immuno-bead test: a survey of 813 consecutive patients. *American Journal of Reproductive Immunology and Microbiology* **7**, 118–123.

Coombs, R.R., Rumpke, P. & Edwards, R.G. (1973) Immunoglobulin classes reactive with spermatozoa in the serum and the seminal plasma of vasectomised and infertile men. In: *Proceedings of the Second International Symposium on the Immunology of Reproduction* (ed. K. Bratamov) pp. 354–359. Bulgarian Academy of Science Press, Bucharest.

El-Demiry, M. & James, K. (1988) Lymphocyte subjects and macrophages in the male genital tract in health and disease. *European Journal of Urology* **14**, 226–245.

Hamerlynck, J.V.T.H. & Rumpke, P. (1968) A test for the detection of cytotoxic antibodies to spermatozoa in man. *Journal of Reproduction and Fertility* **17**, 191–194.

Hendry, W.F. (1982) Bilateral aseptic necrosis of femoral heads following intermittent high-dose steroid therapy. *Fertility and Sterility* **38**, 120 (Letter).

Hendry, W.F., Parslow, J.M., Stedronska, J. & Wallace, D.M.A. (1982b) The diagnosis of unilateral testicular obstruction in subfertile males. *British Journal of Urology* **54**, 774–779.

Hendry, W.F., Stedronska, J., Hughes, L., Cameron, K.M. & Pugh, R.C.B. (1979) Steroid treatment of male subfertility caused by antisperm antibodies. *Lancet* **ii**, 498–501.

Hendry, W.F., Stedronska, J. & Lake, R.A. (1982a) Mixed erythrocyte–spermatozoa antiglobulin reaction (MAR Test) for IgA antisperm antibodies in subfertile males. *Fertility and Sterility* **37**, 108–112.

Jager, S., Kremer, J. & Van Slochteren-Draaisma, T. (1978) A simple method of screening for antisperm antibodies in the male. Detection of spermatozoal surface IgG with the direct mixed antiglobulin reaction carried out on untreated fresh human semen. *International Journal of Fertility* **23**, 12–21.

Jequier, A.M. (1998) Vasectomy-related infertility: a major and costly medical problem. *Human Reproduction* **13**, 1757–1759.

Kremer, J. (1965) A simple sperm penetration test. *International Journal of Fertility* **10**, 209–215.

Kremer, J. & Jager, S. (1980). Characterisation of antispermatozoal antibodies responsible for the shaking phenomenon with special regard to immunological class and antigen reactive sites. *International Journal of Andrology* **3**, 143–152.

Liu, D.Y., Clarke, G.N. & Baker, H.W.G. (1991) Inhibition of human sperm–zona pellucida binding by antisperm antibodies. *Fertility and Sterility* **55**, 440–442.

Mahoney, M.C., Blackmore, P.F., Bronson, R.A. & Alexander, N.J. (1991) Inhibition of human sperm–zona pellucida tight binding in the presence of antisperm antibody positive polyclonal patient sera. *Journal of Reproductive Immunology* **19**, 287–301.

Mancini, R.E., Andrada, J.A., Sarceni, C., Bachmann, A.E., Lavieri, J.C. & Nemirovsky, M. (1965) Immunological and testicular response in men sensitised with human testicular homogenate. *Journal of Clinical Endocrinology and Metabolism* **25**, 859–875.

Markey, C.M., Jequier, A.M., Meyer, G.T. & Martin, G.B. (1994) Testicular morphology and androgen profiles following testicular ischaemia in the ram. *Journal of Reproduction and Fertility* **101**, 645–650.

Mortimer, D. (1994). *Practical Laboratory Andrology*. Oxford University Press, Oxford.

Patrizio, P., Moretti-Rojas, I., Ord, T., Balmaceda, J., Silber, S. & Asch, R.H. (1989) Low incidence of sperm antibodies in men with congenital absence of the vas deferens. *Fertility and Sterility* **52**, 1018–1021.

Rumpke, P. (1954) The presence of sperm antibodies in the serum of two patients with oligozoospermia. *Vox Sang (Basel)* **4**, 135–140.

Schlegel, P.N. & Su, L.-M. (1997) Physiological consequences of testicular sperm aspiration. *Human Reproduction* **12**, 1688–1692.

Shulman, S. (1977) Immune infertility and new approaches to treatment. In: *Immunological Influences on Human Fertility* (ed. B. Boettcher), pp. 281–288. Academic Press, Sydney.

Soffer, Y., Ron, E.R., Golan, A. *et al.* (1990) Male genital mycoplasmas and *Chlamydia trachomatis* culture: its relationship with accessory gland function, sperm quality and autoimmunity. *Fertility and Sterility* **53**, 331–336.

Wilson, L. (1954) Spermagglutinins in human semen and blood. *Proceedings of the Society of Experimental Biology and Medicine* **85**, 652–655.

World Health Organization (1992). *WHO Laboratory Manual for the Examination of Human Semen and Sperm–Cervical Mucus Interaction*, 3rd edn. Cambridge University Press, Cambridge.

16: Genetics and Infertility in the Male

In recent years it has become increasingly clear that genetic abnormalities may be an important cause of infertility in the male and may also be responsible for a number of congenital abnormalities of both the genital tract and of spermatogenesis. As these changes may have considerable implications for any offspring, it is important that the clinician is aware of these anomalies so that the infertile couple can be appropriately counselled.

The detection of genetic abnormalities

Male infertility can be caused by chromosomal aneuploidies and structural anomalies such as translocations, inversions or obvious macrodeletions of portions of an individual chromosome. Male infertility, however, can also be caused by microdeletions that take place at a molecular level and that are not visible by any form of microscopy. These microdeletions can only be detected by chemical means using a technique known as polymerase chain reaction (PCR).

The cytogenetic detection of chromosomal abnormalities

In this technique the individual chromosomes are visualized. The demonstration of these chromosomes depends upon spontaneously dividing cells that are stimulated into division by mitogenic agents and are then held in metaphase so that the individual chromosomes can be visualized and identified. The absence of a chromosome or the presence of an extra chromosome can also result in a disturbance of meiotic division leading an interruption in the process of spermatogenesis. The first of the discoveries that led to the cytogenetic examination of chromosomes occurred in 1938 when Levan demonstrated that colchicine arrested cell division in plants in metaphase (Levan 1938). It is during this stage of cell division that the chromosome pairs separate from each other and can thus each be visualized. During the performance of cytogenetic analysis, white cells are stimulated into cell division by the mitogen phytohaemagglutinin (PHA) and then arrested in metaphase using colchicine.

The most usual cells that are used for the cytogenetic analysis of the chromosomes are the lymphocytes, which make up about 35% of the white blood cells that can be isolated from heparinized plasma. The more commonly used lithium heparin is thought to be toxic to the cells in suspension, and thus all plasma used for the collection of cells for karyotyping must be placed into a solution of sodium heparin rather than lithium heparin.

The blood sample is taken and placed in heparin so that after centrifugation the thin, buff-coloured layer that contains the white cells can be easily identified and drawn off. This plasma–leucocyte suspension is first suspended in around 10 mL of culture medium to achieve a concentration of some 1 million cells per millilitre. This medium contains the PHA that stimulates mitotic division. The presence of red blood cells does not interfere with this process. In the presence of PHA the granulocytes degenerate, leaving only the lymphocytes available for analysis. After culturing these cells for around 48 h at 37 °C, mitotic activity is then arrested using colchicine. The cells are then centrifuged down into a pellet, to which is added a hypotonic solution of potassium chloride. This will cause the red blood cells to lyse, but the lymphocytes will only swell, thus separating the two types of cells. The lymphocytes are then preserved by the suspension in fixative over a period of several hours, after which the cells are mounted on a slide.

Prior to the discovery of Giemsa stain and its application to chromosomes by Moorehead and colleagues (Moorehead *et al.* 1960) chromosomes were stained using standard preparations such as haematoxylin and gentian violet. However, these techniques stained the chromosomes uniformly and left the centromeres colourless. Today the stains used vary in different laboratories, but the most commonly used stains are those of the Romanovsky group and these include Giemsa, Leishman's and Wright's stains. Giemsa remains the most popular stain and provides the so-called G banding of the chromosomes.

After staining, the cells are viewed and photographed using an oil immersion lens and, in this way, any abnormality of the chromosomes can be identified. In larger laboratories today it is possible to use a computer to sort and to identify each pair of chromosomes, and such technology is now even able to identify abnormalities in the banding patterns and the presence or absence of translocations or macrodeletions.

Fluorescence *in situ* hybridization (FISH)

With the recent advances made in molecular cytogenetics, it is now possible to examine the chromosome in more detail and at a level that cannot be visualized by light microscopy. One can now use DNA or RNA to illuminate and identify either the whole chromosome or to identify different parts of it in a technique known as *in situ* hybridization.

Basically, this technique denatures the DNA, or a segment of the DNA, so that the two strands of DNA that make up the helix come to separate from each other. One of the strands of DNA in the chromosome is then replaced by a probe. That probe consists of a similar strand of nucleotide and contains a fluorescent substance. There are a number of different agents that can be used in this technique that, on excitation with ultraviolet light, produce different colours. This technique thus allows one to identify more than one chromosome or chromosomal abnormality at a time. Fluorescent substances such as biotin and acetylaminofluorene can be used for this purpose. This technique can also be used for the identification of abnormal genes within a chromosome or an absence or excess of chromosome numbers within a cell.

As this form of investigation can be completed fairly rapidly, it is the preferred method used in the identification of genetic abnormalities in blastomeres that may be biopsied from the embryo during IVF. It can, however, also be used in examining specific genetic abnormalities in many tissues, including malignant biopsies and even trophoblastic tissue after chorionic villous sampling.

This technique has also been extensively used to study the presence of chromosomal abnormalities in spermatozoa. It is now known that around 0.2–0.35% of sperm from a normal semen sample show some form of chromosomal abnormality, particularly disomy and diploidy (Downie *et al.* 1997), and that these genetic abnormalities are more common amongst sperm that show an abnormal morphology. Using this technique, there is now believed to be an increasing frequency of such abnormalities with advancing paternal age (Wyrobek *et al.* 1996). Unfortunately, all these techniques result in the demise of the sperm under investigation and therefore such a method of selection of sperm cannot be used prior to IVF, or more importantly prior to the injection of these sperm into an oocyte during ICSI.

PCR

This technique is the most sensitive method used to identify abnormalities in DNA. This technique was first described in 1986 by Mullis and colleagues (Mullis *et al.* 1986) and is simple in design (Mullis 1993). It allows one to identify changes, in particular the presence of microdeletions, in a strand of DNA. The technique amplifies this change some 1 million-fold. One is thus able to identify very small changes in a very small strand of DNA. However, in order to be able to identify these changes, the sequence of that particular strand of DNA must of course already be known.

The polymerase chain reaction consists of three main stages. The first step consists of denaturing the DNA into two separate strands and this is achieved by a short heat treatment. The second step consists of the addition of short oligosaccharides, known as primers, that are of exactly the same structure as the dissociated DNA in the normal state. These oligosacharides are annealed to the single-stranded DNA by their addition to the denatured DNA in great excess and by the subsequent cooling of the mixture. In the third step, nucleotide bases are used that extend the primers to complete the double-stranded DNA (Fig. 16.1).

This process is then repeated many times. Where the primer does not 'fit' the original DNA template, there is a greatly reduced generation of the DNA copies while where no abnormality in the DNA sequencing is present,

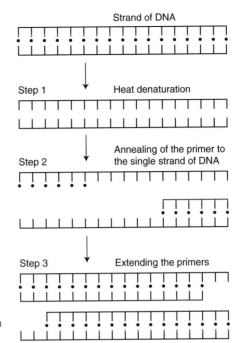

Fig. 16.1 A diagrammatic representation of the polymerase chain reaction (PCR).

the copies increase exponentially. In this way, an area of abnormal chromatin can be identified and an abnormal gene can be positively identified using a primer that 'matches' an abnormal gene.

The technique of PCR has proved to be extremely useful in both the diagnosis of genetic disease and the demonstration of abnormal genotype. It can identify changes in the chromatin that may be as short as 12 basepairs. It can demonstrate changes in the chromatin that are much too small to be identified on a karyotype; indeed, PCR is now more frequently used in genetic diagnosis than is the karyotype. As PCR is effectively *in vitro* cloning of a segment of DNA, it can also be used in mapping areas of chromatin and is thus of great value in mapping the genome as well as in the diagnosis of its abnormalities.

Disorders of the sex chromosomes (gonosomes)

Klinefelter's syndrome

This is a surprisingly common cause of infertility in the human male. This condition was originally described by Klinefelter and colleagues in 1942 (Klinefelter *et al.* 1942). Men with this condition have two X chromosomes, giving them a total complement of 47 chromosomes and a white cell karyotype of 47,XXY (Fig. 16.2). The cause of this condition is not known but it is thought possibly to relate to some form of nondysjunction of the X chromosome at meiotic division.

This condition is a genetically predetermined cause of primary testicular disease. The serum levels of the gonadotrophins are raised and the testosterone levels are reduced in varying degrees.

Infertile men with this condition are usually azoospermic but can occasionally be oligozoospermic. The phenotype of this condition is very variable, as is the degree of androgenization. The libido is often relatively low and there is, because of the low levels of secretion of testosterone, some difficulty with erection at times. The infertile men with this condition may show poor beard growth, a finer than usual skin texture and reduced amounts of androgenically induced hair growth. Testicular size is usually markedly reduced.

Long-term problems for patients with this condition can be identified. Klinefelter's syndrome may be associated with osteoporosis, possibly because of the long-term reduction in testosterone secretion (Horowitz *et al.* 1992) However, testosterone replacement has little effect on the incidence of osteoporosis in this group of patients (Wong *et al.* 1993).

Some patients with many different forms of sex chromosome anomalies as well as those with Klinefelter's syndrome suffer from venous ulceration

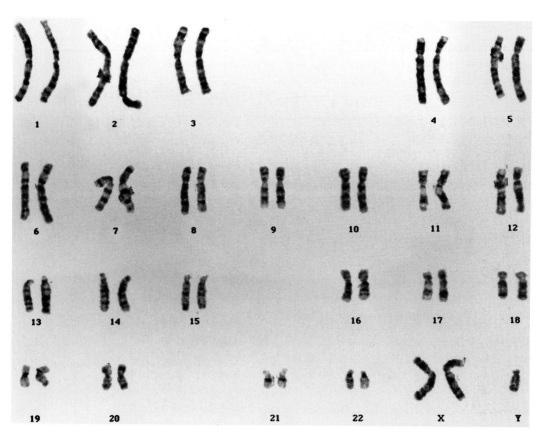

Fig. 16.2 The karyotype seen in men with Klinefelter's syndrome. Note the presence of two X chromosomes. The autosomes in these karyotypes are normal.

and leg ulcers. Patients with Klinefelter's syndrome are also said to be at an increased risk from male breast cancer (Hultborn *et al.* 1997).

The testes in this condition have a somewhat unique appearance characterized by an almost total absence of seminiferous tubules, which have been replaced by sheets of Leydig cells (Fig. 16.3). Although the number of Leydig cells in this condition is probably normal, their function is very abnormal as the levels of testosterone are frequently severely subnormal. However, it is often possible to find small nests of seminiferous tubules that sometimes may contain spermatozoa. These sperm, however, may well contain an increased frequency of diploid sex chromosome content (Guttenbach *et al.* 1997).

There is of course no treatment for this condition, but it is sometimes possible to find spermatozoa in a testicular biopsy which can be used to generate a pregnancy by means of IVF and ICSI. Interestingly, the pregnancies that have been produced in this way tend not to show the presence of an abnormal karyotype suggesting that a pregnancy is only generated by normally haploid spermatozoa (Bourne *et al.* 1997; Palermo *et al.* 1998).

XYY males

This disorder was at one time associated with the presence of antisocial behaviour amongst young men but this has now been disproved. Whether or not this disorder is truly associated with infertility is not known, but the incidence of this disorder amongst infertile males does not appear to be

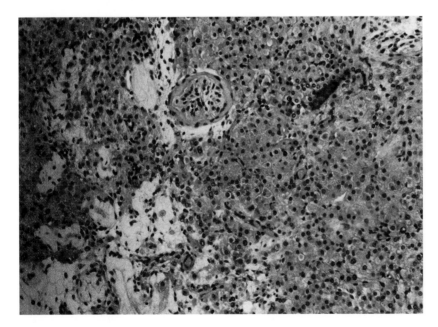

Fig. 16.3 Testicular histology taken from a man with Klinefelter's syndrome. Note the sheets of Leydig cells seen in this condition, together with the occasional tubule that can contain small numbers of spermatozoa.

increased. Changes in testicular histology have, however, been described in men with this chromosomal anomaly (Jequier *et al.* 1979).

XX males

In this disorder a portion of the Y chromosome that carries the *SRY* gene has been translocated and thus such patients appear to only have two X chromosomes. Using FISH, it is now simple to demonstrate the presence of all or part of the Y chromosome cytogenetically. This condition is thus a variant of Klinefelter's syndrome and thus this condition is usually found among a population of both azoospermic and oligozoospermic men.

Balanced translocations involving one of the sex chromosomes

This chromosomal anomaly is very rare but it can be found in studies of infertile male patients (Faed *et al.* 1979). It is almost certainly a cause of infertility and results in a reduction in sperm production. There are many examples of such translocations, which are often but not invariably associated with a reduced sperm count and infertility.

Pericentric inversion of the Y chromosome, i.e. inv(Y)

This is also a very rare genetic event but is one that is unlikely to be associated with infertility as its incidence among a fertile population is the same as that among men attending an infertility clinic (Dutrillaux *et al.* 1982).

The Y chromosome microdeletions and the azoospermic factors (AZF)

This is one of the most exciting recent findings in relation to male infertility as it may explain infertility in some of the cases with disorders of sperm production whose aetiology is unknown. The first observation that was made to implicate the Y chromosome in male infertility was when Tiepolo and Zuffardi noted the deletion of a large portion of heterochromatin on the long arm of the Y chromosome (Yq12) in six men with azoospermia (Tiepolo & Zuffardi 1976). This observation was of course made on the examination of the Y chromosome in a cytogenetic preparation (Fig. 16.4). This finding was not believed to relate to the patients' infertility as it was thought that heterochromatin did not have any genetic activity, and the idea arose that the Y factors responsible for the development of the male gametes were situated in Yq11. These deletions were loosely termed the azoospermic factors, or AZF. Nevertheless some of the cytogenetic changes on the Y chromosome do correlate with an abnormal phenotype in the patient.

Over the years, the presence of the AZF in Yq11 has been confirmed (Vogt 1992), but it became increasingly clear that deletions in this area and

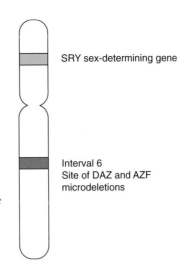

SRY sex-determining gene

Interval 6
Site of DAZ and AZF
microdeletions

Fig. 16.4 A simplified diagram of the Y chromosome showing the relative positions of the *SRY* gene on the short arm, which is responsible for sexual differentiation, and the approximate sites of the microdeletions on the long arm that may give rise to certain forms of male infertility.

their relationship to male infertility was very complex. Many microdeletions are now known to be present in this region of the Y chromosome, many of which are much too small to be seen on a white blood cell karyotype and which can only be demonstrated using the technique of PCR.

It is now believed that there are three loci for deletions in the region Yq11 and these areas have been termed AZFa, AZFb and AZFc. Each microdeletion in these areas appears to relate to a specific phenotype and specific testicular histology.

The deletion that occurs in AZFa is associated with azoospermia and the presence of germinal aplasia (previously known as the Sertoli cell only syndrome) on testicular biopsy (Vogt 1997). It is thus likely that this deletion is affecting the testis prior to puberty, as there is no evidence of any spermatogonia or any maturational change in the germ cells in biopsies from these men.

In men with deletions involving the AZFb region, azoospermia is also seen but their testicular histology shows the presence of a maturational arrest in which the sperm maturation process has been interrupted at a very different stage to that seen in men with the AZFa deletion. These findings suggest that the disruption of spermatogenesis in these patients may occur at or around puberty.

In the third group of men with the AZFc deletions, either azoospermia or severe oligozoospermia may be present. Testicular histology in these patients shows varying stages of maturational arrest but there may be a few tubules that contain mature sperm. Why there are these differences between tubules in the testicular biopsies from these men when only one apparent genetic anomaly is supposed to cause their infertility is at present impossible to explain. However, one must remember that these changes may occur in response to other factors such as age, ischaemia and the effects of toxins (Terada & Hakayama 1991). It is also entirely possible that that these deletions may themselves predispose the testes to damage by these agents.

All these microdeletions may be detected by PCR. They now should be sought among all infertile men with azoospermia or oligozoospermia that has no obvious cause. It is now of course possible to treat successfully patients with very small numbers of sperm in either their ejaculate or in their testicular tissue using ICSI. It is therefore important that the patients are fully informed of the presence of these genetic anomalies, as it is now known that these deletions may be transmitted to a male fetus. The presence of these microdeletions on Yq11 may thus result in a male offspring having the same form of genetically determined infertility as his father (Kent-First *et al.* 1996).

The autosomal anomalies

The *CFTR* gene

The cystic fibrosis transmembrane conductance regulator, otherwise known as the *CFTR* gene, is located on the long arm of chromosome 7 and spans some 230 kilobasepairs. It is responsible for the production of cystic fibrosis transmembrane conductance regulator, a glycoprotein present in the apical membranes of epithelial cells. These substances are found within the organs affected by cystic fibrosis such as the gut, the bronchi and the nasopharyngeal mucosa.

Cystic fibrosis is caused by the homozygous presence of a number of different mutations in the *CFTR* gene. The most common mutation is a deletion known as deltaF508, and it is this mutation that accounts for around 66% of all cases of cystic fibrosis. There are, however, some 65 other mutations that may be found in relation to cystic fibrosis but some of these are very rare. It is of interest that the disease of cystic fibrosis is itself associated with atresia of the vas deferens (Holsclaw *et al.* 1971).

In 1990, Dumur and coworkers (Dumur *et al.* 1990) reported a substantial increase in the incidence of the deltaF508 gene in men with bilateral congenital absence of the vasa deferentia. In a large number of different studies involving patients with congenital absence of the vas, this increased incidence of the deltaF508 mutation, present in a heterozygous form, was confirmed (Anguiano *et al.* 1992; Patrizio *et al.* 1993; Culard *et al.* 1994). However, it became clear that the genital tract anomaly of congenital absence of the vas was not the sole reason for this abnormality but had to be present alongside another as yet unidentified mutation on another chromosome (Patrizio *et al.* 1993).

The mutations that have now been identified to be in association with the genital anomaly of congenital absence of the vas deferens are numerous but, after the deltaF508 deletion, the other three most common mutations are termed G542X, R553X and W1282X. The mutation W1282X is especially common amongst the Ashkenazi Jewish population.

The expression of *CFTR* has been studied and can be detected in the human fetus at 18 weeks' gestation (Trezise & *et al.* 1993). The level of this expression is high in the head of the epididymis, low in the vas deferens and cannot be detected in the seminal vesicles (Tizzano *et al.* 1994). A low level of expression is detected in the testes but there is not thought to be any major effect of cystic fibrosis on sperm production or function. The pathogenesis of this relationship between the mutations of the *CFTR* gene and congenital absence of the vas thus remains unclear.

What is clear, however, is that as 1 in 30 of the population carry one of the *CFTR* mutations, these mutations will also be present in 1 in 30 of the female partners of the men with congenital absence of the vas. As such a partnership could provide a 1 in 4 risk of an offspring with the disease of cystic fibrosis, it is important that these female partners are also screened for the more common mutations of the *CFTR* gene. These couples must also be given good genetic counselling concerning the possible occurrence of this disorder in any offspring. It is also very possible that the condition of bilateral congenital absence of the vasa deferentia could be given to any male child.

Until recently, congenital absence of the vasa deferentia was impossible to treat as no anastomotic connection could be made between the upper epididymis and any part of the vas deferens. However, with the advent of IVF and in particular the development of ICSI, fertility can now be achieved after collection of the sperm from the upper epididymis or the testis (Patrizio & Asch 1988).

Robertsonian translocations

These balanced translocations can be found among infertile men (Fig. 16.5). These autosomal anomalies may be found in men with azoospermia or oligozoospermia. This abnormality of the karyotype is around eight times more common among infertile men than in the general population (Dutrillaux *et al.* 1982; Pandiyan & Jequier 1997).

Translocations as a cause of infertility have been studied in the past and appear to result in an arrest of sperm maturation at the secondary spermatocyte stage (Matsuda *et al.* 1991). However, it must be remembered that these anomalies may not be the sole cause of a male patient's abnormal semen analysis, but they may also be a cause of miscarriage in any pregnancy generated by such a couple.

It must, however, be remembered that these translocations, although balanced in the parent, can result in an unbalanced karyotype in the fetus. Such a problem can produce a miscarriage, a nonviable fetus or a congenital abnormality in a live-born child (Meschede *et al.* 1997). As it is now possible to generate pregnancies using ICSI in men with very low sperm

counts, it is always important to exclude these anomalies prior to this form
of treatment or if such anomalies are present that appropriate genetic counselling is provided for the patients (Testart *et al.* 1996).

An unbalanced translocation

From the point of view of fertility, an unbalanced translocation is much
more likely to be associated with spermatogenic abnormalities as disturbance in chromosomal balance is enhanced at meiotic cell division (Fig.
16.6).

The mitochondrial genome and its possible relationship to infertility in the male

Over the past 5 years, there has been increasing interest in the possible role
of the mitochondrial genome and its relationship to infertility in the male.

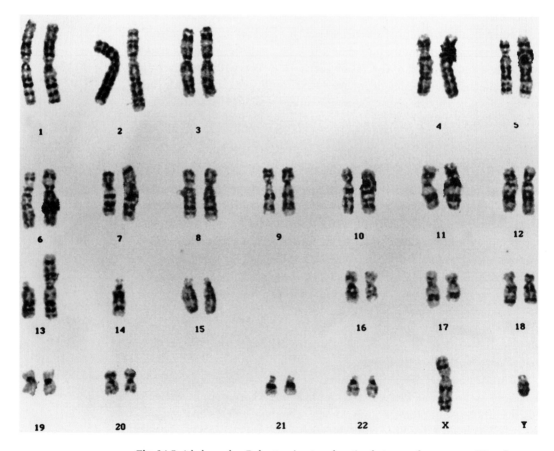

Fig. 16.5 A balanced or Robertsonian translocation between chromosome 13 and
chromosome 14.

The mitochondrial genome is unique in that it has no partner, and unlike nuclear DNA it is circular in structure.

The mitochondria control oxidative phosphorylation and thus play a very important role in the protection of the cell from oxidative damage (Wallace 1992). It is known that, unlike the nuclear genome, mitochondrial DNA has no repair mechanism. Thus, should a deletion occur, it will persist throughout cell division, introducing this abnormality into increasing numbers of cells throughout the body. Indeed, there are a number of different disorders, albeit rare, that are known to be associated solely with deletions of portions of the mitochondrial genome. Examples of purely mitochondrial disease that relate to abnormalities in the mitochondrial genome include myoclonic epilepsy and red ragged fibres (MERRF), Leber's hereditary optic neuropathy (LHON) and mitochondrial encephalopathy, lactic acidosis and stroke-like symptoms (MELAS) (Fig.

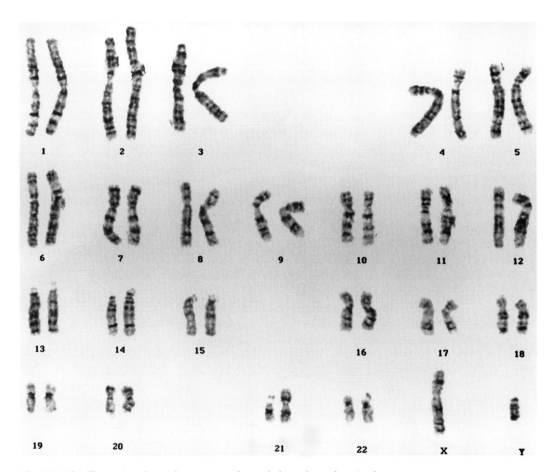

Fig. 16.6 This illustration shows the presence of an unbalanced translocation between the long arm of chromosome 10 and the short arm of chromosome 21. Such a problem might again give rise to both infertility and recurrent miscarriage. However, such a karyotype could also give rise to an offspring with the features of Down's syndrome, making this a difficult problem to manage in an infertility clinic.

16.7). These disorders are the result of either microdeletions or of point mutations.

It is now known that ageing has a profound effect on mitochondrial function and this loss of protection from oxidative damage makes up a major portion of the changes that relate to old age. These changes are associated with the occurrence of a major 4999 basepair deletion in the mitochondrial genome that results in a major reduction in protection of the cell against oxidative damage (Fig. 16.7).

In 1994, it was found that both testicular tissue and spermatozoa that had been taken from infertile males showed an increase in the numbers of mitochondria exhibiting this major deletion (Cummins *et al.* 1994). It is likely that these changes in the degree of protection of the cell against oxidative damage relate to the presence of the reactive oxygen species that are known to be present in the semen of infertile men. However, the exact role played by the mitochondrial genome in the causation of infertility in the male is yet to be elucidated.

Kartagener's syndrome

This is an uncommon condition in which there are normal numbers of sperm in a semen sample but where all motility is absent. It is also frequently known as the immotile cilia syndrome (Eliasson *et al.* 1977). This loss of movement is due to the lack of the dynein arms in the

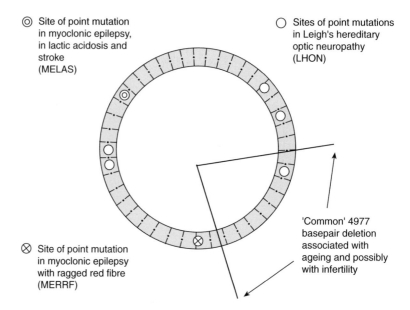

Fig. 16.7 The mitochondrial genome showing the site of the major 4999 basepair deletion that is associated with ageing and possibly with male infertility. The sites of other mitochondrial diseases are also indicated.

axonemes of the spermatozoa. Although Kartagener's syndrome clearly has a genetic basis, neither the site nor the nature of that genetic abnormality is known.

Among patients with this form of infertility, bronchiectasis and sinusitis is the rule, as is the axonemal abnormality that is found in all cilia in every tissue. There may also be a number of congenital anomalies present in these patients including dextrocardia and other cardiac abnormalities.

Because of its association with other congenital abnormalities, the immotile cilia syndrome is likely to be genetically predetermined, although the site of this abnormality has not yet been described.

Attempts have been made to achieve pregnancies using IVF and ICSI but none has been generated and thus little is known about the transmission of this disorder to the offspring. The seriousness of the respiratory and cardiac abnormalities associated with this syndome should be a deterrent to clinicians in carrying out assisted reproduction in men with this condition.

References

Anguiano, A., Oates, R.D., Amos, J.A. *et al.* (1992) Congenital bilateral absence of the vas deferens. A primarily genital form of cystic fibrosis. *Journal of the American Medical Association* **267**, 1794–1797.

Bourne, H., Stern, K., Clarke, G., Pertile, M. & Baker, H.W. (1997) Delivery of normal twins following the intracytoplasmic injection of sperm from a patient with 47, XXY Klinefelter's syndrome. *Human Reproduction* **12**, 2447–2450.

Culard, J., Desgeorges, M., Costa, P. *et al.* (1994) Analysis of the whole CFTR regions and splice junctions in azoospermic men with congenital bilateral aplasia of epididymis or vas deferens. *American Journal of Human Genetics* **93**, 467–470.

Cummins, J.N., Jequier, A.M. & Kan, R. (1994) Molecular biology of male infertility: links with aging, mitochondrial genetics and oxidative stress. *Molecular Reproduction and Development* **37**, 345–362.

Downie, S.E., Flaherty, S.P. & Mathews, C.D. (1997) Detection of chromosomes and estimation of human spermatozoa using fluorescence *in-situ* hybridisation. *Molecular Human Reproduction* **3**, 585–598.

Dumur, V., Gervais, R., Rigot, J.M., Lafitte, J.J. *et al.* (1990) Abnormal distribution of CF Delta F508 allele in azoospermic men with congenital aplasia of epididymis and vas deferens. *Lancet* **336**, 512.

Dutrillaux, B., Rotman, J. & Gueguen, J. (1982) Chromosomal factors in the infertile male. In: *International Persectives in Urology*, Vol. 4, *Aspects of Male Infertility* (ed. R. de Vere White), pp. 89–102. Williams & Wilkins, Baltimore.

Eliasson, R., Mossberg, B., Camner, P. & Afzelius, B.A. (1977) The immotile cilia syndrome. A congenital abnormality as an aetiologic factor in chronic airway infections and male infertility. *New England Journal of Medicine* **297**, 1–6.

Faed, M.J.W., Robertson, J., Lamont, M.A. *et al.* (1979) A cytogenic survey of men being investigated for subfertility. *Journal of Reproduction and Fertility* **56**, 209–216.

Guttenbach, M., Michelmann, H.W., Hinney, B., Engel, W. & Schmid, M. (1997) Segregation of sex chromosomes into sperm nuclei in a man with 47,XXY Klinefelter's karyotype: a FISH analysis. *Human Genetics* **99**, 474–477.

Holsclaw, D.S., Lobel, B., Jockin, H. & Schwackman, H. (1971) Genital abnormalities in male patients with cytic fibrosis. *Journal of Urology* **106**, 568–574.

Horowitz, M., Wishart, J.M., O'Loughlin, P.D., Morris, H.A., Need, A.G. & Nordin, B.E. (1992) Osteoporosis and Klinefelter's syndrome. *Clinical Endocrinology* **36**, 113–118.

Hultborn, R., Hanson, C., Kopf, I., Verbiene, I., Warnhammar, E. & Weimarck, A. (1997) Prevalence of Klinefelter's syndrome in male breast cancer patients. *Anticancer Research* **17**, 4293–4297.

Jequier, A.M., Crich, J.P. & Ansell, I.D. (1979) Testicular histology in an infertile man with 47,XYY karyotype. *Infertility* **2**, 257–260.

Kent-First, M.G., Kol, S., Muallem, A. *et al.* (1996) The incidence and possible relevance of Y-linked microdeletions in babies born after intracytoplasmic sperm injection and their infertile fathers. *Molecular Human Reproduction* **2**, 943–950.

Klinefelter, H.R., Reifenstein, E.C. & Albright, F. (1942) Syndrome characterised by gynaecomastia, aspermatogensis without A-Leydigism and increased secretion of follicle stimulating hormone. *Journal of Clinical Endocrinology* **2**, 615–627.

Levan, A. (1938) The effect of colchicine on root mitosis in *Allium. Heredity* **24**, 167–172.

Matsuda, T., Horii, Y., Hayashi, K. & Yoshida, O. (1991) Quantative analysis of seminiferous epithelium in subfertile carriers of chromosomal translocations. *International Journal of Fertility* **36**, 344–351.

Meschede, D., Louwen, F., Eiben, B. & Horst, J. (1997) Intracytoplasmic sperm injection pregnancy with fetal trisomy 9p resulting from a balanced translocation. *Human Reproduction* **12**, 1913–1214.

Moorehead, P.S., Nowell, P.C., Mellman, W.J., Battips, D.M. & Hungerford, D.A. (1960) Chromosome preparations of leukocyte cultures from human peripheral blood. *Experimental Cell Research* **20**, 613–616.

Mullis, K. (1993) The unusual origin of the polymerase chain reaction. *Scientific American* **262**, 36–43.

Mullis, K., Faloona, F., Scharf, S., Saiki, S.R., Horn, G. & Erlich, H. (1986) Specific enzymatic amplification of DNA *in vitro*: The polymerase chain reaction. *Cold Spring Harbor Symposia on Quantitative Biology* **51**, 263–273.

Palermo, G.D., Schlegel, P.N., Sills, E.S. *et al.* (1998) Births after intracytoplasmic injection of sperm obtained by testicular extraction from men with nonmosaic Klinefelter's syndrome. *New England Journal of Medicine* **338**, 588–590.

Pandiyan, N. & Jequier, A.M. (1997) Mitotic chromosomal anomalies among 1210 infertile men. *Human Reproduction* **12**, 2604–2608.

Patrizio, P. & Asch, R.H. (1988) Epididymal sperm in assisted reproduction. *Annals of Academic Medicine* **21**, 533–537.

Patrizio, P., Asch, R.H., Handelin, B. & Silber, S.J. (1993) Aetiology of congenital absence of vas deferens: genetic study of three generations. *Human Reproduction* **8**, 215–230.

Testart, J., Gautier, E., Brami, C., Sedbon, E. & Thebault, A. (1996) Intracytoplasmic sperm injection in infertile patients with structural chromosomal abnormalities. *Human Reproduction* **11**, 2609–2612.

Tiepolo, L. & Zuffardi, O. (1976) Localisation of factors controlling spermatogenesis in the non-fluorescent portion of the human Y chromosome long arm. *Human Genetics* **34**, 119–124.

Tizzano, E.F., Silver, F.M., Chitayat, D., Benichou, J.C. & Buchwald, D.C. (1994) Differential cellular expression of cystic fibrosis transmembrane regulator in human reproductive tissues. Clues for the infertility in patients with cystic fibrosis. *American Journal of Pathology* **144**, 906–914.

Trezise, A.E., Chambers, J.A., Wardle, C.J., Gould, S. & Harris, A. (1993) Expression of the cystic fibrosis gene in human foetal tissue. *Human Molecular Genetics* **2**, 213–218.

Vogt, P.H. (1992) Y chromosome function in spermatogenesis. In: *Spermatogenesis–Fertilization–Contraception. Molecular, Cellular and Endocrine Events in Male Reproduction* (eds E. Nieschlag & U.F. Habenicht), pp. 226–257. Springer, Heidelberg.

Vogt, P.H. (1997) Genetics of idiopathic male infertility: Y chromosomal azoospermia factors (AZFa, AZF, AZFc). *Baillière's Clinical Obstetrics and Gynaecology* **11**, 773–795.

Wallace, D.C. (1992) Mitochondrial genetics: a paradigm for aging and degenerative diseases? *Science* **256**, 628–632.

Wong, F.H., Pun, K.K. & Wang, C. (1993) Loss of bone mass in patients with Klinefelter's syndrome despite sufficient testosterone replacement. *Osteoporosis International* **3**, 3–7.

Wyrobek, A.J., Aardema, M., Eichenlamb-Ritter, U., Ferguson, L. & Marchetti, F. (1996) Mechanisms and targets in maternal and paternal effects on numerical aneuploidy. *Environmental and Molecular Mutagenesis* **28**, 254–264.

17: Testicular Cancer and Fertility in the Male

Testicular cancer is an uncommon disease and accounts for around 1% of all male cancers (Forman 1991). It does, however, mainly affect young men between the ages of 16–35 years and its management may cause infertility. It is thus of importance to all the clinicians involved in the treatment of infertility.

Its incidence appears to be rising in many European countries, in particular in Denmark (Osterlind 1986). As testicular cancer can have a pivotal position in relation to infertility in the male, it should thus be considered when evaluating the management of abnormal sperm counts and childlessness in the male.

Testicular cancer is a disease of young men. It occurs rarely before puberty and is uncommon among men over 45 years of age. There is a close association of testicular tumours with testicular maldescent, and 1 in every 10 testicular cancers will occur in a maldescended testis.

The development of testicular cancer may also be associated with other abnormalities including hypospadias, ectopic kidneys and various forms of intersex. It has even been suggested that mumps orchitis may predispose a patient to the development of a testicular tumour. The presence of a dysplastic testis has a strong relationship with the development of a testicular tumour and all dysplastic testes should therefore be removed.

There may also be a genetic basis to the development of testicular cancer as it is rare in African Americans and much more common amongst the white races (Brown *et al.* 1986). Several testicular tumours can also occur within one family (Oliver *et al.* 1986).

Testicular tumours

It can be seen, however, that testicular tumours occur within a similar age range to those presenting with male infertility. The relationship between testicular maldescent and infertility makes the presentation of a testicular tumour in an infertility clinic a distinct possibility. It is therefore important that the clinicians that manage infertility understand not only the mode of presentation and method of diagnosis of testicular cancer but also the pathology of these tumours.

There are two main types of testicular tumours (Oliver 1994). The first of these two groups are the germ-cell tumours, of which the seminoma and the teratocarcinoma are the most common. The second group arises from tissue other than the germ-cell line.

Germ-cell tumours of the testis

The seminoma

These tumours arise from the spermatocytes and have a wide range of appearances histologically. They can consist of cells that resemble spermatocytes or they can be highly anaplastic (Fig. 17.1).

They respond well to chemotherapy and do not very often give rise to metastases. They can frequently secrete human chorionic gonadotrophin (hCG) and this marker can be useful diagnostically as well as for the tracking of any recurrence or metastases. These tumours also secrete the enzyme placental alkaline phosphatase and this substance can also be used as a tumour marker. The prognosis following treatment of these tumours is good.

The teratocarcinoma

Like the more familiar teratoma that is seen in the ovary, these tumours consist of several different tissues but are thought to arise from the seminiferous epithelium itself. They can also vary greatly in histological appearance from being a fairly benign-looking tumour to a frank choriocarcinoma. These cancers also secrete hCG and alphafetoprotein, and both these substances can thus be used as markers for these tumours. The teratocarcinomata do metastasize mainly via the blood stream and therefore carry a worse prognosis than the seminoma.

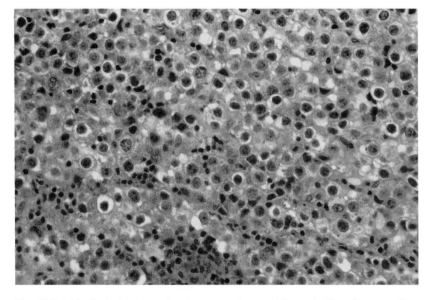

Fig. 17.1 A histological section taken from a seminoma of the testis. Note the generally anaplastic appearance of the cells with the occasional attempt to from rosettes.

Other germ-cell tumours

Examples of other germ-cell tumours are the yolk-sac tumours that may be found in infants and the embryonal carcinomata of the testis. Both these tumours secrete alphafetoprotein, thus demonstrating their origins from the yolk sac.

Nongerm-cell tumours

Leydig cell tumours

These tumours are much less common and are characterized by the secretion of excessive amounts of testosterone. This increase in testosterone production reduces LH secretion almost to nil and thus the contralateral testis that does not contain the tumour will become atrophic. The sperm count will fall to very low levels.

Some of the excess testosterone will be converted to oestrogen and as a consequence many men with these tumours will develop gynaecomastia. The classic presentation of a man with a Leydig cell tumour is an infertile patient with gynaecomastia who has one 'normal'-sized testis (which contains the tumour) and one very small testis (which has atrophied because of the suppression of LH secretion by the high levels of testosterone).

Leydig cell tumours almost never metastasize and can usually be considered to be almost benign. They are clearly easy to diagnose. Occasionally, however, these tumours can indeed demonstrate malignant tendencies (Ober *et al.* 1976).

Sertoli cell tumours

These are very rare. However, as the Sertoli cells secrete small amounts of oestrogen in the normal male, these tumours can occasionally be associated with gynaecomastia if the oestrogen secretions becomes excessive (Davis *et al.* 1981).

The presentation of a testicular tumour

Testicular tumours can present in many ways but can also mimic many other disorders of the testes. As a few of these patients may present with a tumour either initially or during their treatment for infertility, it is important that the clinician has an understanding of the manner in which these tumours may present.

Lump in the scrotum

The most common way in which a testicular tumour will present is as a lump in the scrotum. All lumps in or around the testis need prompt investigation. On palpation, the tumour may form an asymmetrical swelling involving one pole or only part of the testis.

However, tumours such as the Leydig cell tumour can arise centrally within the testis giving the impression of a uniformly enlarged testis or even, owing to the atrophy of the surrounding seminiferous tubules, a testis that is of normal size.

Pain or discomfort

Testicular cancers usually only cause a minor ache in the scrotum and only rarely cause frank pain. However, any discomfort must be investigated and such a symptom must not be ascribed to more minor pathology such as a varicocele without the exclusion of a tumour.

Inflammatory changes

Occasionally a testicular tumour may show signs of inflammation and can thus easily be mistaken for an epididymo-orchitis. If one is in any doubt, then surgical exploration must be undertaken.

It should also be remembered that such changes can occur in an intra-abdominal testis and such pathology may therefore present as an acute abdomen.

Testicular injury

Trauma to the testis often makes the patient seek medical attention. For some reason, there is a high incidence of trauma as a presenting symptom of testicular neoplasms, and thus each patient must undergo careful examination and if necessary investigation in order to exclude a concomitant testicular cancer.

Hydrocele

A hydrocele, although it is often only small, also often accompanies a testicular tumour. If, however, the tumour is large and has invaded the tunica albuginea to extrude out of the testis itself, such a hydrocele can be quite large. In this situation, the diagnosis must be made on ultrasound and if necessary by surgical exploration.

Endocrinopathies

The nongerm-cell tumours of the testis such as the Leydig or Sertoli cell tumours frequently produce hormones. Thus, patients with these tumours can develop gynaecomastia either by the excessive secretion of testosterone, which converts to oestrogen by aromatization, or by the excessive secretion of oestrogen itself.

Backache

Occasionally, testicular tumours that have metastasized to the para-aortic lymph glands can sometimes present with backache. Thus, if a fit young man attends the clinic with such a symptom, it is important that he is examined not only generally but also that the testes are carefully palpated. If there is any doubt about the diagnosis, the patient should undergo testicular and abdominal ultrasound and have the tumour markers in his serum measured.

Investigation of suspected testicular cancer

Knowledge of the investigation of testicular tumours is important as valuable time can be saved by the gynaecologist should one of these patients present in an infertility clinic.

Testicular and abdominal ultrasound

The simplest way to diagnose testicular tumours is by ultrasound (Richie *et al.* 1982). This technique sometimes produces false positive results, but it is better for a young man to undergo an unnecessary exploration than it is for a small malignant tumour of the testis to be missed. The use of magnetic resonance imaging (MRI) may produce more accurate results but its expense may preclude its routine use.

An accurate identification and localization of metastases from these tumours is obtained by the application of a computerized tomography (CT) scan or by MRI. These techniques also provide the urological surgeon with an accurate clinical staging of the tumour and its spread (McLeod *et al.* 1991).

Tumour markers

The serum levels of hCG, alphafetoprotein and placental alkaline phoshatase should also be measured in the serum of any patient who presents with a testicular swelling and is suspected of harbouring a testicular tumour. These testicular tumours can secrete large amounts of hCG; indeed, a testicular tumour is one of the few reasons for achieving a 'positive' pregnancy test in a male patient (Table 17.1).

The pretreatment storage of semen

It is very important that semen is cryopreserved prior to any therapy. However, often in men with testicular cancer, the quality of that semen is poor. If this is the case, the patient should be warned that IVF and ICSI may well be necessary if this semen is to be successfully used in the generation of a pregnancy.

Table 17.1 Testicular tumours and the chemical markers that they secrete. Measurement of these markers is very important diagnostically and will be of value in determining the presence of any recurrence of the tumour

Tumour	Tumour marker
Seminoma	hCG
Teratoma	Alphafetoprotein and hCG
Yolk sac tumours	Alphafetoprotein
Embryonal carcinoma	Alphafetoprotein
Leydig cell tumour	Testosterone
Sertoli cell tumour	Estradiol

As it is now possible, using ICSI, to induce fertilization with only a few dozen sperm, all semen if it contains any sperm at all should be stored if that is the wish of the patient.

Treatment of testicular cancer

The first approach to the treatment of testicular cancer is surgical. An orchidectomy will remove the tumour and also provide the histological diagnosis. An inguinal incision is made and the testis is pulled up out of the scrotum. If the tumour mass is large it may be necessary to enlarge the incision down the neck of the scrotum to avoid bursting the tumour. The cord is then dissected out of the inguinal canal, transected and transfixed at the level of the deep inguinal ring and the testis and the cord are then removed.

If there is CT evidence of spread into the para-aortic nodes then it may be necessary to carry out a retroperitoneal lymph node dissection. During the course of this procedure, especially in situations where the node involvement is extensive, the sympathetic chain may become damaged. This problem can result in either retrograde ejaculation or, more seriously, ejaculatory failure. Patients undergoing this procedure must be warned of this possibility preoperatively.

Radiation and even chemotherapy can also be used in the management of this condition particularly in relation to the treatment of distant metastases. It has been suggested that radiotherapy can be just as effective as surgery in managing para-aortic tumour spread, thus avoiding the damage to ejaculatory function (Hendry *et al.* 1993).

Among patients who have large testicular tumours, irradiation of the scrotum, the groin and the para-aortic nodes may be indicated and chemotherapy may also be required especially in the management of metastases or recurrence. Para-aortic node resection may also be needed for patients who develop recurrences after chemotherapy or radiotherapy (Williams *et al.* 1989).

The problem of carcinoma *in situ* of the testis

More than 25 years ago, it was pointed out that there existed a premalignant form of testicular cancer that preceded the development of tumours (Skakkebaek 1972).

This change, which involves the intratubular gonadocytes, is commonly found in association with and alongside germ-cell tumours of the testis (Fig. 17.2). It is now thought that carcinoma *in situ* of the testis will progress to true tumour formation in almost all postpubertal young men. It is now also believed that the gonadal hormones may play a role in the progression of carcinoma *in situ* of the testis to an invasive tumour (Skakkebaek *et al.* 1987).

It may also be found in the contralateral testis in men with tumours, indicating the great probability of the development of a second tumour in the opposite testis. It is thus suggested that a biopsy of the opposite testis should always be carried out in young men with germ-cell tumours of the testis.

It is clear that if we had an easy and noninvasive way to diagnose the presence of carcinoma *in situ* of the testis, the development of invasive testicular tumours might be avoided. However, sadly, the only way that this preinvasive condition can be diagnosed at present is by testicular biopsy. Attempts have been made to find cells showing *in situ* changes in the ejaculate but this has largely been unsuccessful because of the poor preservation of these cells during the long journey out of the testis and down the epididymal duct.

It is thus important to attempt to identify an 'at risk' subpopulation in

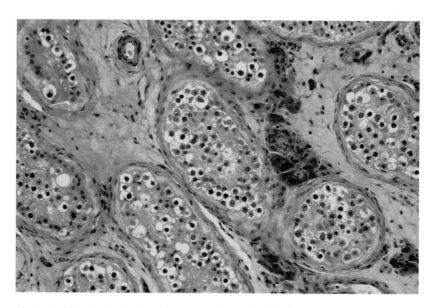

Fig. 17.2 A histological section of carcinoma *in situ* found in juxtaposition to a testicular tumour.

whom testicular biopsy may be a worthwhile procedure. To date these sub-groups include all men with known tumours, men with androgen insensitivity and gonadal dysgenesis. Biopsy is mandatory in these groups. It must be remembered that the biopsy may be positive in both testes.

The incidence of carcinoma *in situ* among men with infertility appears to be 0.4–1.1%, which is only 50% higher than that in the general population. However, its incidence among men with testicular maldescent is between 2% and 3%, which is four times higher than that in the general population (Giwercman *et al.* 1993). However, the incidence of *in situ* carcinoma falls with increasing age and at 45 years of age is considerably less than that of the general population.

Routine testicular biopsy is thus not recommended amongst all men with infertility, but it could be argued that testicular biopsies should be carried out among men with both infertility and a history of testicular maldescent. It is of interest that false negative biopsies seem to be rare. It should also be remembered that damage to the testis may be induced by testicular biopsy and testicular sperm aspiration (Schlegel & Su 1997) and that this damage, together with the effects that it may have on future fertility, must be taken into consideration when deciding upon the merits of a testicular biopsy.

The treatment of carcinoma *in situ*

It is suggested that if the carcinoma *in situ* of the testis is unilateral, a unilateral orchidectomy is indicated. If, however, the changes occur bilaterally (and this is the case in 5–6% of patients), then irradiation of the testes is probably the best therapy. The recommended treatment consists of a total dose of 20 Gy to the testes (2 Gy per day for 10 days) No recurrences have been seen in patients treated in this way (von der Maase *et al.* 1986). Similarly, good results have been obtained using chemotherapy.

However, it must be remembered that these types of treatment will usually render these men azoospermic. Thus, semen cryopreservation prior to therapy is very important.

The implications of testicular cancer for fertility

There are considerable implications for infertility in men with testicular cancer as well as those with a positive biopsy for carcinoma *in situ* of the testis. If an invasive tumour is present, orchidectomy will have to be performed. Should the contralateral testis have been damaged or be atrophic as the result of trauma or some other pathology, then this procedure will render the patient sterile. Storage of semen prior to orchidectomy is very important. If the semen is, at diagnosis of the tumour, already azoospermic it is sometimes possible to retrieve sperm from the testicular tissue itself. Thus, skilled embryologists should be invited to examine such tissue from these patients prior to its immersion in fixative, so that any spermatozoa that are suitable for use in an IVF/ICSI programme can be cryopreserved.

It must be remembered that men with a history of testicular maldescent, which itself is a cause of infertility, have an increased incidence of carcinoma *in situ* of the testis. Such patients can present initially in an infertility clinic and thus the clinicians supervising their infertility must be aware of all the implications of this form of infertility.

The possible presence of *in situ* carcinoma must be considered in each patient with infertility but particularly in those men with a history of maldescent. The merits as well as the disadvantages of a testicular biopsy must be considered by both the clinician and the patient. Many patients with primary testicular disease due to testicular maldescent have a form of infertility that is progressive, and thus storage of semen, even if its quality is poor, is highly recommended.

If the patient has carcinoma *in situ* and particularly if these changes are bilateral, then radiation therapy is recommended. As this treatment will render the patient azoospermic, semen storage must again be undertaken prior to therapy. With the advent of ICSI, pregnancies can now be achieved using very small numbers of spermatozoa, so no matter how poor is the semen quality storage is still advised.

Another problem that can arise from the treatment of invasive carcinoma of the testis is ejaculatory failure that may be the result of para-aortic lymphadenectomy. Patients must be warned of this possible problem and storage of semen in such patients is also recommended.

There are thus many reasons to consider testicular cancer and its many-faceted relationship to male infertility.

References

Brown, L.M., Pottern, L.M., Hoover, R.N., Devesa, S.S., Aselton, P. & Flannery, J.T. (1986) Testicular cancer in the United States: trends in incidence and mortality. *International Journal of Epidemiology* **15**, 164–170.

Davis, S., Di Martino, N.A. & Schneider, G. (1981) Malignant interstitial carcinoma of the testis: report of two cases with steroid synthetic profiles, response to therapy and review of the literature. *Cancer* **47**, 425–431.

Forman, D. (1991) Aetiology of testicular cancers. In: *Urological Oncology: Dilemmas and Developments* (eds A.R. Alderson, R.T.D. Oliver, I.W.F. Hanham & H.J.D. Bloom), pp. 269–282. Wiley, Chichester.

Giwercman, A., von der Maase, H. & Skakkebaek, N.E. (1993) Epidemiological and clinical aspects of carcinoma *in situ* of the testis. In: *Management and Biology of Carcinoma in situ and Cancer of the Testis* (eds N.E. Skakkebaek, K.M. Grigor, A. Giwercman & M. Rorth) pp. 104–110. Karger, Basel.

Hendry, W.F.A., Hern, R.P., Hetherington, J.W., Peckham, M.J., Dearnley, D.P. & Horwich, A. (1993) Para-aortic lymphadenectomy for metastatic non-seminomatous germ cell tumours: prognostic value and therapeutic benefit. *British Journal of Urology* **71**, 208–213.

von der Maase, H., Rorth, M., Walbom-Jorgensen, S. *et al.* (1986) Carcinoma *in situ* in patients with contralateral testicular germ cell cancer. A study of 27 cases in 500 patients. *British Medical Journal* **293**, 1398–1401.

McLeod, D.G., Weiss, R.B., Stablein, D.M. *et al.* (1991) Staging relationships and outcome in early testicular cancer: a report from the testicular cancer inter-group study. *Journal of Urology* **145**, 1178–1183.

Ober, W.B., Kabakow, B. & Hecht, H. (1976) Malignant interstitial cell tumour of the testis: a problem in endocrine oncology. *Bulletin of the New York Academy of Medicine* **52**, 561–583.

Oliver, R.T. (1994) Testicular cancer (review). *Current Opinion in Oncology* **6**, 285–291.

Oliver, R.T., Stephenson, C.A., Parkinson, M.C. *et al.* (1986) Germ cell tumours of the testicle. A model for MHC influence on human malignancy. *Journal of Immunogenetics* **13**, 85–92.

Osterlind, A. (1986) Diverging trends in incidence and mortality of testicular cancer in Denmark 1943–82. *British Journal of Cancer* **53**, 501–505.

Richie, J.P., Birnholtz, J. & Garnick, M.B. (1982) Ultrasonography as a diagnostic adjunct for the evaluation of masses in the scrotum. *Surgery, Gynecology and Obstetrics* **154**, 695–698.

Schlegel, P.N. & Su, L.-M. (1997) Physiological consequences of testicular sperm aspiration. *Human Reproduction* **12**, 1688–1692.

Skakkebaek, N.E., Berthelsen, J.G., Giwercman, A. & Muller, J. (1987) Carcinoma *in situ* of the testis: Possible origin from gonocytes and precursor of all types of germ cell tumours except spermatocytoma. *International Journal of Andrology* **10**, 19–28.

Skakkebaek, N.E. (1972) Possible carcinoma *in situ* of the testis. *Lancet* **ii**, 516–517.

Williams, S.N., Jenkins, B.J., Badenoch, D.F., Fowler, C.G. & Oliver, R.T. (1989) Radical retroperitoneal node dissection after chemotherapy for testicular tumours. *British Journal of Urology* **63**, 641–643.

18: Physical Agents, Drugs and Toxins in the Causation of Male Infertility

Toxic agents are now becoming an important cause of infertility in the male. They may be presented to the patient either as a medication or be the result of pollution. They can act directly on the gonad itself or they may interfere with the normal function of the pituitary–hypothalamic axis.

Some pollutants may also disrupt procreation by their action on the steroid receptors. This activity may occur in the adult when both the transport and the production of the spermatozoa is interrupted or it may impact upon the male fetus *in utero* when development of the reproductive tract may be impaired. Other physical agents may also damage reproduction in the male and these include heat, irradiation and trauma.

Physical agents

Irradiation

Although the effects of radiation on the testis has been known for nearly a century, it was only after the development of atomic energy that this problem received any serious attention.

In 1964, McLeod and associates reported the exposure of men to irradiation after an accident at the Oakridge Nuclear plant and demonstrated azoospermia in more than half of them (McLeod *et al.* 1964). However, some 4 years later, the sperm counts in all of these men had returned to normal.

It is known that low sperm counts may be found in men who have undergone surgery and local irradiation for unilateral testicular tumours. However, at least some of these tumours are likely to be associated with a past history of maldescent and it is thus difficult to separate the effect of the maldescent from that of the therapy. It is now also known that the tumours themselves may interfere with sperm production.

Radiation has its main effect upon the spermatogonia, the B spermatogonia being the most sensitive. Thus, a change in the sperm count will only manifest itself when the more mature spermatozoa have been discharged into the ejaculate. This time lag between the action of the radiation and the loss of sperm from the ejaculate is known as the 'period of maturation depletion'. It would also appear that the more mature is the germ cell in the spermatogenic epithelium, the more resistant it is to the damaging effects of irradiation.

Irradiation also appears to have an effect on the Sertoli cell as damage to the spermatogenic epithelium will result in a rise in the serum FSH levels indicating a reduction in inhibin production by the Sertoli cell. A fall in the FSH level will herald recovery of the spermatogenic epithelium and a return of sperm to the ejaculate.

The effect of any radiation therapy will be dependent upon the dose; the greater the dose applied to the testes, the more rapid and more long lasting will be its effect. In most conditions requiring radiation to the groin area, the dose not exceed 6 Gy and the long-term prognosis is good.

In 1974, Rowley and colleagues (Rowley *et al.* 1974) reported on the effects of different doses of radiation on the spermatogenic epithelium. These authors found that in doses as small as 1–6 Gy damage to the spermatogonia frequently occurred and that in doses of 2–3 Gy loss of maturation of the spermatocytes occurred. This damage was visible on a testicular biopsy when the dose exceeded 4 Gy. Although histological evidence of recovery may be found as early as 6 months after treatment, even using relatively high doses of irradiation, the sperm count may take several years before sperm reappear in the ejaculate, and longer still before the semen analysis becomes normal. Thus, although in most patients their fertility will eventually return, it may be many years before this is achieved.

One of the major concerns about the effects of radiation on the gonad is the possible genetic effect that the radiation may have on the germ cells. However, an examination of the children of victims of the Hiroshima and Nagasaki bombs whose fathers had received around 200 rads of irradiation showed no increased incidence of congenital problems or of the childhood malignancies (Jablon & Kato 1971).

Thus, patients undergoing irradiation therapy that involves the groin area and who receive a radiation dose of below 6 Gy may continue to be fertile for several weeks after therapy. However, as soon as all the mature sperm have been ejaculated, the semen often becomes azoospermic and may remain azoospermic for several years before any recovery takes place.

As many testicular tumours and disorders such as Hodgkin's disease, which also may require irradiation in the lower abdomen, occur in young men who may be desirous of fertility, it is important that semen is cryopreserved prior to the start of any radiation therapy. If, however, such precautions are not taken, then the patient must be warned that provided the dose of radiation is less than 6 Gy recovery usually occurs but it may take several years before any such recovery will be seen.

Trauma

The role of trauma in testicular malfunction is difficult to assess. There is no doubt that trauma may result in a severe reduction in sperm production, but what proportion of abnormal sperm counts from men attending an infertility clinic are indeed induced by trauma is very difficult to assess. Trauma may occur more frequently among sportsmen and those involved in physical lifestyles (e.g. martial arts and team sports such as football).

Trauma may induce testicular ischaemia by either inducing a generalized oedema or by the generation of testicular haematoma. Either of these abnormalities will increase intratesticular pressure and, because of the lack of distensibility of the tunica albuginea, can easily reduce the venous drainage and then the arterial input to the testis. In the ram, even the ligation of a small artery on the surface of the testis can severely compromise the blood supply to the testis (Markey *et al.* 1995). In the human, the removal of a small testicular biopsy can result in the formation of a major haematoma that clearly must interfere with the blood supply to major areas of the testis (Schlegel & Su 1997).

Trauma to the genitalia may result in infertility, even when the injury occurs in children. It is clear that nearly 10% of all male children suffer significant trauma to the gonads prior to puberty (Finkelhor & Wolak 1995). However, how testicular trauma relates to infertility in the adult is not well understood.

It must also be remembered that trauma can also damage the epididymis. Injury may result in the formation of a haematoma around the epididymis resulting in a form of obstructive azoospermia, or to damage to a section of the epididymal duct that may interfere with its function. It would seem, however, that this type of epididymal pathology usually resolves with time and a return to fertility nearly always occurs.

It is, however, important that the occurrence of testicular trauma should be identified from all men attending the clinic with infertility and an abnormal sperm count. Attempts must be made to assess the severity of that injury from the history. Severe testicular trauma, however, may occur in association with multiple injury, when of course its presence may go unnoticed.

Heat

The testes and more importantly the cauda of the epididymis is situated outside the body so that it can be maintained at a temperature that is some 2–3 °C lower that that of the rest of the body. There is evidence in men with febrile illness that spermatogenesis may be reduced. Reduced temperatures in the scrotum are important in maintaining spermatogenesis at a normal level and to promote survival. It is probable that a reduced temperature also reduces the motility of the spermatozoa that are being stored in the cauda of the epididymis, thus increasing their potential lifespan. Increasing the temperature of the testis may thus result in infertility both by reducing sperm production and by interfering with normal sperm function.

There is even evidence now that heat applied to the testis experimentally may even interfere with the quality of any resulting embryo. If the scrotum of a ram is shaved and insulated so that the temperature of the testes is increased, embryo survival appears to be decreased (Mieusset *et al.* 1991).

It has been suggested for many years that tight underpants may result in infertility and that infertile men should convert to the use of boxer shorts. Indeed, there is no doubt that tight underpants, and even trousers, will increase the temperature of the scrotum but whether these factors will induce infertility is much more doubtful. However, many authors have suggested that cooling of the testes will improve fertility and devices based on evaporative cooling have been reported to achieve just that. However, their application has not been popular with the patients and their efficacy is far from proved.

There is, however, one aspect of testicular damage that may be associated with prolonged increase in temperature and that of course is the maldescended or cryptorchid testis. A maldescended testis is almost always abnormal, at least in terms of sperm production. There is no doubt that in experimental cryptorchidism, spermatogenesis is quickly impaired but in naturally occurring testicular maldescent other factors, including the presence of an inherently abnormal testis, may also play a role in the abnormal sperm production by these testes.

Chemotherapeutic agents

The use of chemotherapeutic agents in the treatment not only of cancer but of other conditions, including autoimmune disorders and a wide variety of other conditions, makes the use of these drugs increasingly common.

Cyclophosphamide

This is probably the most commonly prescribed chemotherapeutic agent of all. It is an alkylating agent that acts to inhibit tumour growth and also passes the blood–brain barrier as well as the blood–testis barrier. It also is markedly immunosuppressive. It is thus used in the treatment of many autoimmune diseases, especially systemic lupus erythematosus, as well as in the management of a wide variety of malignancies. It may also be used in children in the treatment of Type 1 nephritis. Cyclophosphamide may also be used as a component of combination chemotherapy in the treatment of conditions such as the lymphomas and leukaemia.

The damage done to the testis by this agent is dose dependent. In daily doses of 3.7 mg/kg, damage to spermatogenesis always occurs (Etteldorf *et al.* 1976; Hsu 1979) resulting in oligozoospermia or azoospermia and at this dose these changes may be permanent. Cyclophosphamide may also interfere with Leydig cell function and thus induce a reduction in the serum testosterone. However, it must be remembered that patients with many forms of cancer may already have an abnormal sperm count prior to treatment and this is of particular importance in men with testicular tumours.

Chlorambucil (Leukeran)

This agent is an aromatic nitrogen mustard that acts also as a bifunctional alkylating agent. It is used in the treatment of the lymphomas and the lymphatic leukaemias as well as in the control of the macroglobulinaemias. It may also be used as an agent in several regimes of combination chemotherapy.

This agent can also interfere with spermatogenesis and at doses of greater than 400 mg per day will frequently cause azoospermia. Recovery of spermatogenesis is variable and may occur. The time taken for a return to fertility is impossible to predict.

Doxorubicin (Adriamycin)

This chemotherapeutic agent acts by inhibiting nucleic acid synthesis and mitosis. It is used most commonly in the management of the haematological malignancies. It is also powerfully immunosuppressant. It is of particular use in tumours of the lung, stomach and liver. It may also be used in combination with other chemotherapeutic agents.

A total of 160–625 mg/m^2 will always induce oligozoospermia or even azoospermia (da Cunha *et al.* 1983). Recovery of spermatogenesis following this treatment does occur but it may take several years to reach completion.

Vinblastine

This is an alkaloid that is obtained from the plant *Vinca rosea*. It arrests cell growth at metaphase. It is used in the treatment of Hodgkin's disease, in mycosis fungoides, as well as Kaposi's sarcoma and even testicular cancer. Its use has been indeed shown to be associated with the development of azoospermia but the recovery rate of this infertility after cessation of treatment is unknown.

Vincristine

This is an alkaloid salt that is also obtained from a plant but this time from the periwinkle (*Cantharanthus roseus*). Its precise mechanism of action of this agent is unknown. Vincristine is used in the treatment of the acute leukaemias, both Hodgkin's disease as well as non-Hodgkin's lymphoma. It may also be used in the management of childhood cancers such as Wilms' tumour. Its effect on fertility has never been studied formally but, like vinblastine, it is known to induce azoospermia. Recovery of fertility occurs in some patients but it may take many months before any sperm reappear in the semen. When vincristine has been given to a prepubertal child, recovery in terms of future fertility is less likely than that seen in an adult.

Cisplatin and carboplatin

This agent is commonly used in the treatment of many different tumours including the lung, gastrointestinal tract, the liver and the testis. Its analogue, known as carboplatin, acts in a similar manner. These agents are heavy metal complexes with a central atom of platinum. Their action is not fully understood but they probably act as bifunctional alkylating agents. These drugs are administered intravenously as a single slowly administered bolus in doses of 400 mg/m².

Their action on the testis is not clear, but as they are powerfully nephrotoxic it is likely that these agents will seriously damage the testis and spermatogenesis.

Paclitaxil (Taxol)

This is a natural product that has antitumour activity and is used in the treatment of a wide variety of different cancers. When given in doses of 300 mg/m², paclitaxil will induce infertility. It is also known to induce chromosomal abnormalities in human lymphocytes. It thus may also be mutagenic in other mammalian cells and it is indeed known to be highly fetotoxic.

Docetaxol (Taxotere)

This antineoplastic substance is used in the treatment of several cancers including lung cancer. It promotes the assembly of tubulin into stable microtubules, thus reducing the amount of free tubulin needed in newly formed cells. It is known to induce testicular atrophy and Leydig cell hyperplasia in mice, and in total doses of around 100 mg/m² it will induce infertility and azoospermia in the human. Taxotere is also known to be fetotoxic.

Ifosfamide (Holoxan)

This is a synthetic alkylating agent that is an analogue of cyclophosphamide and it is also chemically related to the nitrogen mustards. It is used in the treatment of the lymphomas and the sarcomata. It will induce infertility and a severe reduction in the sperm count after a total dosage of 8–10 g/m².

Etoposide

This substance is extracted from the plant *Podophyllum peltatum* and its antitumour effect is based on its ability to arrest the cell cycle at late S or G2 phases. It is used in the treatment of lung cancer, the lymphomas and also the leukaemias.

Etoposide is known to interfere with spermiogenesis in the monkey and reduces testis weight in the rat. It is also highly embryotoxic.

319

Bleomycin sulphate

The antitumour activity of this substance depends upon the single- and double-stranded breaks that it induces in DNA. It is thus an antineoplastic antibiotic. It is used in the treatment of the lymphomata, in renal tumours and in the management of mycosis fungoides. It may well reduce the sperm count and interfere with sperm maturation but its effect on fertility is unclear.

Melphalan (Alkeran)

This is an alkylating agent that is employed in the treatment of metastatic malignant melanoma. This agent is highly mutagenic and induces chromosomal aberrations. It is known to reduce spermatogenesis and this effect can result in temporary or even permanent sterility.

Methotrexate

This antineoplastic substance acts as an antimetabolite because of its anti-folate activity. Although it is best known for its use in the treatment of trophoblastic disease, methotrexate is also of value in the management of the leukaemias and in Burkitt's lymphoma. It is also commonly used in the control of the skin condition psoriasis.

Methotrexate is known to induce chromosomal damage and these aberrations may persist long after the cessation of treatment. There is little information concerning its effects on fertility and spermatogenesis.

Estramustine (Estracyte)

This is a compound made up of a molecule of estradiol and a nitrogen mustard. It was at one time widely used in the treatment of prostate cancer but has now largely been superseded by the antiandrogens and the gonadotrophin-releasing hormone analogues. Its actions on spermatogenesis are not clearly defined but it will reduce gonadotrophin secretion and thus is very likely to have an effect on sperm production. It has had a reputation in the past of inducing impotence and it may also produce gynaecomastia.

Azothiaprine

The exact mode of action of azothiaprine is not clear but it probably acts as an alkylating agent. It is also a powerful immunosuppressant that is used in the treatment of autoimmune disease, in particular in the management of lupus erythematosus and in the control of organ rejection following transplantation.

It is highly teratogenic in the rabbit but does not appear to have any such effects in the human. Its effect on fertility in the human appears to be minor.

Combination chemotherapy

A number of regimes are at present in use and these include CVP (cyclophosphamide, vincristine and prednisone) and MOPP (estramustine, procarbazine, vincristine and prednisolone). The combination known as MVPP (estramustine, vincristine, prednisolone and procarbazine) is, however, hardly ever used today. All these combinations will result in infertility by interfering with spermatogenesis. The sperm count will fall and the serum FSH and even the serum LH may be raised. As more than one agent is involved, infertility is the rule after treatment with these combinations and recovery is much less frequent.

Overall, the damage sustained by the testes as the result of this form of treatment relates not only to the agent used but also to the dose of drug used and its duration.

Chemotherapy in prepubertal boys

Some years ago, the testes of prepubertal boys were believed to be much less sensitive to the damaging effects of chemotherapeutic agents (Schalet 1980). Such results suggested that protection of the adult gonad might be achieved by the use of gonadotrophin-releasing hormone analogues (Glode *et al.* 1981).

However, more recently these suggestions have been disputed as no consistent reduction in spermatogenic damage by chemotherapy can be detected in young boys. The administration of these analogues to beagle dogs did not protect these animals from the testicular damage induced by chemotherapy; indeed, the analogues appeared to enhance these changes (Goodpasture 1987). It would seem therefore that the testes in children are just as susceptible to chemotherapeutic damage in the same way as those of the adult. In children under treatment with vincristine, the resultant testicular damage may in fact be even more severe than that in the adult.

The abuse of drugs and their effect on fertility in the male

Fertility is dependent upon a large number of different factors including the many hormonal changes that are influenced and induced by many of the commonly used illicit drugs.

Marijuana

The active ingredients in the smoke of the dried marijuana plant are a group of agents known as the cannabinoids. The major psychoactive ingredient of this group of chemicals is δ9-tetrahydrocannabinol (THC). A single marijuana cigarette will contain some 20 mg of THC.

Smoking a marijuana cigarette will cause a reduction in the secretion of the gonadotrophins as well as inducing a reduction in the levels of prolactin within 60–90 min of its inhalation (Smith & Asch 1987). This action is thought to take place at the hypothalamus rather than at the level of the pituitary as, at least in women, smoking marijuana reduces LH secretion (Mendelson *et al.* 1986). As a consequence, THC may reduce the levels of testosterone in serum, especially in heavy users (Kolodny *et al.* 1974), and these workers have also demonstrated that such individuals showed sperm counts that were below 30 million per mL.

Studies in both the rat and the dog demonstrate that chronic treatment with THC will result in decreased testis size and abnormal sperm morphology. The cannabinoids have also been shown to reduce protein and nucleic acid synthesis and also inhibit glucose metabolism in the testis. There is also some evidence in nonvertebrate sperm that the cannabinoids may inhibit the acrosome reaction.

Thus, heavy users of marijuana are likely to induce some degree of infertility in the male, but it would appear that infertility of any severity such as azoospermia is not likely to be caused by THC.

Heroin and morphine

It is known that individuals who are addicted to the opiates are often infertile and the men may also suffer from sexual dysfunction of varying severity.

A number of different effects of the opiates have been described in relation to reproduction. The opiates will reduce the levels of FSH and LH in serum and these depressions of gonadotrophin secretion will last for 2–3 h (Wang *et al.* 1978). This will lead to a reduction in serum testosterone, which can be counteracted by the administration of hCG, thus suggesting that there is no direct effect of these narcotics on the testis itself. The opiates will also stimulate the production of prolactin, which may interfere with testosterone production (Van Vugt *et al.* 1979).

Cocaine

Cocaine is a central nervous system stimulant. As it is frequently used alongside heroin, it can be difficult to predict its activity in an individual. Cocaine in moderate doses will reduce both the serum LH and the serum prolactin in the primate. There are, however, no major studies on the reproductive effects of cocaine in the human. However, it has been suggested that abnormal sperm counts twice as common among cocaine users than among nonusers (Bracken *et al.* 1990).

Alcohol

Alcohol will also have an effect on reproductive function. The primary effect of alcohol appears to be on the testis itself, as alcohol does not appear to reduce gonadotrophin secretion. The major endocrine effect of alcohol is on Leydig cell function, which results in a reduction in testosterone synthesis. Both alcohol and its metabolites inhibit testicular enzymes involved in testosterone production (Johnston *et al.* 1981).

Once the alcohol addiction has induced cirrhosis of the liver, then the effects of unmetabolized oestrogen start to have an effect resulting in the suppression of gonadotrophin secretion and the generation of oestrogen effects such as gynaecomastia. The reduction in testosterone secretion will also be manifest in the altered function of the accessory glands of the male genital tract.

Alcohol can also induce impotence and disordered ejaculation by its direct action on the spinal reflex centres. Chronic alcoholism can lead to permanent impotence.

Alcohol may also induce changes in the morphology of spermatozoa (Dixit *et al.* 1976), and semen samples from alcoholic men will also show a greatly increased incidence of abnormal forms (Lester & Van Thiel 1977).

Caffeine

Caffeine may also interfere with fertility but its mode of action is unclear. Caffeine is thought to have an unfavourable effect upon reproduction (Gerhard & Runnebuam 1992), but how this effect is brought about is unclear.

Nicotine

Nicotine is also known to have an adverse effect on fertility and it may act in several different ways.

First, it may reduce the sperm count and increase the frequency of morphologically abnormal sperm in a semen sample. Nicotine may also worsen infertility due to other causes, an example of which is the 'cofactor' effect between the presence of a varicocele and cigarette smoking (Peng *et al.* 1990).

Second, cigarette smoking also has an important relationship with the incidence of erectile failure (Gilbert *et al.* 1986). This effect is a result of the direct action of nicotine on the erectile tissue but in the long term is also likely to act by the induction of arteriosclerosis, causing a reduction of the blood flow in the penile artery.

Anabolic steroids

These agents are frequently used by athletes to increase muscle bulk and are predominately used by individuals involved in weightlifting and power sports. The incidence of their use among men who attend gymnasia appears to be high (Korkia & Stimson 1997). As these agents are scheduled drugs that can only be obtained with a prescription, there is an extensive black market in such drugs, and athletes often use veterinary preparations and preparations that may have been 'cut' or that contain additives such as testosterone itself.

For reasons that are not entirely clear, the anabolic steroids induce hypogonadotrophic hypogonadism and at times the suppression of gonadotrophin secretion can be both profound and prolonged. Uncommonly, the suppression of gonadotrophin secretion can be permanent.

Such men therefore often attend infertility clinics, where they are frequently found to be azoospermic or severely oligozoospermic with unmeasurable serum gonadotrophins and very low serum testosterone levels. These men may thus also complain of reduced libido and even of erectile failure.

Some of these men may also show complications of the injection procedures themselves, and they may also present with infected injection sites or nerve palsy (Evans 1997) from faulty siting of the injection. Anabolic steroid abuse can also result in cardiomyopathy (Ferrara *et al.* 1997) and other forms of cardiac disease (Palatini *et al.* 1996) and more rarely can also give rise to mononeuropathies of the upper body (Mondelli *et al.* 1998). Prolonged use of anabolic steroids may also give rise to abnormal personality traits (Cooper *et al.* 1996). As testosterone is converted to estradiol, gynaecomastia is a common complication of this form of drug abuse.

The best treatment of the infertility associated with this condition is by the use of hCG. A dose of hCG of 2000 U intramuscularly twice weekly will restore spermatogenesis in most patients, but the time taken to achieve a normal sperm count and fertility is very variable.

As the suppression of the secretion of the endogenous gonadotrophins is prolonged, these men will need testosterone replacement when fertility is not needed as testosterone therapy is much cheaper and much less demanding in time than the continued use of hCG. These patients may be given subcutaneous testosterone pellets or intramuscular injections of testosterone enanthate at monthly intervals. The gynaecomastia may also need surgical correction.

Central nervous system stimulants

There are a variety of agents that stimulate the central nervous system and which are subject to abuse. These include lysergic acid diethylamide (LSD), the amphetamines and the drug known as Ecstasy. The action of these drugs is frequently life threatening and, as a consequence, their effects on fertility have never been studied.

Commonly used drugs that may cause infertility

Nitrofurantoin

In the past, a reduction in sperm count in response to the administration of nitrofurantoin has been demonstrated in the rat as well as in the human. However, the reduction in sperm numbers after such treatment is short lived and is unlikely to result in any significant degree of infertility.

Cimetadine

Cimetadine is an H_2 receptor antagonist that is commonly used in the treatment of peptic ulcer. This drug is capable of binding to cytosolic androgen receptors, thus antagonizing the action of dihydrotestosterone. Any infertility caused by this agent is short lived and is quickly reversed after withdrawal of this drug.

Sulfasalazine (Salazopyrine)

This agent is now a very common treatment for various forms of inflammatory bowel disease, in particular in the control of ulcerative colitis. It was first identified as a possible cause of infertility more than 10 years ago (Levi *et al.* 1979). This agent will reduce the sperm concentration together with changes in both sperm motility and morphology in around 70% of all those receiving this therapy (Birnie *et al.* 1981). The drug may also alter the head size of the sperm (Hudson *et al.* 1982). Very long-term therapy may also be associated with a reduction in the serum testosterone (Ragni *et al.* 1984). It appears that it is the sulfapyridine moiety of the sulfasalazine that is the cause of the changes in the semen analysis (O'Morain *et al.* 1984). It may act as an antifertility agent, both by its antiprostaglandin effect on sperm motility, and its antifolate action on spermatogenesis.

However, removal of the drug will rapidly restore the sperm count and the patient's natural fertility to normal. Among patients with severe ulcerative colitis for whom therapy is essential, the sulfasalazine may be replaced with treatment using mesalazine, which seems to have less effect on spermatogenesis.

Phenytoin

This anticonvulsant is known to reduce sperm counts probably by its action in reducing FSH levels (Stewart-Bentley *et al.* 1976). The other anticonvulsants such as phenobarbital and valproate do not have such effects.

Sex steroids

Both oestrogen and testosterone when administered in large doses will suppress gonadotrophin secretion and thus will greatly interfere with spermatogenesis. Indeed, therapy with intramuscular testosterone compounds such as testosterone proprionate (Sustenon, Organon Australia) will render a patient azoospermic within a few weeks.

GnRH analogues and the antiandrogens

These agents, which are frequently used in the treatment of metastatic prostate cancer, will reduce gonadotrophin secretion and thus will ablate sperm production. Examples of the gonadotrophin-releasing hormone analogues include goserelin and leuprolide acetate while antiandrogens that are used in this context include flutamide and cyproterone acetate. As the majority of patients with prostate cancer are not in need of fertility, these side effects are of little consequence.

Gossypol

This agent is a phenolic compound that is extracted from the cotton plant. It has been used, particularly in China, as a male contraceptive for many years. The manner in which this substance reduces the sperm count remains uncertain, although it is known to reduce the testicular production of testosterone by the Leydig cells. Its major side effect is the induction of hypokalaemia.

The heavy metals

The heavy metals are also toxic to the testis and poisoning with these metals may result in infertility. Most frank poisonings with heavy metals are today either the consequence of industrial accidents or the result of a suicide attempt.

Lead

Lead has been known to reduce fertility for many years and indeed has been blamed for the fall of the Roman civilization. In those times, the Romans used lead salts as sweeteners in food and drinks.

Today, most frank lead poisoning is acquired in the workplace. In a report in which men exposed to lead in their occupation were studied, it was clear that increasing lead levels correlated with decreased libido and increasing abnormalities of the semen analysis (Lancranjan *et al.* 1975). Interestingly, no change in serum testosterone was noted in these men. However, in severely lead-poisoned men, the serum testosterone level can indeed be reduced (Braunstein *et al.* 1978). Lead poisoning may also have other endocrine effects and these include reduced glucocorticoid secretions and defects in thyroid function (Cullen *et al.* 1984). As a consequence of these changes, changes in the semen analysis may also occur (Lerda 1992).

Animal studies would seem to confirm the toxic effect of lead upon the reproductive system. Excess lead ingestion may result in a reduction in sperm production, testicular weight and give rise to reduced sexual activity (Eyden *et al.* 1978). Lead may have an action on the FSH receptors, thus interfering with spermatogenesis (Weibe *et al.* 1983). In animal studies, major endocrine changes have been observed, especially in relation to a reduction in both LH and testosterone secretion (Thoreux-Manley *et al.* 1995) as well as FSH (Sokol *et al.* 1985).

Today great care is taken to avoid exposure to lead and thus infertility due to frank lead poisoning is likely to be rare.

Cadmium

Cadmium is well known as a testicular toxin and the various salts of cadmium will induce severe damage to the spermatogenic epithelium in the experimental animal (Boscolo *et al.* 1985). The effect of cadmium on the testis appears to be manifest in the Sertoli cells, which show major changes on electron microscopy. Cadmium may also interfere with the normal functions of the mitochondrial enzymes.

Poisoning with cadmium is a rare event and it would probably cause similar damage to the spermatogenic epithelium in the human as it does in the rodent or the guinea-pig (Suzuki *et al.* 1978).

Mercury

Following the heavy mercury pollution of Minamata Bay in Japan that took place in 1968, a considerable amount is known about the distribution of mercury both in the rat but also in the human.

Mercury is a metal that concentrates in the kidney, the cerebellum and the testes. Mercury poisoning will therefore result in neurological disturbances, renal failure and of course infertility (Eto 1997). In Victorian times hat makers used mercury to clean the felt used in hat making, and hatters thus frequently became poisoned. The shaking disorder that the mercury induced in these unfortunate individuals has been immortalized by the Mad Hatter in Lewis Carroll's *Alice's Adventures in Wonderland*.

Mercury will interfere with spermatogenesis but may also have an effect upon the epididymis as well. The disorder known as 'Pink disease' was a form of mercury poisoning in children that gave a red coloration to their gums. It has been suggested that this may have caused the condition known as Young's syndrome, which is associated with an obstructive lesion in the upper epididymis (Hendry *et al.* 1993).

Other heavy metals

There are also a number of heavy metals in some forms of folk medicines, especially those from the Indian subcontinent; indeed, in India one local medicine which is supposed to resolve infertility contains significant quantities of both arsenic and antimony, both of which are toxic to the spermatogenic epithelium.

Welding and infertility

It has been suggested that the incidence of infertility may be increased in men who use arc-welding as a livelihood (Bonde 1990). Indeed, arc-welding appears to induce a reduction in semen quality (Mortenson 1988). Whether this infertility relates to the inhalation of unburnt acetylene in the gas mixture or whether it relates to the presence of heavy metals in a gaseous form that are chronically inhaled or ingested by the individual performing the welding is quite unknown.

Drug-induced hyperprolactinaemia

Many drugs have the ability to inhibit the secretion of dopamine or antagonize its action. The major effect of prolactin production is to reduce LH secretion, and for this reason hyperprolactinaemia will result in reduced secretion of testosterone. Drugs that markedly elevate serum prolactin include the opiates, the opiate antagonists, the hypotensive agents and chlorpromazine.

Insecticides

The insecticides such as the organochlorides and carbamate, although they cause serious neurological problems, have no known gonadal effects. However, the nematocide dibromodichloropropane (DBCP), which is used particularly to protect the pineapple from a weevil that attacks the roots of this plant, is very toxic to the gonad and may even cause azoospermia after very long-term exposure (Biava *et al.* 1978).

Other agents such as polychlorinated biphenyls (PCB) and dimethyl-2-dichlorvinyl phosphate (DDVP) are also known to be highly gonadotoxic and exposure to these agents has been shown to produce marked testicular changes in the experimental animal (Dikshith *et al.* 1974; Krause & Homola 1974).

The commonly used insecticide dichlorodiphenyltrichloroethane (DDT) may itself have little effect on sperm function but its oestrogenic metabolite dichlorodiphenylethane (DDE) may suppress the spermatogenic epithelium in the human and certainly has had a major effect on wildlife where, in the environment, it has become concentrated in certain parts of the food chain. Other oestrogenic agents, such as chlordecone, dioxin and some of the combustion products of the polycarbonate plastics, may also affect sperm production.

Solvents

The ethylene glycols used in the printing industry and also found in paints may also interfere with spermatogenesis. Indeed an increased incidence of oligozoospermia was demonstrated in a group of shipyard painters whose paints contained these solvents (Hardin 1983).

Exposure to perchlorethylene (PCE) used in the dry cleaning industry may also be a cause of a reduced sperm count, although this effect is not likely to be severe.

It is thus clear from the above that there are many agents that interfere with spermatogenesis and will reduce the sperm count, often to a point where infertility or even sterility is the result. It is thus important that drug therapy together with the occupational details of each male patient form a very important part of the clinical history.

References

Biava, C., Smuckler, E. & Whorton, D. (1978) The testicular morphology of individuals exposed to dibromochloropropane. *Experimental Molecular Pathology* **29**, 448–458.

Birnie, G.G., McLeod, T.I. & Watkinson, G. (1981) Incidence of suphasalazine-induced male infertility. *Gut* **22**, 452–455.

Bonde, J.P. (1990) Subfertility in relation to welding. A case reference study among male welders. *Danish Medical Bulletin* **37**, 195–108.

Boscolo, P., Sacchettoni-Logroscino, G., Ranelletti, F.O., Gioia, A. & Carmignani, M. (1985) Effects of long term cadmium exposure on the testes of rabbits: ultrastructural study. *Toxicology Letters* **24**, 145–149.

Bracken, M.B., Eskanazi, B., Sachse, K., McSharry, J.-E., Hellenbrand, K. & Leo-Summers, L. (1990) Association of cocaine use with sperm concentration, motility and morphology. *Fertility and Sterility* **53**, 315–322.

Braunstein, G.D., Dahlgren, J. & Loriaux, D.L. (1978) Hypogonadism in chronically lead poisoned men. *Infertility* **1**, 33–51.

Cooper, C.J., Noakes, T.D., Dunne, T., Lambert, M.I. & Rochford, K. (1996) A high prevalence of abnormal personality traits in chronic users of anabolic–androgenic steroids. *British Journal of Sports Medicine* **30**, 246–250.

Cullen, M.R., Kayne, R.D. & Robins, J.M. (1984) Endocrine and reproductive dysfunction in men associated with occupational inorganic lead intoxication. *Archives of Environmental Health* **39**, 431–440.

da Cunha, M.F., Meistrich, M.L. & Ried, H.L. (1983) Acute active sperm production after cancer chemotherapy with doxirubicin. *Journal of Urology* **130**, 927–930.

Dikshith, T.S., Rockwood, W. & Coulston, F. (1974) Effects of polychorinated biphenyl (Aroclor 254) on rat testes. *Experimental Molecular Pathology* **22**, 376–385.

Dixit, V.P., Agarwal, M. & Lohiya, N.K. (1976) Effects of a single ethanol injection into the vas deferens on the testicular function of rats. *Endokrinologie* **67**, 8–13.

Eto, K. (1997) Pathology of Minamata disease. *Toxicologic Pathology* **25**, 614–623.

Etteldorf, J.N., West, C.D., Pitcock, J.A. & Williams, D.L. (1976) Gonadal function, testicular histology and meiosis following cyclophosphamide therapy in patients with nephrotic syndrome. *Journal of Paediatrics* **88**, 206–212.

Evans, N.A. (1997) Local complications of self administered anabolic steroid injections. *British Journal of Sports Medicine* **31**, 349–350.

Eyden, B.P., Maisin, T.R. & Mattelin, G. (1978) Long term effects of dietary lead acetate on survival, body weight and seminal cytology in mice. *Bulletin of Environmental Contamination and Toxicology* **19**, 266–272.

Ferrara, P.C., Putnam, D.L. & Verdile, V.P. (1997) Anabolic steroid use as the possible precipitant of dilated cardiomyopathy. *Cardiology* **88**, 218–220.

Finkelhor, D. & Wolak, J. (1995) Nonsexual assaults to the genitalia in the youth population. *Journal of the American Medical Association* **274**, 1692–1697.

Gerhard, I. & Runnebuam, B. (1992) Harmful substances and infertility. Substances of abuse. *Geburtshilfe und Frauenheilkunde* **52**, 509–515.

Gilbert, D.G., Hagen, R.L. & D'Agostino, J.A. (1986) The effects of cigarette smoking on human sexual potency. *Additive Behaviours* **11**, 431–434.

Glode, L.M., Rolinson, J. & Gould, S.F. (1981) Protection from cyclophosphamide-induced testicular damage with an analogue of gonadotropin-releasing hormone. *Lancet* **1**, 1132–1134.

Goodpasture, J.C. (1987) Potentiation of the gonadal toxicity of cyclophosphamide in the dog by adjuvant treatment with an LRH agonist. *Journal of Andrology* **8**, 30–35.

Hardin, B.D. (1983) Reproductive toxicity of the glycol ethers. *Toxicology* **27**, 91–102.

Hendry, W.F.A., Hern, R.P. & Cole, P.J. (1993) Was Young's syndrome caused by exposure to mercury in childhood? *British Medical Journal* **307**, 1579–1582.

Hsu, A.C. (1979) Gonadal function in males treated with cyclophosphamide for nephrotic syndrome. *Fertility and Sterility* **3**, 173–177.

Hudson, E., Dore, C., Sowter, C., Toovey, S. & Levi, A.J. (1982) Sperm size in patients with inflammatory bowel disease on sulfasalazine therapy. *Fertility and Sterility* **38**, 77–84.

Jablon, S. & Kato, H. (1971) Sex ratio in offspring of survivors exposed prenatally to the atomic bombs in Hiroshima and Nagasaki. *American Journal of Epidemiology* **93**, 253–258.

Johnston, D.E., Chiao, Y., Gavaler, J.S. & Van Wiel, D.H. (1981) Inhibition of testosterone synthesis by ethanol and acetaldehyde. *Biochemistry and Pharmacology* **30**, 1827–1831.

Kolodny, R.C., Master, W.H., Kolodner, A.B. & Toro, G. (1974) Depression of plasma testosterone levels after chronic intensive marijuana use. *New England Journal of Medicine* **290**, 872–874.

Korkia, P. & Stimson, G.V. (1997) Indications of prevalence, practice and effects of anabolic steroid use in Great Britain. *International Journal of Sports Medicine* **18**, 557–562.

Krause, W. & Homola, S. (1974) Alteration of the seminiferous epithelium and the Leydig cells of the rat testes after IM application of dichlorvos (DDVP). *Bulletin of Environmental Contamination and Toxicology* **2**, 429–247.

Lancranjan, I., Popescu, H.I., Gavanescu, O., Klepsch, I. & Serbanescu, M. (1975) Reproductive ability of workman occupationally exposed to lead. *Archives of Occupational Health* **30**, 396–401.

Lerda, D. (1992) Study of sperm characteristics in persons occupationally exposed to lead. *American Journal of Industrial Medicine* **22**, 567–571.

Lester, R. & Van Thiel, D.H. (1977) Gonadal function in chronic alcoholism. *Advances in Experimental Medicine & Biology* **85A,** 399–413.

Levi, A.J., Fisher, A.M., Hughes, L. & Hendry, W.F. (1979) Male infertility due to sulphasalazine. *Lancet* **2**, 276–278.

Markey, C.M., Jequier, A.M., Meyer, G.T. & Martin, G.B. (1995) Relationship between testicular morphology and sperm production following ischaemia in the ram. *Reproduction, Fertility and Development* **7**, 119–128.

McLeod, J., Hotchkiss, R.S. & Sitterson, B.W. (1964) Recovery of male fertility after sterilisation by nuclear radiation. *Journal of the American Medical Association* **187**, 637–641.

Mendelson, J.H., Mello, N.K., Ellingboe, J., Skupny, A.S.T., Lex, B.W. & Griffin, M. (1986) Marihuana smoking suppresses Luteinizing Hormone in women. *Journal of Pharmacology and Experimental Therapeutics* **237**, 862–866.

Mieusset, R., Quintana-Casares, P., Sanchez-Partida, L.G., Sowerbutts, S.F., Zupp, J.L. & Setchell, B.P. (1991) The effects of moderate heating of the testes and epididymides of rams by scrotal insulation on fertility and embryonic mortality in ewes inseminated with frozen semen. *Annals of the New York Academy of Sciences* **94**, 445–458.

Mondelli, M., Cioni, R. & Federico, A. (1998) Rare mononeuropathies of the upper limb in bodybuilders. *Muscle and Nerve* **21**, 809–812.

Mortenson, J.T. (1988) Risk for reduced sperm quality among metal workers, with special reference to welders. *Scandinavian Journal of Work, Environment and Health* **14**, 27–30.

O'Morain, C., Smethurst, P., Dore, C.J. & Levi, A.J. (1984) Reversible male infertility due to sulphasalzine: studies in man and rat. *Gut* **25**, 1078–1084.

Palatini, P., Giada, F., Garavelli, G. *et al.* (1996) Cardiovascular effects of anabolic steroids in weight-trained subjects. *Journal of Clinical Phamacology* **36**, 1132–1140.

Peng, B.C., Tomashevsky, P. & Nagler, H.M. (1990) The co-factor effect: varicocele and infertility. *Fertility and Sterility* **54**, 143–148.

Ragni, G., Bianchi Porro, G., Ruspa, M., Barrattini, G., Lombardi, C. & Petrilli, M. (1984) Abnormal semen quality and low serum testosterone in men with inflammatory bowel disease treated for a long time with sulfasalazine. *Andrologia* **16**, 162–167.

Rowley, M.J., Leach, D.R., Warner, G.A. & Heller, C.G. (1974) Effect of graded doses of ionising radiation on the human testis. *Radiation Research* **59**, 665–678.

Schalet, S.M. (1980) Effects of cancer chemotherapy on gonadal function of patients. *Cancer Treatment Reviews* **7**, 141–152.

Schlegel, P.N. & Su, L.-M. (1997) Physiological consequences of testicular sperm aspiration. *Human Reproduction* **12**, 1688–1692.

Smith, C.G. & Asch, R.H. (1987) Drug abuse and reproduction. *Fertility and Sterility* **48**, 355–373.

Sokol, R.Z., Madding, C.E. & Swerdloff, R.S. (1985) Lead toxicity and the hypothalamic-pituitary-testicular axis. *Biology of Reproduction* **33**, 722–728.

Stewart-Bentley, M., Virgi, A., Chang, S., Hiatt, R. & Horton, R. (1976) Effect of dilantin on FSH and spermatogenesis. *Clinical Research* **24**, 101A.

Suzuki, A., Kajimoto, N., Yanagawa, T., Sugimoto, J. & Nagata, M. (1978) A possible mechanism of infertility by acute cadmium intoxication. *Journal of Toxicological Sciences* **3**, 313–323.

Thoreux-Manley, A., Velez de la Celle, J.F., Olivier, M.F., Souffir, J.C., Masse, R. & Pinon-Lataillade, G. (1995) Impairment of testicular endocrine function after lead intoxication in the adult rat. *Toxicology* **100**, 101–109.

Van Vugt, D.A., Bruni, J.F., Sylvester, P.W., Chen, H.T., Iliri, T. & Meites, J. (1979) Interaction between opiates and hypothalmic dopamine on prolactin release. *Life Sciences* **24**, 2361–2367.

Wang, C., Chan, V. & Yeung, R.T.T. (1978) The effect of heroin addiction on pituitary-testicular function. *Clinical Endocrinology* **9**, 455–461.

Weibe, J.P., Salhanick, A.I. & Myers, K.I. (1983) On the mechanism of action of lead in the testis: *in vitro* suppression of FSH receptors, cyclic AMP and steroidogenesis. *Life Sciences* **32**, 1997–2005.

19: Donor Insemination in the Treatment of Male Infertility

The use of sperm to achieve a pregnancy without the occurrence of coitus has been used for some time: it is said that a pregnancy was achieved using sperm from a dead soldier during (or more likely after) the Battle of Waterloo. This, however, does, at this distance in time, seem somewhat fanciful and is likely not to be true. The ability to store semen by cryopreservation was first achieved by Polge and colleagues in 1949 who demonstrated the value of glycerol as a cryoprotectant of fowl spermatozoa (Polge *et al.* 1949). Glycerol and like substances dehydrate the spermatozoa and protect the cells from damage by ice crystals during the freezing process. However, the first pregnancy generated from cryopreserved semen was not reported until 1953 (Bunge & Sherman 1953).

Over the last 30 years, the use of donated sperm to achieve a pregnancy in a couple in whom there was an untreatable form of male infertility has become common.

However, over the last 5 years and with the development of the technique known as ICSI (Palermo *et al.* 1992), it is now possible to achieve pregnancies with only a few dozen sperm. For this reason, donor insemination is being used less and less frequently. However, there are also of course a number of men with primary testicular disease, particularly those with germinal aplasia, in whom no spermatozoa can be found either in the ejaculate or in a testicular biopsy. For such men, donor insemination is still the only option.

It must not be forgotten that some infertile couples, for personal or religious reasons, do not wish to undergo the process of IVF. Treatment by IVF is a prolonged, relatively invasive and expensive process and thus couples may choose the simpler option of donor insemination as a means of resolving their infertility. It must also be remembered, however, that there are individuals who, for personal or religious reasons, may find donor insemination unacceptable. The feelings of each couple on this matter must therefore be carefully evaluated by the clinician in the fertility clinic before coming to a decision concerning treatment.

Acceptability of donor insemination

The acceptability of donor insemination varies greatly between different ethnic groups on the world. Donor insemination is totally unacceptable to Muslim patients and is also banned by the Roman Catholic Church. However, many patients who do not have these religious restrictions frequently prefer, if possible, to use their own partner's sperm for the generation of a pregnancy, and with the advent of reproductive technology, this is becoming increasingly possible. Where IVF and ICSI are acceptable, the use of these techniques is becoming much more common and the use of donor insemination is also clearly becoming less frequent.

Motivation of the sperm donor

The motivation for a man to become a sperm donor varies greatly in different countries. In Australia, one cannot pay an individual to donate sperm but the clinics are allowed to provide him with generous token payments that are euphemistically called 'expenses'. In Australia therefore there is little doubt that the main motivation for sperm donation is financial. For individuals such as university students who exist on meagre grants, sperm donation may even be a means of survival and there is little doubt that payment does appear to assist in the recruitment of donors, especially when this donor programme is established in a university town or city.

Only in the United States is sperm donation run on a frankly commercial basis. Indeed, in one well-known clinic, famous people, including Nobel Prize winners, are recruited to be donors from which the recipients can select their own donor.

In many countries, however, no such commercial system exists. In France, donor insemination is controlled by a central government funded body know as the Fédération Française de Centres d'Etudes et de Conservation du Sperme Humain (CECOS). This organization only accepts sperm from men who already have fathered children and thus common sources of sperm for donation include vasectomy clinics and family planning clinics. Thus in France, no homosexual can act as a donor and there is no financial reward of any sort for a sperm donation in that country.

Until recently, the identity of the donor was in most places kept secret from the recipient. Indeed, for donor insemination there has been a longheld view that secrecy about sperm donation was not only essential but beneficial. Occasionally, the act of donation was also kept secret from the spouse but these attitudes are now clearly changing.

With the advent of the much more accurate identification of paternity as occurs with DNA testing, paternity can no longer be hidden; using this technology, a child can find out whether or not his social father is in fact his biological father. Some sad discoveries have now been made concerning paternity when an apparent biological parent has been approached to act as an organ donor only for the child to discover that his father is not his biological parent.

For such reasons, in the last 15 years, Sweden has insisted that donors are identified. Interestingly, this does not seem to have reduced the number of sperm donors that are being recruited (Daniels & Lalos 1995). However, it would seem that, although the donors do not appear to mind too much about being identified, it is indeed the potential parents and not the sperm donor who is desirous of anonymity. Many couples requiring donor insemination in Sweden now go to neighbouring countries such as Denmark or Belgium for treatment, where, as in most of the other countries in Europe, the identification of either the donor or the recipient does not occur. Likewise in Australia, it is becoming clear that couples who have successfully achieved a pregnancy by donor insemination are failing to report that conception so as to ensure anonymity for themselves.

The recruitment of sperm donors

Almost everywhere, sperm donors are recruited by some form of advertisement, and such inducements can be found in magazines, newspapers or even on television. Notices are often placed in universities and colleges to attract students and even members of the university staff.

Only in the US are members of the public approached personally, and these approaches often only involve famous people. Intellectual prowess seems to be highly valued in the US and hence the recruitment of Nobel laureates.

The assessment of a potential sperm donor

When a man offers his services as a sperm donor, he must first go through a fairly rigorous process of assessment.

The clinical history and examination

The individual is asked to attend the clinic where he undergoes a history taking and a clinical examination. From the clinical history, it is important to try to exclude any major genetic disorder in the donor or in his family. Lifestyle factors are now included in the clinical history and, because of the increased risk of human immunodeficiency virus (HIV) infection, sexually active homosexuals are usually excluded from acting as donors.

Any past history of sexually transmitted disease also usually excludes a man from acting as a sperm donor. The presence of genital herpes or genital warts, or a history of painful micturition or urethral discharge, must make a potential donor unacceptable. Such a history, which could suggest the past presence of a chlamydial infection, should also exclude sperm donation.

The clinical examination includes a general and neurological examination as well as a clinical examination of the genitalia. Testicular size together with the normality of the shape and consistency of the epididymis is ascertained. The presence of the vas must also be confirmed and in any donor who is over 40 years of age a rectal examination may be indicated.

Microbiological screening

Some clinics take urethral swabs to test for the possible presence of chlamydial infection (Nagel *et al.* 1986), *Trichomonas* or *Neisseria* infection in the genital tract in the donor. All these disorders can be transmitted to a woman during donor insemination.

The American Society of Reproductive Medicine now recommends that sperm donors are also screened for the presence of antibodies to the cytomegalovirus in their serum (American Fertility Society 1990), as this infection, if transmitted to a pregnant woman, can induce fatal lesions in the baby. The incidence of cytomegalovirus antibody among both the semen donors and the recipients also seem to be high (Prior *et al.* 1994).

All donors also need to be tested for HIV (Stewart *et al.* 1985), for the presence of antigens of hepatitis B (Berry *et al.* 1987) and of hepatitis C (McKee *et al.* 1996). In many donor insemination programmes, a white blood cell karyotypic analysis is also performed (Matthews *et al.* 1983).

Semen analysis and 'test' freeze

The next step is to carry out a semen analysis. It is also useful to carry out some sperm freezing tests on the semen. Some semen samples do not result in a very good post-thaw motility, and as all semen samples have to be cryopreserved today it is important to test each semen sample for a good motility after cryopreservation.

The quarantine of the semen samples

In the past, it was common to use fresh semen for donor insemination but after the onset of the acquired immune deficiency syndrome (AIDS) pandemic this practice clearly became dangerous. However, there persisted a belief that fresh semen was more fertile than frozen semen and gave an improved pregnancy rate. There is in fact little evidence that fresh semen in donor insemination has any advantage over semen that has been cryopreserved (Mortimer & Richardson 1982). However, the use of fresh semen persisted long after HIV had been identified as a major problem and as a result a number of women became unnecessarily infected with the HIV.

Today only frozen semen that has undergone a period of quarantine is used for donor insemination. After the initial hepatitis tests and the HIV test are found to be negative, several samples of semen are collected and cryopreserved. Most clinics have a special quarantine Dewar in which these samples are stored prior to their clearance. Until around 1988, these semen samples were held in quarantine, prior to use, for 3 calendar months. However, after a case was reported in the United Kingdom where an HIV-infected patient took 11 weeks to seroconvert, the quarantine period was extended to 6 months. It is likely that such a prolonged period prior to sero-conversion is very rare.

At the end of the 6-month period, i.e. 6 months after the last sample of semen from the donor has been cryopreserved, the donor is recalled and the HIV and the hepatitis B and C antigen tests are repeated. If these tests remain negative, the semen can then be released for use in a donor insemination programme.

The cryopreservation of semen

The cryopreservation of semen became a reality when in 1949, Polge and coworkers discovered that glycerol protected fowl spermatozoa from the otherwise lethal effects of freezing in liquid nitrogen. By applying a variety of different protocols based upon the use of glycerol, it became possible to cryopreserve the sperm of domestic animals and finally to achieve the cryopreservation of human sperm. The first human births using cryopreserved human sperm within a donor insemination programme were in fact reported in the 1950s, long before the onset of the AIDS epidemic.

Uses of cryopreservation of semen other than for donor insemination

The cryopreservation of semen can be used in contexts other than donor insemination.

'Absentee husbands'

There are many women whose husbands may work at some distance from home and may be away from their partners for several weeks at a time. This makes for great difficulties in the treatment of their infertility and for this reason, the semen can be cryopreserved and used either as an inseminate or within an IVF programme. This problem may produce difficulties when the semen is of poor quality as the cryopreservation will considerably reduce the viability of semen. This deterioration in semen quality following cryopreservation is particularly marked when the initial quality of the semen is poor; indeed, the cryopreservation of such abnormal semen may necessitate the application of ICSI rather than classic IVF.

Associated female disorders necessitating artificial insemination

In some female patients, such as those with hostile mucus intrauterine insemination may be needed to achieve conception. It is of course much better to use fresh semen for this purpose, but sometimes there are men who find the production of samples to order very difficult. Thus, the use of frozen semen may help in this respect.

Disorders and difficulties with ejaculation

In male patients with disorders of ejaculation or with difficulties in relation to the production of a semen sample, production of semen for artificial insemination may be unreliable. For this reason, it may be of value to store semen prior to its use.

Storage of semen prior to chemotherapy and/or radiation treatment

Tumours in the testis tend to occur in young men and these may, following surgery need treatment with either chemotherapy or radiation or even with both of these modalities. These treatments may render the patient azoospermic. Storage of semen samples prior to this type of therapy and their use for either insemination or IVF would avoid the need for the use of donated sperm to achieve a pregnancy.

Storage of semen prevasectomy

The incidence of unwanted vasectomy as a cause of infertility is now common, and it has been suggested that storage of semen by cryopreservation would avoid the need for a reversal and would overcome the infertility induced by failure of a vasectomy reversal. However, as vasectomy is now a very common procedure, the cost involved in storing semen and the storage space that would be needed to preserve semen from every man with vasectomy-related infertility would be enormous. Thus, the use of cryopreservation of semen in the prevention of vasectomy-related infertility is thus probably not feasible.

Oligozoospermia

At one time prior to the advent of assisted conception, the freezing of sperm was used in an attempt to increase the number of spermatozoa in the ejaculate from men with very low sperm counts. Such a procedure is, however, of no real value as sperm from severely oligozoospermic semen rarely survive the process of cryopreservation.

It must also be remembered that some conditions that cause male infertility, in particular primary testicular disease, are progressive. In such patients, the semen quality may gradually worsen, and if the disorder is severe, it may eventually render the patient azoospermic. Storage of sperm prior to this disaster may avoid the need for any surgical intervention or the collection of sperm from a testicular biopsy. It may even prevent the possible risk of failure to identify any sperm in a testicular biopsy.

The process of cryopreservation

Many regimes for freezing semen have been used in the past but the methods that are most commonly used should be both simple and cheap. Some clinics make use of complex and expensive equipment while others make use of much simpler methodology.

Cryoprotectants

These substances protect the spermatozoa from the effects of ice crystals by the osmotic extraction of the water from the cell. The first agent that was used for this purpose was glycerol and this substance remains the best agent for the cryopreservation of sperm. There have, however, been a number of cryoprotectants that have been used and these include propanediol (PROH) and dimethylsulphoxide (DMSO), but none is as good as glycerol in the cryoprotection of spermatozoa.

In the early days of sperm cryopreservation, cryoprotectants contained egg yolk, and examples of these preparations include TEST yolk buffer and TEST yolk–citrate medium. However, because of the need for fresh egg yolk in the preparation, these agents have now largely been abandoned. A well-known cryoprotective medium also containing egg yolk was a preparation known as the Carlberg–Matheson–Gemzell mixture. However, this has now also been superseded by a glycerol solution containing a number of different nutrients but without the presence of any egg yolk.

The cryoprotectant used by the author is relatively simple and consists of a medium containing glycerol and antibiotics (Table 19.1).

Semen containers used in sperm cryopreservation

As the rate of freezing must be uniform throughout the sample, the semen containers must have a small diameter and only hold a small volume of the semen–cryoprotectant mixture. Glass vials may be used in which 0.25–0.5 mL of the semen mixture may be frozen and stored.

Alternatively, straws may be used. These arrive from the manufacturers with one end sealed with a cotton-wool plug containing some dehydrated

Table 19.1 The formulation of the cryoprotectant used by the author in the cryopreservation of semen. No egg yolk is used in this preparation

Product	Quantity
Analar water	850 mL
Glycerol	150 mL
NaCl	5.8 g
KCl	0.4 g
Calcium lactate	0.76 g
Magnesium sulphate	0.12 g
Sodium dihydrogen phosphate	0.05 g
Sodium bicarbonate	2.6 g
Glucose	8.59 g
Fructose	8.59 g
Glycine	10.0 g
Hepes	4.77 g
Streptomycin	0.05 g
Penicillin	0.05 g

concrete powder. This plug allows air to pass through it that will facilitate the drawing up of the semen–cryoprotectant mixture. The powder fully seals the end of the straw on contact with fluid.

Each of these straws will hold some 0.25 or 0.5 mL of the cryoprotectant–semen mixture. These straws have the advantage that they are easy to handle and to store. They are manufactured in 10–15 different colours. Each straw is filled with the semen–cryoprotectant mixture using a 1-mL syringe attached to a small length of silastic tubing that is attached to each individual straw.

After loading with the semen–cryoprotectant mixture, the open end of each straw is sealed. This can be done by using a polyvinyl powder that polymerizes and seals the end of the straw on contact with moisture. These powders are also available in different colours, thus providing a second colour code that can make identification of individual straws within a Dewar of liquid nitrogen somewhat easier. Alternatively, each straw can be sealed using the proprietary preparation Cha-Seal (Chase Instruments, Georgia, USA), which seals the ends of the straw on freezing. An average semen sample, when diluted with cryoprotectant, will fill around 20 straws.

Preparation of the semen for cryopreservation

The sample of semen to be cryopreserved is placed in an incubator at 37 °C for 15–30 min to ensure total liquefaction and reduce viscosity. With samples that are very viscous, time in the incubator should be increased to 60 min.

The sample is then mixed in equal volume with the cryoprotectant solution. In order to avoid osmotic shock, which can cause death of the sperm, the cryoprotectant mixture must only be added drop by drop and gently swirled after each addition. When all the cryoprotectant has been added, gentle mixing is continued to ensure that the sperm have all achieved contact with the mixture.

A syringe is now attached to the concrete end of the straw and 0.5 or 0.25 mL of the semen–cryoprotectant mixture is drawn up into the straw. One must make sure that the semen mixture comes in direct contact with the closed end of the straw, i.e. there is no air bubble at the end of the straw. This will ensure wetting of the powders so producing an efficient seal. The distal end of the straw is now sealed with polyvinyl powder (or the Cha-Seal) and the straw accurately labelled. The straw and its contents are now ready for cryopreservation.

Labelling the straws for storage

It is of course very important that the straws are labelled very carefully and very accurately. This can be achieved in several different ways. Each straw can be labelled using special adhesive tags that are resistant to damage by the liquid nitrogen. The straws can also be bar-coded or the straws can also be identified using the colour-coding system provided by the straws themselves and the coloured polyvinyl powder.

Newer straws are now available that are double coated, allowing the label to be inserted within the straw itself. This innovation may help prevent any loss of labels from straws.

The freezing protocols that are used in the cryopreservation of sperm

The rate of freezing is very important in the cryopreservation of sperm. Complex equipment will do this very accurately but it is also possible to cryopreserve sperm using a hand-freezing method that is less controlled but is of course much cheaper to execute. Today in a human donor insemination clinic, controlled, reliable and repeatable methods of freezing are needed in order to maximize sperm survival and pregnancy rates. There are a wide variety of protocols that can be used to freeze sperm but the most commonly used regime is a simple one.

The straws are first placed in some handy container such as a beaker and placed in a refrigerator for 2–10 min. The straws will thus equilibrate to a temperature of 4 °C. The straws are then put in the freezer for a further 5–10 min to reduce their temperature to around –18 °C.

The straws are now suspended over a pool of liquid nitrogen to reduce their temperature to –70 °C, which is that of the vapour phase, for a further 5–10 min. The straws are then plunged into liquid nitrogen, reducing them to a temperature of –196 °C for permanent storage (Table 19.2).

Programmed freezing units

Although there are many complex programmable cryopreservation units that are commercially available today, many of these units are relatively expensive. The cryopreservation of spermatozoa is in fact simple and thus only simple piece of equipment is needed.

However, there are many laboratories that not only cryopreserve sperm but also store embryos, whose freezing protocols are much more complex

Table 19.2 A simple protocol for the cryopreservation of spermatozoa

1 Straws are placed in the refrigerator for 10 min and will equilibrate at 4 °C
2 Straws are placed in the freezer for 10 min and will equilibrate to a temperature of –18 °C
3 Straws are suspended over a pool of liquid nitrogen for 10 min to reduce their temperature to –70 °C
4 Straws are now plunged into liquid nitrogen reducing their temperature to –196 °C for permanent storage.

than are those that are applied to spermatozoa. A good compromise in this respect is the Cryo-Logic equipment (Cryo-Logic Ltd, Victoria, Australia), which is both simple and relatively inexpensive, and which can be used to cryopreseve many different types of tissue (Fig. 19.1).

Storage tanks for cryopreserved sperm

The most suitable tanks for use in a small laboratory are those of 34–40 L in volume. It is important to have narrow-necked tanks as this reduces the loss of liquid nitrogen each time the tank is accessed. In these tanks the straws are placed in small, divided containers within the liquid nitrogen and are suspended from the top of the tank for easy retrieval.

Each 40-L tank will hold around 14 000 straws and thus will be more than adequate for all but the largest donor insemination programmes (Fig. 19.2). For those clinics that run a donor programme where semen is collected prior to use, it is important to have a separate tank where semen that has not completed the quarantine period can be stored prior to its clearance for use within a donor programme. It is also of value to have a smaller Dewar containing only liquid nitrogen, which can be used as a 'top-up' for the main storage tank when necessary.

It is also useful to own a special Dewar known as a 'dry shipper'. These small tanks are lined with a metal mesh that traps the liquid nitrogen in its interstices and this reduces evaporation and also minimizes any spill of liquid nitrogen should the container be accidentally tipped over. The liquid

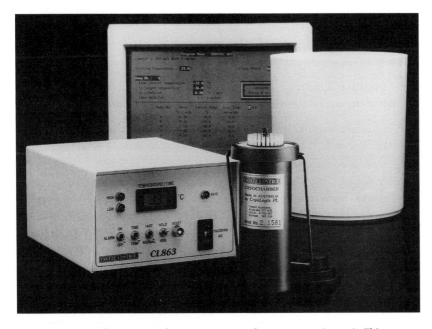

Fig. 19.1 A simple but very satisfactory programmed cyropreservation unit. This apparatus can be used in the cryopreservation of both spermatozoa and embryos.

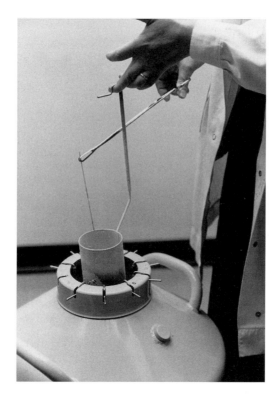

Fig. 19.2 The type of Dewar used by many laboratories for the cryopreservation and storage of semen.

nitrogen in these containers will last for 4–5 days. These containers are ideal therefore for the transport of semen both locally and even internationally. Most dry shippers can also be padlocked to prevent any tampering and damage to the stored semen contained within them.

Thawing the straws and the assessment of cryosurvival

The most commonly used method of thawing the straws either for use in insemination or for assessing the cryosurvival is by simply removing them from the liquid nitrogen and leaving them at room temperature for 10 min. Motility can be enhanced further by placing the straws in the incubator at 37 °C for another 10 min

After freezing any sample of semen it is important to assess its quality after thawing. The main damage done to a semen sample after freezing is the reduction in sperm motility A single straw is thawed in the manner described above, its motility estimated and compared with that prior to the freeze. This can be expressed as a cryosurvival factor, which is calculated as given below:

Cryosurvival factor = % motile sperm post-thaw/% motile sperm prefreeze

Consents in donor insemination

Those patients who can receive donated gametes will vary in different parts of the world. In some countries, sperm donation cannot be provided to unmarried female patients nor to women without male partners, such as lesbian women.

It is of course very important to obtain consent both for donation from the sperm donor and for the receipt of sperm from both the female patient and her spouse. In most countries where donor insemination is carried out, conception confers legal parenthood on the male partner, although interestingly, this was not the case in the UK until recently.

In most European countries, with the exception of Sweden, the anonymity of the donor and the recipient is maintained. In recent years in Sweden, the identity of both the donor and the recipient is known to both parties. This does not, however, seen to be acceptable to some Swedish recipients who appear to travel for donor insemination to other neighbouring countries in Europe. In other countries, Swedish patients can receive their donor insemination without having to reveal their identity to anyone, let alone to the donor.

Another major question in relation to donor insemination is the right (or otherwise) of the child to know of his biological origins. Until recently, children were not told that they were the product of sperm donation and could discover their biological origins in many unfortunate ways. In contrast to the old-fashioned method of paternity testing based on blood types only, it is now possible, using the DNA test, to determine paternity with unfailing accuracy. Children will thus be able to determine their biological paternity if they so wish.

Another time at which children conceived by sperm donation may learn of their paternity is in the area of organ donation and transplantation. Because of their genetic similarity, fathers are often approached to act as kidney donors for their male children. It is at this point that the children can discover the facts concerning their biological paternity. Problems such as these have caused many people to suggest that all children conceived by donor insemination should be informed of their origins, and some even advocate that the donor should meet all the children that his sperm donations have produced. In some countries, access to the identity of the donor is now mandatory and this has caused some difficulties with the recruitment of sperm donors.

Overall, it is likely that in the future there will be much more frankness between both the donor and recipient concerning sperm donation and the biological parentage of any children produced by this method. It is also likely that a small number of patients will continue to use donor insemination as a simple method of treatment of severe forms of male infertility and that the identification of both the donor and the recipient will become a reality in most countries of the world.

References

American Fertility Society (1990) New guidelines for the use of semen for donor insemination. *Fertility and Sterility* **53** (Suppl. 1), 65–71.

Berry, W.R., Gottesfield, R.L., Alter, H.J. & Vierling, J.M. (1987) Transmission of hepatitis B virus by artificial insemination. *Journal of Association* **257**, 1079–1081.

Bunge, R.G. & Sherman, J.K. (1953) Fertilizing capacity of frozen of human spermatozoa. *Nature* **172**, 767.

Daniels, K. & Lalos, O. (1995) The Swedish insemination act and the availability of donors. *Human Reproduction* **10**, 1871–1874.

Matthews, C.D., Ford, J.H., Peek, J.C. & McEvoy, M. (1983) Screening of karyotype and semen quality in an artificial insemination program: acceptance and rejection criteria. *Fertility and Sterility* **40**, 648–654.

McKee, T.A., Avery, S., Majid, A. & Brinsden, P.R. (1996) Risks for the transmission of hepatitis C during artificial insemination. *Fertility and Sterility* **66**, 161–163.

Mortimer, D. & Richardson, D.W. (1982) Sex ratio of births resulting from artificial insemination. *British Journal of Obstetrics and Gynaecology* **89**, 132–135.

Nagel, T.C., Tagetz, G.E. & Campbell, B.F. (1986) Transmission of *Chlamydia trachomatis* by artificial insemination. *Fertility and Sterility* **46**, 956–960.

Palermo, G., Joris, H., Devroey, P. & Van Steirteghem, A.C. (1992) Pregnancies after intracytoplasmic injection of a single spermatozoon into an oocyte. *Lancet* **340**, 17–18.

Polge, G., Smith, A.I.U. & Parkes, A.S. (1949) Revival of spermatozoa after vitrification and dehydration at low temperatures. *Nature (London)* **164**, 666.

Prior, J.R., Morroll, D.R., Birks, A.G., Matson, P.L. & Lieberman, B.A. (1994) The screening for cytomegalovirus in semen donors and recipients within a donor insemination programme. *Human Reproduction* **9**, 2076–2078.

Stewart, G.J., Tyler, J.P., Cunningham, A.L. *et al.* (1985) Transmission of human T-cell lymphotrophic virus type II (HTLV-II) by artificial insemination. *Lancet* **14**, 581–585.

20: The Role of IVF and Microassisted Fertilization in the Management of Male Infertility

With the discovery of IVF as a treatment of infertility, it was realized that far fewer sperm were required to fertilize an egg than were needed for insemination and for the generation of a natural pregnancy. It was thus not long after the first successful use of IVF in the management of tubal infertility that it became clear that this technology could be used in the management of infertility in the male (Trounson *et al.* 1981).

These techniques indeed seemed to be more successful than the other almost totally ineffective methods of management that were then available, particularly in attempting to overcome the problems associated with primary testicular disease, which is likely to be the most common cause of male infertility. Indeed, IVF was used for the management of infertility caused by reduced numbers of sperm or by abnormal sperm function. This did in fact produce pregnancies that would otherwise not have been generated but the overall results were, at least by today's standards, relatively poor.

There then appeared the first reports concerning the various techniques now known collectively as 'microassisted' fertilization (Fischel *et al.* 1994). Attempts were initially made to thin the zona pellucida and thus facilitate sperm penetration by techniques known as zona 'drilling' and zona 'cutting'. In the first of these, 2–3 μL of acid Tyrode's solution was injected onto a point on the surface of the zona causing the partial dissolution of the zona at that point. The second technique that was used to thin the zona involved slicing off a portion of the zona using a fine glass needle in a technique known as zona 'cutting' (Fig. 20.1). Although these techniques were quite successful in the mouse allowing good fertilization rates using only 5000 sperm per oocyte, the results in the human were poor.

Nearly 10 years ago, Fischel and colleagues devised the technique known as subzonal sperm injection (SUZI) (Fischel *et al.* 1990). In this procedure, sperm are injected into the perivitelline space using a micromanipulator. As many sperm are not functionally normal, the results of this technique were not good. As a consequence, more than one sperm was injected into the perivitelline space, and therefore this technique frequently resulted in polyspermic fertilization. Thus, what one gained in relation to fertilization was to some extent lost by the generation of polyspermic embryos.

The major change in success rates occurred in 1992 when Palermo and colleagues described the technique now known as intracytoplasmic sperm injection (ICSI) (Palermo *et al.* 1992). As the result of this advance

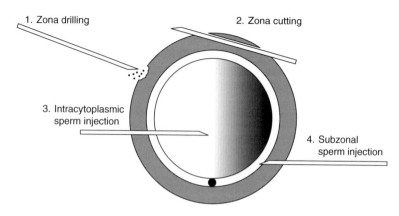

1. Zona drilling

2. Zona cutting

**3. Intracytoplasmic
sperm injection**

**4. Subzonal
sperm injection**

Fig. 20.1 A diagrammatic representation of the techniques of microassisted fertilization.

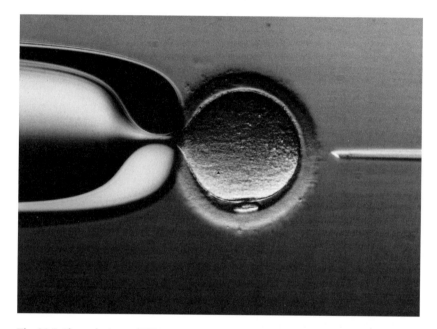

Fig. 20.2 The technique of ICSI.

(Fig. 20.2) there occurred a very major improvement in both fertilization rates and pregnancy rates in microassisted fertilization.

So successful has this treatment been that Palermo and colleagues have suggested that this technique could be used to treat all forms of male infertility (Palermo *et al.* 1995). Pregnancies are achieved using very few sperm in an ejaculate, and it is now of course possible to generate pregnancies using sperm that are taken from the upper regions of the epididymis (Silber 1998) and even using sperm harvested from the seminiferous tubules of the testis (Schoysman *et al.* 1993).

It now also seems possible to generate pregnancies from very abnormal sperm such as those with globozoospermia (Lundin *et al.* 1994; Liu *et al.*

1995) as well as using testicular sperm taken from the testes of men with Klinefelter's syndrome (Bourne *et al.* 1997). ICSI is also proving to be a very successful treatment for immunological infertility in the male whose spermatozoa show heavy binding to antisperm antibodies (Nagy *et al.* 1995a).

At present, it appears that it may also be possible to generate pregnancies using immature sperm in the form of both round and elongated spermatids. This has been performed with great success in the mouse (Kimura & Yanagamachi 1995a) but has not yet been so effective in generating pregnancies in the human (Tesarik 1996). Indeed, in the mouse, it has even been possible to produce live offspring following injection of the oocytes with only the nuclei of secondary spermatocytes (Kimura & Yanagamachi 1995b).

The impact of ICSI on the management of infertility, particularly in the male, has been enormous. The temptation, however, to use this technique for all forms of infertility has been very great. As a consequence, the more conventional approach to male infertility, namely the identification of the cause of the infertility and the application of simpler forms of treatment, is rapidly being abandoned. The lack of any form of diagnosis and with the absence of any idea about the aetiology of a particular patient's problem makes the identification of the many causes of male infertility virtually impossible and thus interferes with any attempt to prevent this disorder (Cummins & Jequier 1994).

The use of ICSI in this way may also result in medicolegal problems: if a patient finds at a later date that his infertility could have been treated in a simpler and less costly way, it may initiate a complaint against the clinician that leads to resolution through the courts.

Indications for the use of ICSI in the management of male infertility

There are now many reasons to use ICSI in overcoming the problems associated with an abnormal sperm count.

Primary testicular disease

This is likely to be the most common cause of infertility in the male and will present clinically with reduced testicular size and, not infrequently, with a raised serum FSH level. However, in some patients with this condition, these two parameters may be normal. The semen analysis may contain reduced sperm numbers, poor sperm motility or increased numbers of sperm showing an abnormal morphology. These abnormalities may be the sole cause of the infertility or may simply be contributing to a couple's childlessness by interacting with other problems in the female partner.

There is no known way of improving the semen analysis in men with this disease, and thus one must use the semen in the best way to achieve fertilization and embryogenesis. If the condition is severe enough, the only way to achieve pregnancy is by means of ICSI.

It must also be remembered that primary testicular disease is frequently progressive and thus the patients may have semen analyses that decline in quality so that eventually these men are azoospermic. Although it is usually best to use fresh semen in any IVF/ICSI attempt, it is not uncommon for a patient with primary testicular disease to unexpectedly produce an azoospermic semen sample. Should this happen at the time of the treatment by IVF/ICSI, the frozen samples can then be used without any problem to the patient.

When the primary testicular disease is severe enough, there may be too few sperm being produced to appear in the ejaculate. In this situation it may, however, be possible to find an occasional seminiferous tubule containing sperm that can be used within an IVF/ICSI cycle. These tubules may be difficult to find and it may require several biopsies before any sperm can be retrieved and indeed if the testes are very small and the serum FSH very raised, no sperm may be found. The damage that may be done to the testes by repeated biopsies in the past must not be forgotten (Schlegel & Su 1997).

It is in these patients that immature sperm, such as elongated or round spermatids, have been injected into the oocytes in an attempt to generate a pregnancy. The round spermatids are, however, very difficult to differentiate from lymphocytes. It is the problem in finding the round spermatids within a testicular biopsy that probably greatly contributes to the high failure rate associated with the injection of immature sperm in men with primary testicular disease.

Obstructive lesions of the male genital tract

This is today a very common reason to use IVF/ICSI. In these conditions, the sperm may have to be retrieved from the testes, the epididymis or from the vas deferens.

In men with rete testis obstruction, testicular sperm must be collected by means of a testicular biopsy, but in this condition and in the absence of a second pathology copious numbers of sperm can usually be harvested.

In men with epididymal lesions, the sperm may have to be collected from the upper epididymis where the ability of sperm taken from this site to fertilize an egg is very reduced. Interestingly, among patients with obstructive lesions involving the epididymis, reasonable sperm motility may be present.

Among patients with vasal or ejaculatory duct obstruction, it is often possible to collect sperm by washing out the vas deferens via a vasotomy incision (Hirsh *et al.* 1993). These techniques are also used in men with ejaculatory failure. As many of these sperm that are behind an obstruction in the vas are immotile, better results are obtained with IVF/ICSI than with IVF alone.

Regretted vasectomy is now a frequent cause of infertility. There are several ways in which vasectomy and its unsuccessful reversal may result in infertility. After a reversal, the damage to the epididymis may be so severe that the sperm in the ejaculate remain immotile even after their passage down the whole of the epididymal duct. It is usually best to manage this form of infertility by IVF/ICSI.

Failure of a reversal of the vasectomy is also a common problem in an infertility clinic. The presence of epididymal 'blow-outs' is a common cause of failure of these operations and in this situation it will be necessary to collect sperm from the upper epididymis.

Interestingly, many patients today are unwilling to undergo reversal of vasectomy but still wish to achieve a pregnancy while leaving the vasectomy in place. In such men, the sperm may be collected from the vas deferens or, if a 'blow-out' is present, sperm may need to be collected from the epididymis. This option allows for fertility in the presence of otherwise permanent contraception!

Disorders of ejaculation

Disorders of ejaculation are another important reason for the application of IVF/ICSI to the management of the infertility. In retrograde ejaculation, it is often not possible to obtain an antegrade ejaculate. Alternatively, the antegrade ejaculate that is obtained from these patients may be heavily contaminated with urine, which will greatly reduce sperm motility (Crich & Jequier 1978).

In men with ejaculatory failure whose semen samples may be collected by electroejaculation, the quality of the ejaculate is frequently poor with poor motility and reduced sperm numbers (Gerig et al. 1997). In these patients fertilization failure in standard IVF can be a risk, and IVF/ICSI often provides a much higher fertilization and pregnancy rate (Hultling et al. 1997). In men with ejaculatory failure due to spinal cord injury, the incidence of obstructive and partial obstructive lesions is high (Jequier et al. 1998) and thus epididymal, or even testicular, sperm may have to be used to achieve fertilization, for which ICSI will be essential.

Autoimmune infertility in the male

In men with high titres of antibody in their semen that is sufficient to cause infertility, the application of IVF/ICSI is now the most effective way in which to achieve a pregnancy (Clarke et al. 1997). Fertility is impaired by the inability of antibody-coated sperm to bind to the zona pellucida. Although many authors continue to use steroids in both high and low doses as a standard treatment for this type of infertility, many of the studies published are not adequately randomized and their validity must thus be questioned. The treatment of these men with high-dose steroid therapy (Shulman 1977) is, in comparison with the results achieved by IVF/ICSI, no longer acceptable and neither is the danger of avascular necrosis of the hip, which has been reported following this form of treatment (Hendry 1982).

Thus, IVF/ICSI has now become the standard therapy for all severe forms of autoimmune male infertility (Nagy *et al.* 1995a), particularly where the presence of antisperm antibodies of the immunoglobulin A (IgA) subgroup predominate in the seminal fluid.

Abnormalities of sperm morphology

It has long been known that abnormal morphology of the spermatozoon may be associated with an abnormal complement of chromosomes. This relates particularly to the presence of bulbous heads in an ejaculate. There are, however, certain specific abnormalities in sperm structure that cause absolute infertility, and recent work suggests that pregnancies may be generated by the application of IVF/ICSI to these particular anomalies.

Abnormalities of the axoneme

Many disorders of the axoneme may occur in spermatozoa. The axoneme extends from just below the head down to the tip of the tail and is made up of the classic 9 + 2 configuration. The axoneme also includes the proximal centriole, which lies just below the head and which is known to be essential for the initiation of the intraooplasmic fertilization process, being responsible for the formation of the sperm aster (Van Blerkom & Davis 1995). There is also a defect of spermatozoa where the head is functionally separated from the flagellum (Zanefeld & Polakowski 1977) and in sperm with this condition the sperm show very small heads or a 'pin-head' deformity. This condition is likely to be genetically inherited.

A well-known but nevertheless uncommon abnormality of the axoneme is that seen in a condition known as Kartagener's syndrome, in which there is total loss of sperm motility because of an absence of the dynein arms of the axoneme (Afzelius *et al.* 1975). This abnormality is present in all the ciliary tissue of the body and as a consequence results in considerable respiratory abnormalities such as bronchiectasis and abnormal absorptive patterns in the gut. There is likely to be a major genetic basis for this condition as it is also associated with dextrocardia and other cardiac abnormalities. The technique of IVF/ICSI has also been applied to the infertility caused by this condition but, although fertilization can be achieved, very few pregnancies have been reported to date (von Zumbusch *et al.* 1998). Great care must be taken when applying any form of assisted conception to this condition as the respiratory problems that may be associated with this disorder are not only distressing but can also be life threatening. Occasionally, patients with this condition may be in such severe respiratory failure to necessitate heart–lung transplantation.

In a semen sample, there can also be many different types of axonemal abnormalities that can be present in a single ejaculate. The diagnosis of an axonemal disorder can only be made using transmission electron microscopy and should be applied to all semen samples that show severe asthenozoospermia for which an explanation cannot be found.

It must be remembered that total asthenozoospermia does not necessarily indicate the presence of an axonemal abnormality. Such a situation can be seen in semen samples that lack fructose or have been produced by patients with severe epididymal pathology.

Abnormalities of the head of the sperm

The most common anomalies that are seen involving the sperm head are those related to the acrosome. In spermatozoa, the acrosome can be totally absent or it can be hypoplastic or degenerate.

The most well-known abnormality that is seen in the sperm head is a condition known as globozoospermia, a condition that was described by Schirren and colleagues in 1971 (Schirren *et al.* 1971). It is of interest to note that in sperm with an absence of an acrosome, the shape of the nucleus within the sperm head alters in shape and the condition of globozoospermia is no exception to this rule. The sperm in this condition totally lack an acrosome and the head assumes a round shape. Thus, in men with this condition, no penetration of the zona pellucida can occur and the infertility is absolute. A number of reports have now shown that normal fertilization and even pregnancies can occur after the application of IVF/ICSI to this condition (Liu *et al.* 1995). However, this abnormality is also likely to have a genetic basis, but whether or not this condition is passed on to male offspring conceived in this way is at present unknown.

Other structural defects of the head include the presence of vacuoles within the nucleus as well as an incomplete condensation of the chromatin; this may indicate the presence of abnormalities within the sperm head. The implications that these abnormalities may have for any offspring that are generated by using such spermatozoa within an IVF/ICSI programme is unknown.

Nonviable spermatozoa

One problem that may face the clinicians in an IVF clinic is the patient who presents with immotile spermatozoa that are nonviable on an Eosin Y test. There is now good evidence that pellets of DNA that have been stripped of all of their coverings can generate normal pregnancies, at least in the mouse (Kimura & Yanagamachi 1995b).

There is also some circumstantial evidence that nonviable sperm, at least nonviable according to the Eosin Y test, can generate normal human pregnancies when injected into human oocytes. What effects such abnormalities when used in an ICSI programme can have on the future fertility or even on the phenotype of the offspring is totally unknown.

351

These findings thus beg the question as to whether any of the investments of the chromatin or indeed even the proximal centriole are strictly necessary for the generation of an embryo. As many such 'dead' sperm are now being injected into oocytes in IVF/ICSI programmes all over the world, doubtless the answer to this question will be demonstrated in the not too distant future.

A negative acrosome ionophore challenge (ARIC) test

This test identifies spermatozoa that appear to be unable to undergo the acrosome reaction and this defect may in fact relate to the problem of failed fertilization that can occur in routine IVF (Cummins *et al.* 1991). In the laboratory, the sperm are subjected to the action of a calcium ionophore that mimics the effects of the zona pellucida protein that stimulates an influx of calcium into the sperm and initiates the acrosome reaction.

If there is an increase in the occurrence of this induced acrosome reaction over the spontaneous acrosome reaction of less than 10%, there is a significant reduction in the fertilization rate and an increase in the incidence of total fertilization failure (Cummins *et al.* 1991). Indeed, if the increase in the induced acrosome reaction is zero, there is a very significant increase in the incidence of total fertilization failure among these patients. This test is thus useful in predicting fertilization failure and can be of value to the patient prior to a standard cycle of IVF. Such a fertilization problem appears to be totally resolved by the application of IVF/ICSI (Liu *et al.* 1997).

Unexpected failed fertilization in classic IVF

Another important use for IVF/ICSI is when there is unexpected failed fertilization after a standard cycle of IVF. It must be remembered that there are frequently female causes of this disaster, such as an absence of sperm-head receptor proteins on the zona pellucida, recurrent polyspermy and even an increased diameter of the zona itself, which interferes with penetration of the zona by the sperm. However, many of these failures of fertilization may relate to abnormal sperm function, but it is frequently a problem whose exact nature cannot today be determined.

Whatever the cause of this fertilization failure, the use of IVF/ICSI usually resolves the problem. However, despite this therapeutic success, it is stressed that as the genetic implications of the use of IVF/ICSI have not yet been evaluated, an uncritical use of ICSI for all forms of infertility cannot yet be condoned.

Methods of collection of sperm other than from the ejaculate for ICSI

As has already been discussed, sperm that have been collected from many different parts of the male genital tract can be used within an IVF/ICSI programme.

The collection of testicular sperm

The method of collection of sperm from testicular tissue will depend upon the pathology present and the reason for the testicular sperm collection.

Collection of sperm in patients with primary testicular disease

Where there may be difficulty in collecting sperm and where the sperm may be very few and far between in the testicular tissue, the biopsy is best taken as an open procedure. Where difficulty in finding sperm is predicted, it is a good idea to carry out this biopsy 1 day prior to the egg pick-up. Culturing testicular tissue for 24h can generate sperm from biopsy samples which, on initial examination of the testicular tissue, appear to contain no sperm.

A general anaesthetic is given to the patient and the scrotum is opened. It is best to start with the larger of the two testes, should indeed such a difference in size exist. A small incision is made in the tunica albuginea, after which the seminiferous tubules bulge out through this incision. The bulging tissue is removed preferably with a knife and given to the embryologist who teases out the tubules with needles under a low-power microscope. It may be necessary to take several biopsies in this circumstance and indeed one will frequently fail to find any sperm in many patients with a marked reduction in testis size or where the serum FSH is raised. Culture of the tissue in medium may reveal the presence of sperm tails on the following day.

It has been suggested that the retrieval of sperm can be facilitated by the careful dissection of individual tubules with the use of the operating microscope. However, this will greatly increase the time taken for the collection of the testicular sperm and consequently greatly increase the cost. This technique may be of value in men with primary testicular disease where there is very severe suppression of sperm production.

It is also of value in these patients to take a small testicular biopsy that is to be examined histologically. These biopsies must be fixed in special fixative such as Bouin's or Stieve's solutions prior to histological examination.

The tunica albuginea is best closed using a fine suture of either polydiaxonone (PDS, Ethicon Ltd) or polyglactin 910 (Vicryl, Ethicon Ltd). After very careful haemostasis (the scrotum and its contents are extremely vascular), the skin is closed, usually using some form of subcuticular suture. The patient can go home later that day and will be more comfortable wearing some form of light scrotal support over the next 2–3 days.

Collection of testicular tissue from patients with normal testicular histology

This type of sperm collection is only carried out for patients with a very high obstruction in the epididymis such as nonjunction of the efferent ductules with the epididymis or in men who are known to have rete testis obstruction. One must remember, however, that the condition of germinal aplasia where no sperm whatever are present in semen can mimic obstructive disease very closely (Jequier *et al.* 1984).

However, where a biopsy has been taken in the past and the state of sperm production has been shown to be normal, a biopsy can be taken using a simple aspiration needle. Either a general or a local anaesthetic can be used. If local anaesthesia is used, a spermatic cord block is most effective, after which aspiration of testicular tissue is carried out using fine needle aspiration. The diameter of the needle should be around 18 gauge. A butterfly needle can be used for this purpose. On removal of the needle from the testis, pressure should be placed on the site of puncture to aid haemostasis.

It is of course perfectly feasible to take an open biopsy even from patients with a past biopsy that is known to be normal, and this is indeed the author's preference. An open biopsy allows for the avoidance of any blood vessels on the surface of the testis and this is likely to avoid the development of haematomata within the testis, which is a common occurrence of any of these biopsies (Schlegel & Su 1997).

In testes with copious numbers of spermatozoa, the testicular tissue can be very satisfactorily cryopreserved (Nagy *et al.* 1995b), thus avoiding the need for repeated collection of sperm from the testis.

The collection of epididymal sperm

Sperm must be collected from different parts of the epididymis when there is an obstructive lesion present either in the epididymal duct or in the very proximal portion of the vas deferens. Common indications for such a procedure include a failed vasectomy reversal, where vasectomy reversal would be inappropriate or past infective disorders have induced epididymal obstruction. It must, however, be remembered that in men who have had a severe epididymitis or epididymo-orchitis, sperm production may also have been damaged.

Percutaneous collection of epididymal sperm

This procedure has the advantage that it can easily be carried out under local anaesthesia (Craft *et al.* 1995). As for a testicular biopsy, it is best to use a block of the spermatic cord to anaesthetize the area for this procedure. The percutaneous collection of epididymal sperm has, however, the disadvantage that the exact nature of the lesion causing the problem cannot be visualized.

The distended tubules can be palpated and aspirated using a butterfly needle to which is attached a small insulin syringe containing a small quantity of medium. It is important to aspirate a reasonable number of sperm so that some of the spermatozoa can be cryopreserved and thus the procedure does not have to be repeated at each attempt at IVF/ICSI.

Open epididymal aspiration

For this procedure, the scrotum is opened in the same manner as that used to collect testicular sperm and the whole testis is delivered out through the wound. It must be remembered that among patients with a past history of epididymo-orchitis, there may be considerable adhesions present around both the epididymis and even around the testis itself. Such adhesions may have to be dissected off the epididymis in order to visualize the distended tubules. The tubules are then opened under direct vision and the trapped rete testis fluid oozes out as a grey–white coloured opalescent fluid. This fluid is aspirated into a small syringe that contains medium. The fluid is then examined microscopically for the presence of spermatozoa.

There will also be some tubules close to the obstructed portion of the epididymis that contain yellow-coloured inspissated material. These tubules should not be opened as they often only contain dead sperm as well as plentiful number of macrophages. Such macrophages generate reactive oxygen species that can damage sperm, and the sperm in these tubules are best avoided during an epididymal sperm collection.

It is usually possible to collect relatively large numbers of sperm this way and repeat collections are rarely necessary using the open technique. Open collection also allows for a more selective collection of sperm from the individual tubules above the site of the obstruction in the epididymis.

Vasal sperm collection

This procedure is largely used in men with disorders of ejaculation where there are no other pathologies present in the genital tract. This procedure can be carried out under local anaesthesia. However, it is also the author's preferred method of collecting sperm from men with anejaculation due to spinal injury as in these men there is a considerable risk of autonomic hyperreflexia. For this reason, either a general or a regional anaesthetic is preferred.

In this procedure, the vas is located in the same manner as that used in performing a vasectomy. A small incision is made in the overlying scrotal skin and a loop of vas is pulled out through the wound. The vas is then hemisected and a small 21 gauge cannula is inserted into the lumen of the vas towards the testis. Around 3–4 mL of medium is now forcibly injected into the vas while the cauda of epididymis is milked by palpation from outside the scrotum. After about 30 s, the vas is aspirated. If the genital tract is normal, large numbers of sperm can be collected which can be cry-opreserved if required. The vas is then closed using some form of fine absorbable suture such as polyglactin 910 (PDS, Ethicon Ltd). The vas is then dropped back into the wound and the skin closed with a small sub-cuticular stitch.

Collection of sperm from the bladder in men retrograde ejaculation and in men with ectopic ejaculatory ducts

The collection of sperm from the bladder is usually relatively simple and large numbers of sperm can usually be obtained provided the genital tract is otherwise normal.

An antegrade ejaculate can be produced using a number of different techniques, but the ejaculate so obtained is more often than not contaminated with urine, as of course are any samples of semen that are flushed from the bladder. The low osmolality of the urine together with an inhospitable pH frequently reduces the motility of sperm and make the application of ICSI of benefit.

The semen may also be contaminated with urine if the sperm emerge into the renal tract from ectopically sited ejaculatory ducts such as the ureters (Redman & Suleiman 1976).

The problem of totally immotile sperm in IVF/ICSI

One of the problems that now face clinicians and scientists involved in IVF/ICSI is when an ejaculate, or more particularly sperm, aspirated from the proximal ducts of the genital tract shows no motility. The importance of this problem is that it can thus be very difficult to tell the difference between sperm that are simply immotile and sperm that are in fact dead.

Although there is little doubt that the injection of immotile sperm leads to a reduction in fertilization rate, especially where the Eosin Y test shows severely reduced sperm vitality, it does indeed seem possible to achieve fertilization among human sperm that show a very low percentage vitality (Nagy *et al.* 1995c). As has already been stated, there is now some circumstantial evidence that nonmotile human sperm that show zero vitality can provide both a normal fertilization rate with the generation of both embryos and on-going pregnancies.

Despite these apparently reassuring results, many feel that only live sperm should be used to generate human pregnancies and thus it is recommended that the hypo-osmotic swelling (HOS) test (Jeyendran *et al.* 1984) should be carried out on immotile sperm prior to their selection for injection at ICSI (see Chapter 5). The HOS test is carried out on the spermatozoa to be used for ICSI and those sperm whose tail swells in response to the hypo-osmotic solution selected. These sperm with swollen tails are placed into a normo-osmotic solution and time is allowed for the tails to be restored to their normal shape. These sperm that have been proved to be vital are then used for intracytoplasmic sperm injection.

The use of immature male gametes in IVF/ICSI

It has indeed now been shown that male gametes prior to completion of maturation can successfully be used in the generation not only of embryos (Tesarik 1996) but of viable pregnancies (Fischel *et al*. 1995; Barak *et al*. 1998). Both round as well as elongated spermatids have been used for this purpose. Despite much work on this aspect of IVF/ICSI, the pregnancy rate using these immature forms of the male gamete remains poor (Fig. 20.3). However, the major problem that faces the embryologist in this situation is the identification, especially of the round spermatids as they are of similar size to cells such as lymphocytes. It is thus likely that at least some of the apparent fertilization failure in this technique is caused by the injection of cells into the oocyte that are not sperm precursors.

The advantages and the disadvantages of IVF/ICSI

The advent of ICSI into the realms of assisted reproduction has brought great improvements in our ability to generate pregnancies from situations where, even with IVF, the results of treatment in terms of pregnancies were very poor. It can indeed truly be considered as one of the major break-

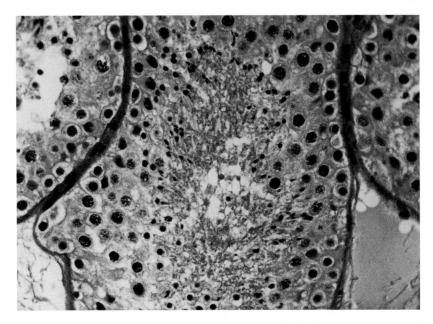

Fig. 20.3 A histological section of a human seminiferous tubule showing the presence of both elongated and round spermatids. These immature forms have been used in an IVF/ICSI programme in an attempt to overcome infertility in men in whom no mature spermatozoa can be found.

throughs in the management of infertility of this century. Not only is ICSI of value in overcoming infertility in the male but also in a variety of different types of infertility in the female. Also, whether we like it or not, ICSI is being used more and more frequently: in 1996 microassisted fertilization accounted for around 30% of all assisted reproduction (Hurst *et al.* 1996) while today in the author's clinic it probably exceeds 50%.

The technique of ICSI has also allowed us to examine many aspects of fertilization, a good example being the beautiful demonstration of the many changes in the sperm head and of the oocyte itself after ICSI (Payne *et al.* 1997). The technique of ICSI has thus provided a great 'learning experience' not only for the clinicians involved in the management of infertile patients but also for those scientists interested in the whole process of gamete interaction and fertilization.

One problem with ICSI that has already been alluded to is that because of its great success as a means of overcoming infertility, it is being used to treat all forms of infertility. Frequently, no regard is paid to the aetiology of this problem; indeed, even Palermo and colleagues have suggested its application to all forms of male infertility (Palermo *et al.* 1995).

The technique of ICSI can also be used to overcome causes of infertility that were previously untreatable, but which are today also known to have a genetic basis. An example of one of these conditions is Klinefelter's syndrome, in which at best a few dozen sperm may now be sufficient to generate a pregnancy (Bourne *et al.* 1997). Interestingly, the transmission of an extra sex chromosome to the fetus does not seem to occur. Another genetically predetermined disorder that ICSI has allowed us to overcome is bilateral congenital absence of the vas deferens.

Thus, today IVF/ICSI allows us to treat genetic forms of infertility which in the past have been self-limiting because of the impossibility of any form of therapy. As has now been demonstrated in relation to the microdeletions on the long arm of the Y chromosome that are related to disturbances in sperm production, these problems can be transmitted to male offspring by the application of IVF/ICSI (Kent-First *et al.* 1996). It is thus possible that IVF/ICSI is, at least in some circumstances, providing the IVF clinicians with a self-generating cause of infertility.

Today ICSI is also being applied to the use of immature sperm from a man in whom no mature sperm can be found, either in the ejaculate or in the testis, in attempts to achieve a pregnancy. The implications of these techniques for the offspring that may be conceived in this way are still unknown.

One important and very real concern about ICSI is the possibility that its use will generate abnormalities in the offspring. So far there is little evidence that this is a problem. In several studies carried out by Bonduelle and colleagues, the major malformation rate among children conceived by IVF/ICSI is no greater than that in children conceived naturally (Bonduelle *et al.* 1996a), but there appeared to be a slight increase in *de novo* chromosomal abnormalities among children generated from cryopreserved ICSI embryos (Bonduelle *et al.* 1996b). However, the number of children in all these studies is still small and further studies are needed to confirm or refute these findings. There has also been a suggestion that ICSI may relate to the presence of certain alterations in development in children conceived by ICSI and that this procedure was associated with delays in mental development at the age of 1 year (Bowen *et al.* 1998). There is, however, no evidence that there is any alteration in mental development among children conceived by ICSI, at least at 2 years of age (Bonduelle *et al.* 1998). Again much greater numbers are needed before we can be sure that conception by ICSI does not carry these risks.

Although there will doubtless be some problems in relation to the use of ICSI in the management of infertility, it is very clear that the advantages of the technique of ICSI continue to outweigh its disadvantages. It is, for sure, a technique that will be increasingly used in the management of both female as well as male infertility.

References

Afzelius, B.A., Eliasson, R., Johnson, O. & Lindholmer, C. (1975) Lack of dynein arms in immotile human spermatozoa. *Journal of Cell Biology* **66**, 225–232.

Barak, Y., Kogosowski, A., Goldman, S., Soffer, Y., Gonen, Y. & Tesarik, J. (1998) Pregnancy and birth after transfer of embryos that developed from single-nucleated zygotes obtained by injection of round spermatids into oocytes. *Fertility and Sterility* **70**, 67–70.

Bonduelle, M., Joris, H., Hofmans, K., Liebaers, I. & Van Steirteghem, A.C. (1998) Mental development of 201 ICSI children at 2 years of age. *Lancet* **351**, 1553.

Bonduelle, M., Legein, J., Buysse, A. *et al.* (1996a) Prospective follow up of 423 children born after intracytoplasmic sperm injection. *Human Reproduction* **11**, 1558–1564.

Bonduelle, M., Willikens, J., Buysse, A. *et al.* (1996b) Prospective study of 877 children born after intracytoplasmic sperm injection, with ejaculated, epididymal and testicular spermatozoa and after replacement of cryopreserved embryos obtained after ICSI. *Human Reproduction* **11** (Suppl. 4), 131–152.

Bourne, H., Stern, K., Clarke, G., Pertile, M., Speirs, A. & Baker, H.G. (1997) Delivery of normal twins following the intracytoplasmic injection of spermatozoa from a patient with 47,XXY Klinefelter's syndrome. *Human Reproduction* **12**, 2447–2450.

Bowen, J.R., Gibson, F.L., Leslie, G.I. & Saunders, D.M. (1998) Medical and developmental outcome at 1 year for children conceived by intracytoplasmic sperm injection. *Lancet* **351**, 1529–1534.

Clarke, G.N., Bourne, H. & Baker, H.W.G. (1997) Intracytoplasmic injection for treating infertility associated with sperm autoimmunity. *Fertility and Sterility* **68**, 112–1176.

Craft, I., Khalifa, Y., Boulos, A., Pelekanos, M., Foster, C. & Tsirigotis, M. (1995) Factors influencing the outcome of *in-vitro* fertilization with percutaneous aspirated epididymal spermatozoa and intracytoplasmic sperm injection in azoospermic men. *Human Reproduction* **10**, 1791–1794.

Crich, J.P. & Jequier, A.M. (1978) Infertility in men with retrograde ejaculation. The action of urine on sperm motility and a simple method for achieving antegrade ejaculation. *Fertility and Sterility* **30**, 572–576.

Cummins, J.M. & Jequier, A.M. (1994) Treating male infertility needs more clinical andrology, not less. *Human Reproduction* **9**, 1214–1219.

Cummins, J.M., Pember, S.M., Jequier, A.M., Yovich, J.L. & Hartmann, P.E. (1991) A test of the human acrosome reaction following ionophore challenge. Relationship to fertility and other seminal parameters. *Journal of Andrology* **12**, 98–103.

Fischel, S., Green, S., Bishop, M. *et al.* (1995) Pregnancy after intracytoplasmic injection of spermatid. *Lancet* **345**, 1641–1642 (letter).

Fischel, S., Jackson, P., Antinori, S., Johnson, J., Grossi, S. & Versaci, C. (1990) Subzonal insemination for the alleviation of infertility. *Fertility and Sterility* **54**, 828–835.

Fischel, S., Timson, S., Lisi, F., Jacobson, M., Rinaldi, L. & Gobetz, L. (1994) Micro-assisted fertilization in patients who have failed subzonal insemination. *Human Reproduction* **9**, 2444–2445.

Gerig, N.E., Meacham, R.B. & Ohl, D.A. (1997) Use of electroejaculation in the treatment of ejaculatory failure secondary to diabetes mellitus. *Urology* **49**, 239–242.

Hendry, W.F. (1982) Avascular necrosis of the femoral heads following intermittant high-dose steroid therapy. *Fertility and Sterility* **38**, 120. (letter).

Hirsh, A.V., Mills, C., Tan, S.L., Bekir, J. & Rainsbury, P. (1993) pregnancy using spermatozoa aspirated from the vas deferens in a patient with ejaculatory failure due to spinal injury. *Human Reproduction* **8**, 89–90.

Hultling, C., Rosenlund, B., Levi, R., Fridstrom, M., Sjoblom, P. & Hillensjo, T. (1997) Assisted ejaculation and *in-vitro* fertilization in the treatment of infertile spinal cord-injured men: the role of intracytoplasmic sperm injection. *Human Reproduction* **12**, 499–502.

Hurst, T., Shafir, E. & Lancaster, P. (1996) Assisted conception in Australia and New Zealand 1996. *AIHW National Perinatal Statistics Report*. The Australian Institute of Health and Welfare.

Jequier, A.M., Ansell, I.D. & Bullimore, N.J. (1984) Germinal aplasia: how it may mimic obstructive azoospermia. *British Journal of Urology* **56**, 537–539.

Jequier, A.M., Barblett, H.C. & Sainty, C.A. (1998) Infertility among men with spinal cord injury: genital tract pathology and the results of ART. *Proceedings of the Annual Meeting of the Fertility Society of Australia* (1998) (Abstract).

Jeyendran, R.S., Van der Ven, H., Perez-Palaez, M., Crabo, B. & Zanefeld, L.J.D. (1984) Development of an assay to assess the functional integrity of the human sperm membrane and its relationship to other semen characteristics. *Journal of Reproduction and Fertility* **70**, 219–228.

Kent-First, M.G., Kol, S., Muallem, A. *et al.* (1996) The incidence and possible relevance of Y-linked microdeletions in babies born after intracytoplasmic sperm injection and their infertile fathers. *Molecular Human Reproduction* **2**, 855–862.

Kimura, Y. & Yanagamachi, R. (1995a) Development of normal mice from oocytes injected with testicular sperm or round spermatids can develop into normal offspring. *Development* **121**, 2397–2405.

Kimura, Y. & Yanagamachi, R. (1995b) Development of normal mice from oocytes injected with the secondary spermatocyte nuclei. *Biology of Reproduction* **53**, 855–862.

Liu, D.Y., Bourne, H., Baker, H.W. & G. (1997) High fertilization and pregnancy rates after intracytoplasmic sperm injection in patients with disordered zona pellucida-induced acrosome reaction. *Fertility and Sterility* **67**, 955–958.

Liu, J., Nagy, Z., Joris, H., Tournaye, H., Devroey, P. & Van Steirteghem, A.C. (1995) Successful fertilization and establishment of pregnancies after intracytoplasmic sperm injection in patients with globozoospermia. *Human Reproduction* **10**, 626–629.

Lundin, K., Sjogren, A., Nilsson, L. & Hamberger, L. (1994) Fertilization and pregnancy after intracytoplasmic microinjection of acrosomeless spermatozoa. *Fertility and Sterility* **62**, 1266–1267.

Nagy, Z.P., Verheyen, G., Liu, J. *et al.* (1995a) Results of 55 intracytoplasmic sperm injections in the treatment of male-immunological infertility. *Human Reproduction* **10**, 1775–1780.

Nagy, Z., Liu, J., Janssenswillen, C., Silber, S., Devoey, P. & Van Steirteghem, A.C. (1995b) Using ejaculated, fresh and frozen–thawed epididymal and testicular spermatozoa gives rise to comparable results after intracytoplasmic sperm injection. *Fertility and Sterility* **63**, 808–815.

Nagy, Z.P., Liu, J., Joris, H. *et al.* (1995c) The result of intracytoplasmic sperm injection is not related to any of the three basic sperm parameters. *Human Reproduction* **10**, 1123–1129.

Palermo, G.D., Cohen, J., Alikani, M., Adler, A. & Rosenwaks, Z. (1995) Intracytoplasmic sperm injection: a novel treatment for all forms of male factor infertility. *Fertility and Sterility* **63**, 1231–1240.

Palermo, G., Joris, H., Devroey, P. & Van Steirteghem, A.C. (1992) Pregnancies after intracytoplasmic injection of a single spermatozoon into an oocyte. *Lancet* **340**, 17–18.

Payne, D., Flaherty, S.P., Barry, M.F. & Matthews, C.D. (1997) Preliminary observations on polar body extrusion and pronuclear formation in human oocytes using time-lapse video cinematography. *Human Reproduction* **12**, 532–541.

Redman, J.F. & Suleiman, J.S. (1976) Bilateral vasal–ureteral communications. *Journal of Urology* **116**, 808–809.

Schirren, C.G., Holstein, A.F. & Schirren, C. (1971) Uber die Morphogenese rundkopfigur Spermatozoen des Menschen. *Andrologia* **3**, 117–125.

Schlegel, P.N. & Su, L.-M. (1997) Physiological consequences of testicular sperm extraction. *Human Reproduction* **12**, 1688–1692.

Schoysman, R., Van der Zwalman, P., Nijs, M. *et al.* (1993) Pregnancy after fertilization with human testicular sperm. *Lancet* **342**, 1237. (Letter).

Shulman, S. (1977) Immune infertility and new approaches to treatment. In: *Immunological Influences on Human Fertility* (ed. B. Boettcher), pp. 281–288. Academic Press, Sydney.

Silber, S.J. (1998) Intracytoplasmic sperm injection today: a personal review. In: *Human Reproduction* **13** (Suppl. 1), Current Theory and Practice of ICSI (eds P. Devroey, B.C. Tarlatzis & A.C. Van Steirteghem), pp. 208–218.

Tesarik, J. (1996) Fertilization of oocytes by injecting spermatozoa, spermatids and spermatocytes. *Reviews in Reproduction* **1**, 149–152.

Trounson, A.O., Leeton, J.F. & Wood, C. (1981) Successful human pregnancies by *in vitro* fertilization and embryo transfer in controlled ovulatory cycles. *Science* **212**, 681–682.

Van Blerkom, J. & Davis, P. (1995) Evolution of the sperm aster after micro-injection of isolated sperm centrosomes into meiotically mature human oocytes. *Molecular Human Reproduction* **10**, 2179–2182.

Zanefeld, L.J.D. & Polakowski, K.L. (1977) Collection and physical examination of the ejaculate. In: *Techniques of Human Andrology* (ed. E.S.E. Hafez), pp. 147–172. Elsevier-North Holland, Amsterdam.

von Zumbusch, A., Fiedler, K., Mayerhofer, A., Jesberger, B., Ring, J. & Vogt, H.-J. (1998) Birth of healthy children after sperm injection in two couples with male Kartagener's Syndrome. *Fertility and Sterility* **70**, 643–646.

Index

Please note: This index is in letter-by-letter order, where hyphens and space within index headings are ignored in the alphabetization.